49.50

Pancreatic Disease

Springer
Berlin
Heidelberg
New York
Barcelona
Hong Kong
London
Milan
Paris
Singapore
Tokyo

P. G. Lankisch and E. P. DiMagno

Pancreatic Disease

State of the Art and Future Aspects of Research

With 40 Figures and 47 Tables

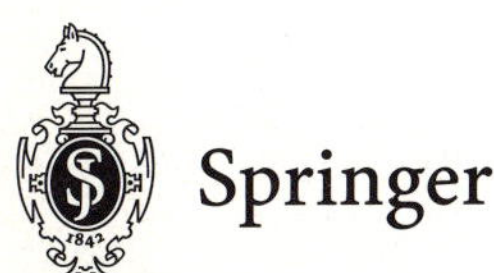

Springer

Prof. Dr. Paul G. Lankisch
Medizinische Klinik
Städtisches Klinikum Lüneburg
Bögelstraße 1
D-21339 Lüneburg

Prof. Dr. Eugene P. DiMagno
Mayo Foundation
Gastroenterology Research Unit
200 First Street, SW
Rochester, Minnesota 55905
USA

ISBN 3-540-65357-0 Springer-Verlag Berlin Heidelberg New York

Cataloging-in-Publication Data applied for
Die Deutsche Bibliothek – CIP-Einheitsaufnahme
Lankisch, Paul, G.: Pancreatic disease: state of the art and future aspects of research; with 47 tables / P.G. Lankisch and E.P. DiMagno. – Berlin; Heidelberg; New York; Barcelona; Hong Kong; London; Mailand; Paris; Singapore; Tokyo: Springer, 1998
ISBN 3-540-65357-0

Cover-Design: Design & Production GmbH, Heidelberg
Satz: K + V Fotosatz GmbH, Beerfelden

SPIN 10686044 18/3134-5 4 3 2 1 0 – Printed on acid-free paper

Preface

In the past several years much progress has been made in understanding the basic mechanisms of pancreatic physiology and the pathogenesis, diagnosis, and treatment of pancreatic disease.

A symposium took place in Munich on 18–19 September 1998 that aimed at summarizing current knowledge of the exocrine pancreas and giving direction to future research. It targeted all practitioners and scientists working in the field of exocrine pancreatic disease. The symposium was also designed to stimulate young persons embarking on a career in this area.

It was an exciting meeting for all of us. We wish to extend our thanks to all participants for their prompt submission of manuscripts and to Springer-Verlag for speedy publication, providing us with an up-to-date volume on pancreatic research.

We would also like to thank G. Beyendorff-Hajda and W. Glöckner, as well as D. Krüger, representatives of Knoll Deutschland GmbH, for their organizational assistance and Knoll itself for its generous sponsorship, which enabled colleagues from other countries to participate and made publication of the symposium possible.

P. G. Lankisch
E. P. DiMagno

Table of Contents

Part I Acute Pancreatitis

1 Acute Pancreatitis: Mechanisms of Cell Injury – Genetics
D.C. WHITCOMB 3

2 Events Inside the Pancreatic Acinar Cell in Acute Pancreatitis: Role of Secretory Blockade, Calcium Release and Dehydration for the Initiation of Trypsinogen Activation and Autodigestion
C. NIEDERAU and R. LÜTHEN 14

3 Immunologic Mechanisms in Acute Pancreatitis
J. SCHÖLMERICH 24

4 Mechanisms in Cellular Injury
CH. HANCK and M.V. SINGER 36

5 Acute Pancreatitis: Bacterial Translocation and Pancreatic Infections
ST. W. SCHMID, W. UHL, and M.W. BÜCHLER 39

6 Staging and Early Nasolateral Feeding in Acute Pancreatitis
C.W. IMRIE 55

7 Acute Pancreatitis: Medical and Endoscopic Treatment
C. LÖSER and U.R. FÖLSCH 66

8 Surgical Treatment of Acute Pancreatitis
H.G. BEGER, B. RAU, J. MAYER, and R. ISENMANN 78

Part II Chronic Pancreatitis

9 Chronic Pancreatitis: Do Different Etiologies (Alcohol, Obstruction) Invoke Different Mechanisms?
J. MÖSSNER 93

10 Exocrine Pancreatic Secretion, Pain, and Malabsorption
G.H. ELTA 102

11 Intestinal Transit of Chyme and its Regulatory Role: Clinical Implications
P. LAYER and J. KELLER 112

12 Treatment of Exocrine Pancreatic Insufficiency in Chronic Pancreatitis
M.J. BRUNO 121

13 Mechanisms of Fibrosis and Potential Antifibrotic Agents
A. MENKE, R. VOGELMANN, M. BACHEM, and G. ADLER 132

14 Mechanisms of Pain and its Medical Management, Including Neurolytic Treatments
L. GULLO 140

15 Endoscopic Treatment of Pain and Complications of Chronic Pancreatitis
R. JAKOBS, D. APEL, and J.F. RIEMANN 146

16 Surgical Treatment of Chronic Pancreatitis
H.G. BEGER, M. SIECH, and W. SCHLOSSER 155

Part III Cystic Fibrosis

17 Genetics and Molecular Pathology of Cystic Fibrosis
B. TÜMMLER 167

18 Treatment of Gastrointestinal Manifestations in Cystic Fibrosis
M. STERN 180

19 Is Idiopathic Chronic Pancreatitis Cystic Fibrosis?
J.A. COHN 193

Part IV Pancreatic Cancer

20 Growth Factors and Transcription Factors in Pancreatic Cancer
H. FRIESS, Z.W. ZHU, L. WANG and M.W. BÜCHLER 205

21 Biological Approaches to the Therapy of Pancreatic Cancer
M.A. TEMPERO 222

22 Pancreatic Cancer: Preclinical Development of an Experimental Treatment Strategy Using Retinoids and Interferon-alpha
St. Rosewicz 230

23 Aspects of Radical Surgery for Exocrine Cancer of the Pancreatic Head
A. Andrén-Sandberg, D. Hoem, and H. Gisslason 238

Part V Epidemiology

24 Lessons Learned about Pancreatitis and Pancreatic Cancer from Epidemiological Studies
A.B. Lowenfels, P. Maisonneuve and P.G. Lankisch 253

Subject Index 263

List of Contributors

ADLER, GUIDO, Prof. Dr. med.
Department of Internal Medicine I, University of Ulm, Robert-Koch-Strasse 8, D-89070 Ulm, Germany

ANDRÉN-SANDBERG, ÅKE, MD PhD
Department of Surgery, Haukeland University Hospital, N-5021 Bergen, Norway

APEL, DARIUS, Dr. med.
Department of Gastroenterology, Klinikum Ludwigshafen gGmbH, Bremserstrasse 79, D-67063 Ludwigshafen, Germany

BACHEM, MAX, MD
Department of Clinical Chemistry, University of Ulm, Robert-Koch-Strasse 8, D-89070 Ulm, Germany

BEGER, HANS G., MD, FACS
Head of the Department of General Surgery, University of Ulm, Steinhövelstrasse 9, D-89075 Ulm, Germany

BRUNO, MARCO J.
Academic Medical Center, Division of Gastroenterology and Hepatology, Meibergdreef 9, 1105 AZ Amsterdam, The Netherlands

BÜCHLER, M.W., PROF. DR.
Department of Visceral and Transplantation Surgery, University Hospital of Bern, Inselspital, CH-3010 Bern, Switzerland

COHN, JONATHAN A., MD
Departments of Medicine and Cell Biology, Duke University Medical Center, Durham, NC 27710, USA

ELTA, GRACE H., MD
University of Michigan Medical Center, 3912 Taubman Center, Box 0362, Ann Arbor, MI 48109, USA

FÖLSCH, U.R., Prof. Dr. med.
I. Medizinische Universitätsklinik, Christian-Albrechts-Universität Kiel, Schittenhelmstrasse 12, D-24105 Kiel, Germany

FRIESS, HELMUT, MD
Department of Visceral and Transplantation Surgery, University Bern, Inselspital, CH-3010 Bern, Switzerland

GISSLASON, HJÖRTUR
Department of Surgery, Haukeland University Hospital, N-5021 Bergen, Norway

GULLO, LUCIO, Prof.
Department of Internal Medicine and Gastroenterology, University of Bologna, S. Orsola Hospital, Via Massarenti, 9, I-40138 Bologna, Italy

Hanck, Christoph, MD
Dept. of Internal Medicine IV (Gastroenterology), University Hospital of Heidelberg at Mannheim, Theodor Kutzer Ufer 1, D-68167 Mannheim, Germany

Hoem, Dag
Department of Surgery, Haukeland University Hospital, N-5021 Bergen, Norway

Imrie, C.W., Prof.
Glasgow Royal Infirmary, Lister Department of Surgery, 16 Alexandra Parade, Glasgow G31 2ER, Great Britain

Isenmann, Rainer
Department of General Surgery, University of Ulm, Steinhövelstrasse 9, D-89075 Ulm, Germany

Jakobs, Ralf, Dr. med.
Department of Gastroenterology, Klinikum Ludwigshafen gGmbH, Bremserstrasse 79, D-67063 Ludwigshafen, Germany

Keller, Jutta, MD
Department of Internal Medicine, Israelitic Hospital, Orchideenstieg 14, D-22297 Hamburg, Germany

Layer, Peter, MD, Prof. of Medicine
Head of Department of Internal Medicine, Israelitic Hospital, Orchideenstieg 14, D-22297 Hamburg, Germany

Löser, Christian, Prof. Dr. med.
I. Medizinische Universitätsklinik, Christian-Albrechts-Universität Kiel, Schittenhelmstrasse 12, D-24105 Kiel, Germany

Lowenfels, Albert B., MD
Department of Surgery, New York Medical College, Valhalla, NY, 10595, USA

Lüthen, Reinhard
Department of Medicine, Heinrich-Heine-University Düsseldorf, Moorenstrasse 5, D-40225 Düsseldorf, Germany

Maisonneuve, Patrick
Clinical Epidemiology Program, European Institute of Oncology, Milan, Italy

Mayer, Jens, MD
Department of General Surgery, University of Ulm, Steinhövelstrasse 9, D-89075 Ulm, Germany

Menke, Andre
Department of Internal Medicine I, University of Ulm, Robert-Koch-Strasse 8, D-89070 Ulm, Germany

Mössner, Joachim, Prof. Dr. med.
Medizinische Klinik und Poliklinik II, University of Leipzig, Philipp-Rosenthal-Strasse 27, D-04103 Leipzig, Germany

Niederau, Claus, MD
St. Josef-Hospital, Academic Teaching Hospital, Department of Internal Medicine, Mülheimerstrasse 83, D-46045 Oberhausen, Germany

Rau, Bettina
Department of General Surgery, University of Ulm, Steinhövelstrasse 9, D-89075 Ulm, Germany

Riemann, J.F., Prof. Dr. med.
Medizinische Klinik C, Klinikum Ludwigshafen gGmbH, Bremserstrasse 79, D-67063 Ludwigshafen, Germany

ROSEWICZ, STEFAN, Prof. Dr.
Virchow-Klinikum,
Medizinische Klinik
mit Schwerpunkt Hepatologie
und Gastroenterologie,
Augustenburger Platz 1,
D-13353 Berlin, Germany

SCHLOSSER, W., MD
Department of General Surgery,
University of Ulm, Steinhövel-
strasse 9, D-89075 Ulm, Germany

SCHMID, STEFAN W., MD
Department of Visceral and Trans-
plantation Surgery, University
Hospital of Bern, Murtenstrasse 35,
CH-3010 Bern, Switzerland

SCHÖLMERICH, JÜRGEN, Prof. Dr.
Klinik und Poliklinik für Innere
Medizin I, Klinikum der Universität
Regensburg, D-93042 Regensburg,
Germany

SIECH, M., MD
Department of General Surgery,
University of Ulm, Steinhövel-
strasse 9, D-89075 Ulm, Germany

SINGER, MANFRED V.,
Prof. Dr. med.
Dept. of Internal Medicine IV
(Gastroenterology), University
Hospital of Heidelberg at Mannheim,
Theodor Kutzer Ufer 1,
D-68167 Mannheim, Germany

STERN, MARTIN, Prof. Dr.
Universitäts-Kinderklinik,
Hoppe-Seyler-Strasse 1,
D-72076 Tübingen, Germany

TEMPERO, MARGARET A., MD
University of Nebraska Medical
Center, Omaha, NE, USA

TÜMMLER, BURKHARD,
Prof. Dr. med.
Klinische Forschergruppe, OE 6710,
Zentrum Kinderheilkunde,
Medizinische Hochschule Hannover,
D-30623 Hannover, Germany

UHL, WALDEMAR, MD
Department of Visceral and
Transplantation Surgery, University
Hospital of Bern, Murtenstrasse 35,
CH-3010 Bern, Switzerland

VOGELMANN, ROGER
Department of Internal Medicine I,
University of Ulm, Robert-Koch-
Strasse 8, D-89070 Ulm, Germany

WANG, L.
Department of Visceral and
Transplantation Surgery,
University of Bern, Inselspital,
CH-3010 Bern, Switzerland

WHITCOMB, DAVID C., MD PhD
Associate Professor of Medicine,
Division of Gastroenterology and
Hepatology, University of Pittsburgh,
Pittsburgh, PA 15261, USA

ZHU, Z.W., MD
Department of Visceral and
Transplantation Surgery,
University of Bern, Inselspital,
CH-3010 Bern, Switzerland

Part I
Acute Pancreatitis

Acute Pancreatitis: Mechanisms of Cell Injury – Genetics

D.C. Whitcomb

Introduction

Acute pancreatitis was defined at the Symposium of Marseilles as an acute condition typically presenting with abdominal pain and usually associated with elevated pancreatic enzymes in blood or urine, due to inflammatory disease of the pancreas. This clinically based definition remains useful for diagnosing and treating most cases of acute pancreatitis. However, it also reflects the limits in identifying and understanding the molecular and cellular pathophysiologic mechanisms that underlie this common disorder. Acute pancreatitis encompasses a variety of processes. The acute injury within the pancreas appears to develop rapidly, and the inciting factors may resolve before diagnosis and therapeutic interventions can be initiated. The injury results in an acute inflammatory response that may itself worsen the injury, causing significant local and systemic complications. Investigative efforts directed toward understanding and limiting the subsequent inflammatory reaction provide some hope of improving the outcome of more severe cases, if instituted early in the disease process. However, research directed at understanding the early molecular mechanisms initiating acute pancreatitis, and developing effective *preventive* strategies may be equally important.

Progress toward understanding the pathophysiology of acute pancreatitis in human beings has traditionally faced several major obstacles. These include the inaccessibility of the human pancreas to observation, the unpredictability of disease onset, the nonspecific nature of abdominal pain early in the course of acute pancreatitis, an inability to safely biopsy the pancreas, difficulty in distinguishing initiating events from the concomitant inflammatory response, and the obvious problems of investigating a tissue that self-destructs during the disease process. Indeed, the pathophysiological process leading to acute pancreatitis has been so difficult to prove that even basic questions continue to be raised as to whether the process begins in the acinar cell or reflects leakage of lipase-rich fluid from the ducts into the interstitial space, resulting in fat necrosis and inflammation [5].

Researchers often turn to animal models to answer fundamental questions about disease processes. The goal of any animal model is to provide meaningful insights into the pathogenesis and pathophysiology of these important disease states in man [56]. Although a variety of animal models of pancreatitis have been developed since Claude Bernard injected bile and olive oil into the pancreatic duct in 1856 [4], each model has significant drawbacks. The underlying concern continues to be the artificial methods used to induce pancreatitis, and therefore their suitability for preventive and therapeutic studies [2, 35]. This problem was clearly illustrated by Steinberg and Schlesselman when they compared the outcomes of therapeutic studies in animal models of acute pancreatitis with similar protocols in human acute pancreatitis [52]. Although 81% of the 25 animal protocols studied had a positive outcome with respect to survival, only 7.7% of the resulting 13 human studies demonstrated a positive outcome. Thus, our ignorance about early events in acute pancreatitis and the corresponding uncertainties in animal models is reflected in the lack of a translational impact of animals studies when applied to the human condition [56]. The critical question to be answered is, what pathways initiate acute pancreatitis in human beings?

Hereditary Pancreatitis

Because of the uncertainty of animal models, our group and others turned to a fascinating *human* model of acute and chronic pancreatitis, known as hereditary pancreatitis. Patients with hereditary pancreatitis develop repeated episodes of acute pancreatitis that are nearly indistinguishable from pancreatitis seen with gallstones, acute alcohol ingestion, drugs, or other causes. However, in hereditary pancreatitis a major provocative insult to the pancreas usually cannot be identified. A single molecular defect that predisposes affected individuals to this disorder was suggested by the clear autosomal dominant inheritance pattern [13, 42, 49, 56]. Furthermore, it was predicted that the mutation in the hereditary pancreatitis gene would disrupt a critical component of the mechanism that protected nonaffected individuals from acute pancreatitis [55]. Using genetic linkage studies, the hereditary pancreatitis locus was independently narrowed to the long arm of chromosome 7 by Le Bodic et al. [33] and Whitcomb et al. [55] in 1996, and later confirmed by Pandya et al. [41]. Within months the disease gene was identified by Whitcomb et al. [54] through mutational analysis of candidate genes within the newly mapped region. A single G to A transition mutation was identified in the third exon of cationic trypsinogen that resulted in an arginine (CGC) to histidine (CAC) substitution at amino acid residue 105 (numbered 117 using the common chymotrypsinogen numbering system for serine proteases). This mutation was observed in all individuals affected by hereditary pancreatitis and the obligate carriers from five kindreds, but not in individuals who married into the families or in 140 unrelated individuals.

However, other kindreds with a similar phenotype tested negative for the cationic trypsinogen R117H mutation. Mapping and sequencing studies demonstrated that the disease gene in these kindreds also mapped to chromosome 7q35 and were associated with a second mutation in the second exon of the cationic trypsinogen gene. A single A to T transversion mutation resulted in the substitution of asparagine (AAC) to isoleucine (ATC) at amino acid 21 (N21I) [21]. These findings have been validated worldwide [16, 17, 25, 26, 38, 39]. Thus, the cationic trypsinogen gene appears to be a central element in the initiation and development of acute and chronic pancreatitis in these families.

The Role of Trypsin in Digestion

Trypsin is the central enzyme in pancreatic exocrine physiology [46]; it is a serine protease that hydrolyzes dietary proteins at internal lysine and arginine amino acids. Thus, it plays an important role in the digestion of dietary proteins. However, at least five additional observations about this enzyme illustrate its importance. First, the proenzyme of trypsin, trypsinogen, is the most abundant protein synthesized by the pancreas. Second, trypsinogen is the only enzyme directly activated by the brush border enzyme enterokinase. Third, trypsin is the driving force in the pancreatic enzyme activation cascade, changing all of the other pancreatic proenzymes to their active form. Fourth, trypsin is synthesized by three similar genes, resulting in cationic trypsinogen (two thirds of pancreatic trypsinogen), anionic trypsinogen (one third of pancreatic trypsinogen), and mesotrypsinogen (~5% of pancreatic trypsinogen). This redundancy again points to the importance of trypsin. Finally, trypsin plays an important role in controlling feedback regulation of pancreatic exocrine secretion through digestion of CCK-releasing factors in the duodenum. However, the factors that illustrate trypsin's importance also highlight some potential dangers of premature trypsinogen activation within the pancreas. These factors include trypsinogen's abundance, the rapid amplification of trypsin activity through trypsinogen activation, and, through the activation of all other proenzymes, the potential for pancreatic autodigestion.

Cationic Trypsinogen

Interestingly, the only mutations identified to date in patients with hereditary pancreatitis are the cationic trypsinogen R117H mutation [54] and the cationic trypsinogen N21I mutation [21, 54]. No pancreatitis-associated mutations have been identified in anionic trypsinogen, or in any of the other digestive enzymes. Therefore, consideration of the unique features of human cationic trypsin may provide clues about the mechanisms of human acute pancreatitis.

Cationic trypsin is a two-domain molecule with the catalytic site in the cleft between the two globular domains. The domains are connected on the opposite side of the molecule by a semi-flexible connecting chain, and R117 is in the center of this chain. The only known significance of R117 in the cationic trypsinogen molecule is that it is the initial hydrolysis site of trypsin, leading to permanent inactivation. Based on this information and on the hypothesis of Rinderknecht et al. [47] that trypsin autolysis may be a self-destruct mechanism preventing pancreatic autodigestion, we proposed that the cationic trypsinogen R117H mutation eliminates this important initial hydrolysis site [55]. This mutation would thereby prevent destruction of trypsin prematurely activated in the pancreas and, in turn, would lead to generalized zymogen activation, autodigestion, and pancreatitis [55]. The importance of this observation is that it provides strong evidence that *premature trypsin activation* plays a central role in *human* acute pancreatitis. The second, and complementary, piece of evidence that trypsin is a central factor in human acute pancreatitis is the effectiveness of the trypsin inhibitor gabexate in preventing endoscopic retrograde cholangiopancreatography (ERCP)-induced acute pancreatitis [8]. These observations also support the use of animal models of acute pancreatitis that involve early activation of trypsinogen.

Premature Trypsinogen Activation

Trypsinogen activation occurs with the hydrolysis of a 7–10 amino acid TAP portion of the N-terminal region of the molecule. The small cleavage fragment, TAP, is immunologically distinct from the same sequence within trypsinogen, thereby allowing for detection of trypsinogen activation in situ. Recently, several laboratories have used TAP to determine the site of trypsinogen activation in a rat model of acute pancreatitis.

Animal Models of Trypsinogen Activation

Trypsinogen is synthesized in the rough endoplasmic reticulum and transported to the Golgi system. No trypsinogen activation appears to occur along this pathway, perhaps because of the co-synthesis of trypsinogen with pancreatic secretory trypsin inhibitor (PSTI) [1]. After reaching the Golgi system, the proteins are sorted [30] and trypsinogen (with other digestive enzymes) moves into condensing vesicles, where the proteins condense into dense-core particles [15]. The condensed enzymes appear to be quite stable, because minimal trypsinogen activation occurs in the zymogen granules [27, 40].

The first detectable site of TAP, and therefore trypsinogen activation, appears to be a supranuclear compartment within small (<1 μm) vesicles [40]. Interestingly, these vesicles contain lysosomal membrane markers and may allow co-localization of trypsinogen and cathepsin B [27, 37, 40]; cathepsin B can activate trypsinogen under experimental conditions [19, 24]. Shortly thereafter, the majority of immunoreactive TAP shifts to a heavier fraction associated with zymogen granules and/or larger vacuoles [27, 31, 37, 40]. It has long been proposed that acute pancreatitis in animals is initiated by lysosomal hydrolases acting on trypsinogen, following fusion of the zymogen granules and lysosomes [50, 51], although this may actually occur in the newly defined compartment noted above. The inhibition of either trypsin [40] or cathepsin B [48] limits the acinar cell injury during cerulean hyperstimulation in the rodents, pointing to the central role of active trypsin in this model. Finally, new evidence suggests that trypsinogen activation may occur as a normal process in a pathway of regulated enzyme secretion that differs from the storage pool (i.e., zymogen granules) [23]. Blockade of secretion of this compartment by cholecystokinin hyperstimulation leads to trypsinogen activation and pancreatitis, whereas bombesin hyperstimulation causes equal trypsinogen activation but neither blocks enzyme secretion nor causes pancreatitis [23]. Thus, trypsinogen activation may be a normal process in this compartment, that is pathological only when secretion is blocked [23, 34]. These studies and others [22, 34, 37, 43, 45] demonstrate the importance of trypsinogen activation and enzyme secretory blockade in some animal models of acute pancreatitis. However, these animal studies must be viewed in the context of human physiology.

Differences Between Human Disease and Animal Models

The first potentially importance difference between human pancreatitis and rodent models lies in the mechanisms responsible for activating trypsinogen. In rodents, initial rat trypsinogen activation may require the action of cathepsin B (above), whereas human trypsinogen *auto*activates without cathepsin B [10, 19]. This factor may also explain the markedly increased difficulty in working with human pancreas compared with rat pancreas that investigators in this field have experienced. Thus the co-localization of cathepsin B and trypsinogen in the same compartment may be necessary only in animals. On the other hand, it is yet to be determined whether inhibition of cathepsin B in human beings will limit the development of acute pancreatitis, as seen with inhibition of trypsin [8].

The Role of Calcium

In individuals affected with hereditary pancreatitis, episodes of acute pancreatitis are the exception. Most of the time, the pancreas appears to function normally. Therefore, variables in addition to the R117 hydrolysis mechanism must also be important. Intracellular calcium may be one of these important factors.

Calcium in Experimental Pancreatitis

In an experimental rat model a calcium infusion that increased serum calcium concentration threefold resulted in elevation of serum amylase levels and tissue TAP levels and in some morphological evidence of pancreatic injury [36]. In another study using isolated rat pancreatic acini stimulated with cerulein or carbachol, intracellular trypsinogen activation doubled in the presence of elevated calcium concentrations in the buffer [20]. On the cellular level, sustained elevations in acinar cell calcium concentrations are associated with changes of acute pancreatitis, and these elevated calcium levels may result from ductal hypertension, alcohol, hypoxia, hypercalcemia, hyperlipidemia, and various drugs [53]. These observations led Ward et al. [53] to suggest that elevated concentrations of acinar cytosolic free ionized calcium may be the trigger for acute pancreatitis [53].

Calcium and Trypsinogen

What is the connection between intracellular calcium concentrations and trypsinogen activation, as suggested by the studies of Mithofer et al. [36] and Frick et al. [20]? One possibility relates to the 20-year-old observations that the activation and stability of human cationic and anionic trypsinogens are modulated by the calcium concentration. For example, Colomb et al. [11] demonstrated that both human cationic and anionic trypsin autoactivate, but in all cases cationic trypsinogen autoactivated more rapidly than anionic trypsinogen. Increasing the calcium concentration increased the rate of cationic and anionic trypsinogen autoactivation. Thus, intracellular calcium elevations may be associated with an increased rate of trypsinogen autoactivation to trypsin.

Colomb et al. [12] also demonstrated that both anionic and cationic trypsin were rapidly autolyzed in the absence of calcium, with a 50% loss of cationic trypsin and a 100% loss of anionic trypsin within 10 min. However, in the presence of 20 m*M* calcium cationic trypsin activity was constant for more than 6 h, whereas anionic trypsin retained up to 60% of its activity for 2 h. These results demonstrate the importance of calcium in stabilizing both cationic and anionic trypsinogens in their active state and preventing hydrolysis, the greatest stability being seen with cationic trypsin. Therefore, experimental hypercalcemia (>10× higher than expected in vivo) results in protection from hydrolysis. The result may be similar to the predicted protection from hydrolysis seen with the cationic trypsinogen R117H mutation. However, the mechanism of cationic trypsinogen protection in hypercalcemic buffers is unknown.

Other Genetic Factors Influencing Acute Pancreatitis

Although the discussion above offers plausible explanations for cases of hereditary pancreatitis in family members with the cationic trypsinogen R117H mutation, many questions remain unanswered. First, what is the mechanism responsible for susceptibility to acute pancreatitis in the cationic trypsinogen N21I mutation? Based on the clinical similarities between kindreds with the trypsinogen R117H and trypsinogen N21I mutations and the location of the N21I mutation on the surface of the trypsinogen molecule opposite the active site and near R117 [28, 29, 44], we speculate that the consequence of this mutation is either to enhance autoactivation of trypsinogen, to alter the binding of pancreatic secretory trypsin inhibitors, or to impair trypsin inactivation by altering the accessibility of R117 to trypsin-like enzymes and/or protecting the adjacent C22-C157 disulfide bond to prolong survival of trypsin after limited hydrolysis [21]. In a preliminary study, Kurth et al. demonstrated that the cationic trypsinogen with the N21I mutation has normal catalytic function, but they have yet to define the pancreatitis-associated changes [32]. Thus, the reason for acute pancreatitis in patients with hereditary pancreatitis remains to be determined.

A second unanswered question is why mutations in the cationic trypsinogen, but not in the anionic trypsinogen, are associated with human hereditary pancreatitis. One explanation may be that the lower level of anionic trypsinogen expression compared with cationic trypsinogen expression is important. Stoichiometrically, the higher ratio of PSTI to anionic minimizes the chance of excessive mutant anionic trypsinogen activation exceeding the inhibitory capacity of PSTI. A more likely explanation is that anionic trypsin is slower to autoactivate and quicker to autolyze under each experimental condition compared with cationic trypsinogen. However, the actual mechanism remains to be determined.

Another interesting and potentially important observation made by our group [3] and others [16] is that several kindreds with hereditary pancreatitis have neither the cationic trypsinogen R117H nor the N21I mutations. In small families, complete sequencing of the cationic and anionic trypsinogen gene failed to identify other mutations in these genes that result in amino acid substitutions or that segregate with the disease. Furthermore, in at least two large families the chromosome 7q35 region has been excluded [3, 16], and we have identified a suggestive linkage of this new hereditary pancreatitis disease gene to a region on chromosome 12 [3]. Since this likely represents a new hereditary pancreatitis-associated gene, new insights into the mechanisms normally protecting the pancreas from autodigestion are likely.

Finally, other genetic and/or environmental factors may also be important. In an ongoing study of identical twins there was a striking similarity in the age of onset between the twin pairs. However, even with twin pairs there appears to be only 80% disease penetrance, as seen with other families. These findings also require further investigation to determine the underlying mechanism.

Genetic Diseases with Acute Pancreatitis as a Feature

Hyperlipidemia

Several varieties of familial hyperlipidemia are associated with recurrent attacks of acute pancreatitis. Hyperlipoproteinemia type I may present with dominant clinical features of pancreatitis, such as episodic abdominal pain, nausea, and vomiting. For example, a family with this disorder was found to be hyperlipidemic because of a deficiency in liproprotein lipase through two different mutations in exon 3 of the lipoprotein lipase gene: a missense mutation, 75Arg→Ser, inherited through the paternal line, and a truncation,

73Tyr→Ter, through the maternal line [57]. Another family had recurrent acute pancreatitis associated with a circulating inhibitor of lipoprotein lipase inhibitor [6]. Members of still another family in England with recurrent episodes of acute pancreatitis were found to have an apolipoprotein C-II deficiency [14]. Apolipoprotein C-II acts as a necessary cofactor for the activation of lipoprotein lipase, and deficiencies result in marked hypertriglyceridemia.

Hyperparathyroidism

Hypercalcemia from familial hyperparathyroidism was reported to result in chronic pancreatitis in one family [7]. Although a number of cases of acute pancreatitis presenting in patients with hyperparathyroidism have been reported, this does not appear to reflect a genetic defect.

Homocystinuria

Collins and Brenton described two children in whom acute pancreatitis was a complication of homocystinuria [9]. This pancreatitis may have resulted from thrombosis of pancreatic blood vessels. Although rare, we screened one child for trypsinogen mutations in whom the final diagnosis of homocystinuria was made by her attending physician.

Conclusion

The discovery of the mutations in the cationic trypsinogen gene responsible for hereditary forms of pancreatitis [21, 54, 55], combined with results from clinical trials in preventing ERCP-associated pancreatitis [8] provides us with strong evidence that cationic trypsinogen plays an important role in human acute pancreatitis. Human cationic trypsinogen is relatively unique among members of the trypsin family in its ability to autoactivate within zymogen granules of pancreatic acinar cells [18]. Although the site and mechanism of trypsinogen activation in man remains a mystery, significant progress is being made toward understanding trypsinogen activation in an animal model. The mechanisms preventing pancreatic autodigestion in normal individuals appears to involve competitive inhibition of trypsin's catalytic domain by PSTI and, in a setting where the amount of autoactivated trypsin exceeds the ability of PSTI to inhibit its own activity by autodigestion [54]. The observation that elevations in intracellular calcium are associated with pancreatitis, and the important role of calcium in enhancing cationic trypsinogen autoactivation [10, 11, 19] and limiting the rate of trypsin autolysis [12] also point to a central role for trypsin in acute pancreatitis. The presence of two separate mutations in the same gene in most unrelated kindreds with hereditary pancreatitis suggests that cationic trypsinogen may play a dominant role in both hereditary and nonhereditary forms of premature protease activation-mediated acute and chronic pancreatitis [54, 55]. The observation that at least one additional gene mutation is associated with hereditary pancreatitis [3, 16] suggests that further insights may be forthcoming.

References

1. Arias AE, Boldicke T, Bendayan M (1993) Absence of trypsinogen autoactivation and immunolocalization of pancreatic secretory trypsin inhibitor in acinar cells in vitro. In Vitro Cell Dev Biol 29:221–227
2. Banerjee A, Galloway S, Kingsnorth A (1994) Experimental models of acute pancreatitis. Br J Surg 81:1096–1103
3. Bartness M, Duerr RH, Ford MA, et al (1998) Potential linkage of a pancreatitis associated gene on chromosome 12. Pancreas 17:426
4. Bernard C (1856) Leçons de physiologie experimentale, vol 2. Bailleire, Paris, pp 278
5. Blackstone M, Whitcomb DC (1998) Premature trypsin activation in hereditary pancreatitis. Gastroenterology 115:796–799
6. Brunzell JD, Miller NE, Alaupovic P, et al (1983) Familial chylomicronemia due to a circulating inhibitor of lipoprotein lipase activity. J Lipid Res 24:12–19
7. Carey MC, Fitzgerald O (1968) Hyperparathyroidism associated with chronic pancreatitis in a family. Gut 9:700–703
8. Cavallini G, Tittobello A, Frulloni L, Masci E, Mariana A, Di Francesco V (1996) Gabexate for the prevention of pancreatic damage related to endoscopic retrograde cholangiopancreatography. N Engl J Med 335:919–923
9. Collins JE, Brenton DP (1990) Pancreatitis and homocystinuria. J Inherit Metab Dis 13:232–233
10. Colomb E, Figarella C (1979) Comparative studies on the mechanism of activation of the two human trypsinogens. Biochim Biophys Acta 571:343–351
11. Colomb E, Figarella C, Guy O (1979) The two human trypsinogens. Evidence of complex formation with basic pancreatic trypsin inhibitor-proteolytic activity. Biochim Biophys Acta 570:397–405
12. Colomb E, Guy O, Deprez P, Michel R, Figarella C (1978) The two human trypsinogens: catalytic properties of the corresponding trypsins. Biochim Biophys Acta 525:186–193
13. Comfort M, Steinberg A (1952) Pedigree of a family with hereditary chronic relapsing pancreatitis. Gastroenterology 21:54–63
14. Cox DW, Breckenridge WC, Little JA (1978) Inheritance of apolipoprotein C-II deficiency with hypertriglyceridemia and pancreatitis. N Engl J Med 299:1421–1424
15. Dartsch H, Kleene R, Kern HF (1998) In vitro condensation-sorting of enzyme proteins isolated from rat pancreatic acinar cells. Eur J Cell Biol 75:211–222
16. Dasouki M, Cogan J, Summar M, et al (1998) Heterogeneity in hereditary pancreatitis. Am J Med Genet 77:47–53
17. Ferec C, Raguenes O, Bignon JD, Georgelin T, Lebodic L (1997) Hereditary pancreatitis gene (in French). M S Med Sci 13:246–249
18. Figarella C, Amouric M, Guy-Crotte O (1984) Proteolysis of human trypsinogen. I. Pathogenic implications in chronic pancreatitis. Biochem Biophys Res Commun 118:154–161
19. Figarella C, Miszczuk-Jamska B, Barrett AJ (1988) Possible lysosomal activation of pancreatic zymogens. Activation of both human trypsinogens by cathepsin B and spontaneous acid activation of human trypsinogen 1. Biol Chem Hoppe-Seylers 369[Suppl]: 293–298
20. Frick TW, Fernandez, del CC, Bimmler D, Warshaw AL (1997) Elevated calcium and activation of trypsinogen in rat pancreatic acini. Gut 41:339–343
21. Gorry M, Gabbaizadeh D, Furey W, et al (1997) Multiple mutations in the cationic trypsinogen gene are associated with hereditary pancreatitis. Gastroenterology 113:1063–1068

22. Grady T, Saluja A, Kaiser A, Steer M (1996) Edema and intrapancreatic trypsinogen activation precede glutathione depletion during cerulein pancreatitis. Am J Physiol 271:G20–G26
23. Grady T, Otani T, Mah'moud M, Rhee S, Learch MM, Gorelick FS (1998) Zymogen proteolysis within the pancreatic acinar cell is associated with cellular injury. Am J Physiol 275:G1010–G1017
24. Greenbaum LM, Hirshkowitz A, Shoichet I (1959) The activation of trypsinogen by cathepsin B. J Biol Chem 234:2885–2890
25. Gress TM, Micha AE, Lacher U, Adler G (1997) Hereditary pancreatitis, caused by mutations in the cationic trypsinogen gene (in German). Dtsch Med Wochenschr 122:1461–1465
26. Gress TM, Micha AE, Lacher U, Adler G (1998) Diagnosis of a "hereditary pancreatitis" by the detection of a mutation in the cationic trypsinogen gene (in German). Dtsch Med Wochenschr 123:453–456
27. Hofbauer B, Daluja A, Learch M, et al (1998) Intra-acinar cell activation of trypsinogen during cerulein-induced pancreatitis in rats. Am J Physiol 275:G352–G362
28. Hubbard S, Eisenmenger F, Thornton J (1994) Modeling studies of the change in conformation required for cleavage of limited proteolytic sites. Protein Sci 3:757–768
29. Hubbard S, Eisenmenger F, Thornton J (1994) Limited proteolysis sites modeling, Hubbard.kin 3.5 (2PTC, 1TGN, 5RSA). Protein Sci [serial online] 3:URL: http://prosci.org/Kinemage/, Filename: Hubbard.kin 3.5
30. Klumperman J, Kuliawat R, Griffith JM, Geuze HJ, Arvan P (1998) Mannose 6-phosphate receptors are sorted from immature secretory granules via adaptor protein AP-1, clathrin, and syntaxin 6-positive vesicles. J Cell Biol 141:359–371
31. Kruger B, Lerch MM, Tessenow W (1998) Direct detection of premature protease activation in living pancreatic acinar cells. Lab Invest 78:763–764
32. Kurth T, Teich N, Kistner S, Mossner J, Keim V (1998) Expression of the N21I-mutation of human cationic trypsinogen in a yeast system. Digestion 59:243 (abstr)
33. Le Bodic L, Bignon JD, Raguenes O, et al (1996) The hereditary pancreatitis gene maps to long arm of chromosome 7. Hum Mol Genet 5:549–554
34. Leach SD, Moldin IM, Sheele GA, Gorelick FS (1991) Intracellular activation of digestive enzymes in rat pancreatic acini: stimulation by high dose of cholecystokinin. J Clin Invest 87:362–366
35. Lerch M, Adler G (1994) Experimental models of acute pancreatitis. Int J Pancreatol 15:159–170
36. Mithofer K, Fernandez-Del Castillo C, Frick TW, Lewandrowski KB, Rattner DW, Warshaw AL (1995) Acute hypercalcemia causes acute pancreatitis and ectopic trypsinogen activation in the rat [see comments]. Gastroenterology 109:239–246
37. Mithofer K, Fernandez-Del Castillo C, Rattner DW, Warshaw AL (1998) Subcellular kinetics of early trypsinogen activation in acute rodent pancreatitis. Am J Physiol 274:G71–G79
38. Nagasaki Y, Koizumi M, Shimosegawa T, et al (1997) Trypsinogen gene mutation in Japanese patients with juvenile or familial pancreatitis. Pancreas 15:447
39. Nishimori I, Adachi K, Kamakura M, et al (1997) Cationic trypsinogen gene mutation in hereditary pancreatitis. Pancreas 14:448
40. Otani T, Chepilko S, Grendell J, Gorelick F (1998) Co-distribution of trypsinogen activation peptide and the granule membrane protein, GRAMP-92, in rat cerulein-induced pancreatitis. Am J Physiol 275:G999–G1009
41. Pandya A, Blanton SH, Landa B, et al (1996) Linkage studies in a large kindred with hereditary pancreatitis confirms mapping of the gene to a 16-cm region on 7q. Genomics 38:227–230
42. Perrault J (1994) Hereditary pancreatitis. Gastroenterol Clin North Am 23:743–52
43. Rao K, Tuma J, Lombardi B (1976) Acute hemorrhagic pancreatic necrosis in mice. Intraparenchymal activation of zymogens, and other enzyme changes in pancreas and serum. Gastroenterology 70:720–726
44. Richardson D (1996) MAGE. Protein Science Kinemages. Available on URL:http://prosci.org/Kinemage/, gopher://gopher.prosci.uci./11/kinemage: The Protein Society, 1992–1996
45. Rinderknecht H (1986) Activation of pancreatic zymogens. Normal activation, premature intrapancreatic activation, protective mechanims against inappropriate activation. Dig Dis Sci 31:314–321

46. Rinderknecht H (1993) Pancreatic secretory enzymes. In: Go VLW, DiMagno EP, Gardner JD, Lebenthal E, Reber HA, Scheele GA (eds) The pancreas: biology, pathobiology, and disease. Raven, New York, pp 219–251
47. Rinderknecht H, Adham NF, Renner IG, Carmack C (1988) A possible zymogen self-destruct mechanism preventing pancreatic autodigestion. Int J Pancreatol 3:33–44
48. Saluga AK, Donovan EA, Yamanaka K, Yamaguchi Y, Hofbauer B, Steer ML (1997) Cerulein-induced in vitro activation of trypsinogen in rat pancreatic acini is mediated by cathepsin B. Gastroenterology 113:304–310
49. Sibert JR (1978) Hereditary pancreatitis in England and Wales. J Med Genet 15:189–201
50. Steer ML (1992) How and where does acute pancreatitis begin? Arch Surg 127:1350–1353
51. Steer ML, Meldolesi J, Figarella C (1984) Pancreatitis. The role of lysosomes. Dig Dis Sci 29:934–938
52. Steinberg W, Schlesselman S (1987) Treatment of acute pancreatitis: comparison of animal and human studies. Gastroenterology 93:1420–1427
53. Ward JB, Petersen OH, Jenkins SA, Sutton R (1995) Is an elevated concentration of acinar cytosolic free ionised calcium the trigger for acute pancreatitis? (review) [42 refs]. Lancet 346:1016–1019
54. Whitcomb DC, Gorry MC, Preston RA, et al (1996) Hereditary pancreatitis is caused by a mutation in the cationic trypsinogen gene. Nat Genet 14:141–145
55. Whitcomb DC, Preston RA, Aston CE, et al (1996) A gene for hereditary pancreatitis maps to chromosome 7q35. Gastroenterology 110:1975–1980
56. Whitcomb DC, Ulrich II CD (1999) Hereditary pancreatitis: new insights, new directions. In: Neoptolemus JP (ed) Balliere's clinical gastroenterology: acute pancreatitis. Blackwell Scientific, Oxford (in press)
57. Wilson DE, Hata A, Kwong LK, et al (1993) Mutations in exon 3 of the lipoprotein lipase gene segregating in a family with hypertriglyceridemia, pancreatitis, and non-insulin-dependent diabetes. J Clin Invest 92:203–211

Events Inside the Pancreatic Acinar Cell in Acute Pancreatitis: Role of Secretory Blockade, Calcium Release, and Dehydration in the Initiation of Trypsinogen Activation and Autodigestion

C. NIEDERAU and R. LÜTHEN

Introduction

Recent studies offer new insight into the processes which may lead to protease activation and cell damage during acute pancreatitis. Several mechanisms which finally lead to cell damage in vitro and to acute pancreatitis in vivo cause a rapid increase of $[Ca^{2+}]_i$ in the acinar cells. This $[Ca^{2+}]_i$ increase is followed shortly thereafter by cell dehydration and a blockade of protein secretion. Recent studies suggest that the cell shrinkage may largely explain the secretory blockade, which is an early characteristic of acute pancreatitis. Several mechanisms that cause $[Ca^{2+}]_i$ increase, cell dehydration, and secretory blockade also result in activation of trypsinogen. Calcium chelators can reduce the trypsinogen activation, and cell dehydration can restore the secretory function. Thus, these cellular events are probably linked in a causal relationship (Fig. 1). Recent studies also show that trypsinogen activation occurs inside the acinar cell and may be the primary step leading to autodigestion. Once trypsin has become activated, its inhibition does not alter the course of pancreatitis, because other proteases which are activated by trypsin finally cause the subsequent cell damage. Clinical studies should therefore focus rather on new protease inhibitors, which more specifically also inhibit elastase and phospholipase in already established pancreatitis. Other studies should analyze means of inhibiting a pathological calcium release and of overcoming the secretory blockade. Re-hydration may be a crucial factor not only in preventing shock but also in restoring cellular functions.

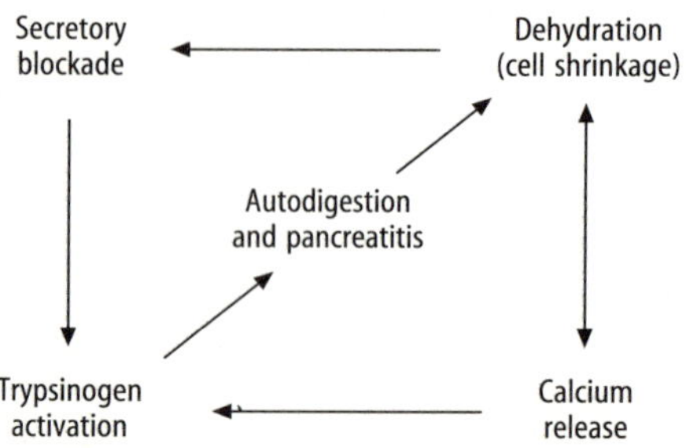

Fig. 1. Potential interactions between important factors in the pathophysiology of acute pancreatitis

Activation of Pancreatic Proteases and Lipases

Almost a century ago, Chiari suggested that acute necrotizing pancreatitis was due to autodigestion of exocrine tissue by proteolytic and lipolytic enzymes [1]. Although it is generally accepted that active digestive enzymes are found in pancreatic tissue during the process of acute pancreatitis, the mechanism that triggers the activation process is still unknown. Once the activation cascade has been initiated by one of various toxic mechanisms (e.g., gallstones, alcohol, ERCP, hyperlipemia), the pathophysiology of pancreatitis probably no longer depends on the initiating factor. Physiologically, activation of trypsinogen to trypsin is the trigger which activates other digestive enzymes in the form of a cascade, except for lipase, which already occurs in its active form inside the pancreatic acinar cell. Previous studies which evaluated the noxious potential of digestive enzymes have focused mainly on trypsin as the major enzyme mediating the autodigestive process. As yet, multiple controlled clinical trials with trypsin inhibitors have failed to alter the course of acute pancreatitis (literature in [2]). Some of the more recently developed protease inhibitors such as gabexate, camostate, and nafamostate are serine protease inhibitors that inactivate various other digestive pancreatic enzymes in addition to trypsin. The inhibitory potential of these antiproteases toward chymotrypsin is considerably smaller, however, than that toward trypsin. Furthermore, these antiproteases are only weak inhibitors of phospholipase A_2 and elastase. Lipase itself is unlikely to play a major role in initiating pancreatitis, because it is already active inside the zymogen granule of the normal cell under physiological conditions. Lipase may cause additional damage, however, when substrates are available from which the enzyme can liberate noxious free fatty acids.

Recent studies show that the noxious potential of various digestive enzymes for pancreatic acinar cells is strikingly different [3]. Elastase, lipase, chymotrypsin, and phospholipase A_2 were several orders of magnitude more potent in damaging acinar cells when compared with trypsin on a molar basis (Fig. 2): At nanomolar concentrations elastase caused a rapid destruction of the cells, whereas micromolar concentrations of trypsin were necessary to cause at least some cell damage. In general, the degree of noxious potential of an enzyme was inverse to the order in which it was activated. Although activation of trypsinogen initiates the activation cascade, this enzyme is the one least harmful to the pancreas in terms of direct damage. Elastase, which is activated late in the cascade of events, is by far the most harmful enzyme in terms of direct cell damage. A comparison of the noxious potential of enzymes produced surprising results. Elastase is generally believed to act mainly on elastin in the vessels, thereby contributing to the hemorrhagic lesions seen in severe pancreatitis. However, elastase appears to have a broad spectrum of action on many proteins, the variety of which is greater than generally assumed. In view of these data, it is not surprising that the clinical studies failed to show any advantageous effects of antiproteases, which cause only moderate inactivation of chymotrypsin and even less (or no) inactivation of phospholipase and elastase. In the clinical situation, the patient usual-

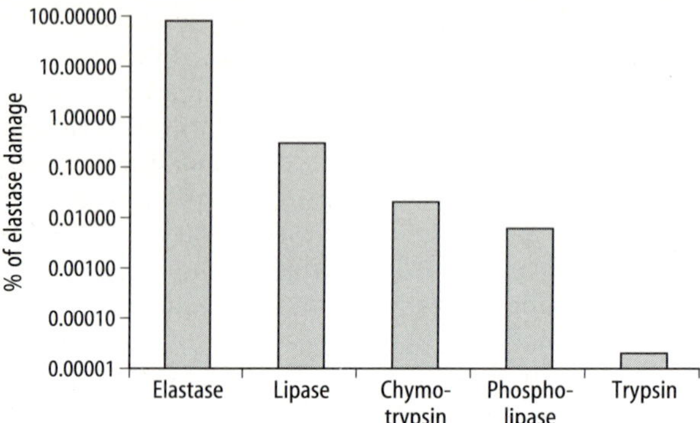

Fig. 2. Noxious potential of pancreatic digestive enzymes in a molar comparison. The results show the relative amount of enzyme necessary to damage 20% of isolated pancreatic acinar cells after 90 min exposure (i.e., 20% cells taking up trypan blue) when compared with the damage caused by a specific elastase concentration. (Adapted from [3])

ly presents at least several hours after the onset of symptoms, at a time when the initial activation of trypsinogen has probably already occurred. Although it is theoretically still useful to prevent any further activation of trypsinogen, the recent results clearly show that the main effort should be aimed at inhibiting those enzymes which have a greater noxious potential, such as elastase.

In several animal models of acute pancreatitis, activation of trypsinogen has been demonstrated to occur early in the course of the disease (literature in [4, 5]). It has also been shown that the prophylactic administration of a protease (trypsin) inhibitor (prior to the onset of pancreatitis) prevented both the increase in active trypsin and the development of pancreatitis. The therapeutic administration of a trypsin inhibitor was only able to decrease the amount of active trypsin but did not prevent pancreatitis [2]. These studies predicted the outcome of several later clinical controlled studies in which trypsin inhibitors failed to alter the course of already established pancreatitis (literature in [2]). In contrast, a trypsin inhibitor was able to reduce the incidence of ERCP-induced pancreatitis when given prophylactively, i.e., prior to ERCP [6]. These clinical and experimental results both fit to the hypothesis that, although the activation of trypsin triggers the activation cascade, other digestive enzymes are mainly responsible for tissue damage in the following pathophysiological process of pancreatitis.

Our studies in isolated cells [3] confirm previous work by Mössner's group [7] showing that lipase and triolein exert only moderately noxious effects in pancreatic acini when given alone. The admixture of enzyme and substrate, however, caused marked cellular damage. Incubation with oleic acid, the free acid which is liberated from triolein by the enzyme lipase, led to a degree of damage similar to that caused by the combination of lipase and triolein. Thus, lipase probably causes its damage via the release of free fatty acids. Similar results were obtained for the action of phospholipase A_2 and lecithin. The product of the action of phospholipase A_2 on lecithin is lysolecithin, which caused marked cell damage in the present experiments as well as in previous studies. Again, the noxious potential of phospholipase A_2 was enhanced when its substrate lecithin was added to the incubation solution. In the clinical situation active digestive enzymes including phospholipase A_2 and lipase will exit the damaged or necrotic cell to enter the interstitium, where they have access to various sources of fat and fat tissue.

Other recent studies strongly support the concept that acute pancreatitis begins as an autodigestive process within the pancreatic gland and within the pancreatic acinar cell (literature in [7]). These studies include the identification of mutations in the trypsinogen gene in kindreds with hereditary pancreatitis [8] and the identification of early trypsinogen activation inside the pancreatic acinar cells using the detection of trypsinogen activation peptide (TAP) [9, 10].

Trypsinogen Activation: TAP Studies

It was shown only recently that trypsinogen activation is one of the earliest events in this process and that it may lead to subsequent activation of the other proteolytic enzymes [9, 10]. The measurement and quantification of activated trypsin in pancreatic tissue and serum has been hampered by methodological problems caused by binding of the activated protease to a variety of protease inhibitors. A better understanding of the autodigestive process has become possible with the characterization of a small cleavage product which is generated during trypsinogen activation. This pentapeptide, termed trypsinogen activation peptide, can be measured more reliably than active trypsin itself [11]. Measurement of TAP generation recently showed that trypsinogen activation occurs a few minutes after experimental damage to pancreatic acinar cells in vitro and in acute experimental pancreatitis in vivo [9] (Fig. 3). Our own recent results for the first time present direct morphological

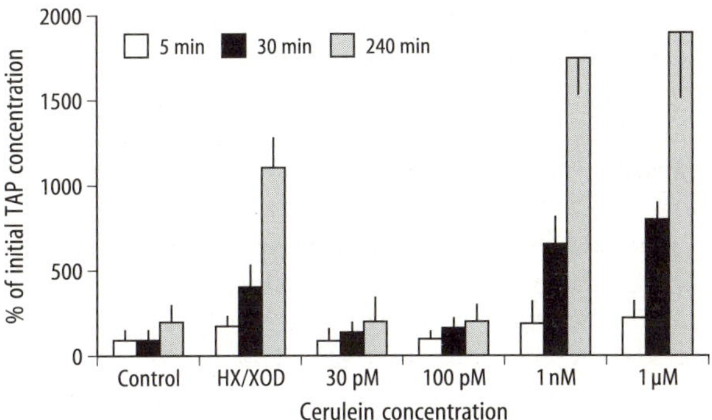

Fig. 3. Concentration of trypsinogen activation peptide (TAP) in isolated pancreatic acini after stimulation with various concentrations of the CCK analogue cerulein or after exposure to a radical-generating solution containing xanthine oxidase and hypoxanthine; for details of methods see [9]

evidence of trypsinogen activation inside pancreatic acinar cells during experimental acute pancreatitis [10]. Therefore, the autodigestive process is likely to originate inside acinar cells, rather than in the interstitium or duct lumen as suggested by others (literature in [10]). Previous studies showed that acinar vacuolization and autophagic phenomena in the vicinity of zymogen granules and the Golgi region coincided with zymogen activation, suggesting that these cellular compartments are likely candidates for the site of this activation process (literature in [10]). Intracellular location of the activation of digestive zymogens following in vitro stimulation with high doses of CCK was also suggested by others (literature in [10]). Subcellular fractionation studies implicated secretory granules and vacuoles as possible intracellular sites of serine protease activation (literature in [10]). These findings are substantiated by our results, which show TAP staining at the luminal side of the acinar cell, apparently along the secretory pathway of digestive enzymes, probably labeling Golgi apparatus and zymogen granules. Studies at a higher level of resolution using immune EM are currently being undertaken to further elucidate the location of zymogen activation during acute pancreatitis.

Colocalization Hypothesis

Studies in several models of pancreatitis and in the clinical situation show that large vacuoles form inside the acinar cells which partly fuse with zymogen (a process termed either autophagocytosis or crinophagy; for literature see [12]). The admixture of digestive and lysosomal enzymes in such vacuoles ("colocalization") is proposed to be important because the lysosomal enzyme cathepsin B can activate trypsinogen in vitro and may thereby initiate the activation cascade of proteolytic enzymes to trigger autodigestion. Our own recent studies, however, showed that complete inhibition of cathepsin B did not prevent trypsinogen activation caused by cerulein hyperstimulation of the pancreatic acinar cell in vitro. Similarly, treatment with cathepsin B inhibitors failed to ameliorate acute experimental pancreatitis in vivo. Thus, to us it appears unlikely that cathepsin B is the main trigger for activation of trypsinogen in acute pancreatitis.

Secretory Blockade

During the past 30 years, numerous clinical trials have failed to improve the course of acute pancreatitis using drugs aimed at inhibiting exocrine pancreatic secretion (literature in [2, 13]). The rationale for such treatment is "to set the pancreas at rest". The list of substances which all failed in prospective randomized trials includes glucagon, calcitonin, atropine, pancreatic polypeptide, H2-antagonists, and somatostatin, as well as the application of a nasogastric tube (literature in [13]). During the past 10 years experimental cell biology has presented unequivocal evidence that exocrine secretion is markedly impaired during the early course of acute pancreatitis [13]. The inability to discharge secretory proteins, including proteases, may increase the risk of trypsinogen activation inside the pancreatic acinar cell. The latter event is generally thought to trigger the autodigestive process. Thus, it does not make any sense to inhibit exocrine pancreatic secretion early in the course of pancreatitis by the administration of drugs or other measures. Rather, further studies should look into the possibility of overcoming the secretory blockade in early acute pancreatitis.

In spite of the failure to treat pancreatitis by inhibiting exocrine secretion, oral food intake should not be allowed during the initial course of pancreatitis. A marked stimulation of the gland may have many deleterious cell biological effects, in addition to stimulating exocrine secretion (literature in [13]). Oral food intake is also contraindicated in patients with motility dysfunction and ileus.

Cell Dehydration

Recent data also show that oxidative stress induced by various mechanisms causes a marked inhibition of enzyme secretion in isolated rat pancreatic acinar cells. This secretory blockade is probably mediated to a large degree by cell dehydration [14]. These findings are not only of cell physiological interest; they may also have clinical implications. Pancreatic secretory function is markedly reduced in acute pancreatitis [13] due to as yet largely unknown mechanisms. Acute pancreatitis is associated with muscle cell dehydration (cell shrinkage) [15]. One might speculate that the marked general cell dehydration in pancreatitis is also present in other organs, such as the liver. On the other hand, it has been shown that rehydration improves the prognosis of acute pancreatitis [16]. The present results show that cell shrinkage itself is sufficient to markedly inhibit the secretory capacity of pancreatic acinar cells [14]. Thus, cellular dehydration may at least partly explain the secretory blockade seen in acute pancreatitis.

The Role of Calcium

Hypercalcemia is associated with an increased risk of developing acute and chronic pancreatitis (literature in [17]). This association was first established in patients with hypercalcemia due to hyperparathyroidism. Acute pancreatitis has been noted as the first symptom of hyperparathyroidism. It was recently reported that intravenous administration of calcium during cardiac bypass surgery may be responsible for the frequent development of acute pancreatitis after this type of intervention. Previous studies have also shown that hypercalcemia may alter pancreatic exocrine secretion. However, the role of intracellular calcium in mediating pancreatic damage, in acute pancreatitis for example, has only recently been investigated.

Intracellular calcium plays a fundamental role in regulating numerous enzyme activities and mediating effects of hormones and growth factors that control a wide variety of cellular processes, such as muscle contraction, metabolism, cell secretion, differentiation, and growth. A large and sustained increase of $[Ca^{2+}]_i$ in the acinar cells also plays a key role in mediating cell damage in general [18] and is involved in the pathogenesis of acute pancreatitis [17]. Many mechanisms which lead to pancreatic cell damage in vitro and pancreatitis in vivo, such as free radicals or supraphysiological concentrations of the CCK analogue cerulein, cause a rapid intracellular $[Ca^{2+}]_i$ increase. It is also noteworthy that the toxins of special types of scorpions and some organophosphorous insecticides cause prolonged elevations of $[Ca^{2+}]_i$ via an anti-cholinesterase effect and, thereby, acute pancreatitis (literature in [17]). Other drugs which are associated with an increased risk of pancreatitis have been shown to cause release of $[Ca^{2+}]_i$, e.g., estrogens and thiazides (literature in [17]). Both hyperlipidemia and ethanol may also interact with $[Ca^{2+}]_i$; the latter factors are associated with a significant risk of pancreatitis (literature in [17]). Lipoproteins have been shown to cause oscillations of $[Ca^{2+}]_i$ in some cell types (literature in [17]). Ethanol may exert its effect of cell calcium rather indirectly, either by potentiating the calcium increase due to cholinergic stimulation or by generating free radicals, which are known to increase $[Ca^{2+}]_i$ (literature in [17]).

The $[Ca^{2+}]_i$ increase precedes all the other functional and morphological alterations in the acinar cells investigated and may therefore be the cause, or at least an important mediator, and not the result of cell damage [17] (Fig. 4). The inhibitor of intracellular calcium release TMB-8 almost completely inhibited the increase in $[Ca^{2+}]_i$, whereas the calcium channel blocks and depletion of extracellular calcium did not. Therefore, the increase in $[Ca^{2+}]_i$ is due to a release from intracellular stores and not to an influx of extracellular $[Ca^{2+}]_i$ supporting the idea of $[Ca^{2+}]_i$ as an intracellular signal molecule for cell death after exposure to free radicals. The increase in $[Ca^{2+}]_i$

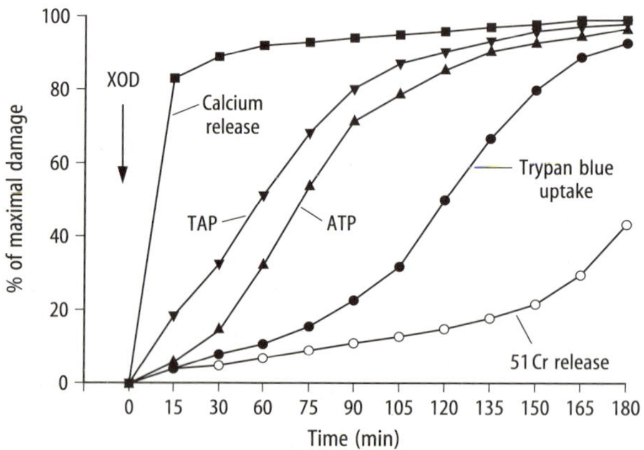

Fig. 4. Biochemical and morphological damage to isolated pancreatic acinar cells after xanthine oxidase (*XOD*) was added to a solution containing hypoxanthine; for details of solutions and subsequent release of free radicals see [9]. The results show the percentage of maximal damage after addition of XOD for various tests; for details of measurements see [9]

may also lead to activation of trypsin inside the pancreatic acinar cells. Little is known, however, about why an increase in $[Ca^{2+}]_i$ stimulates physiological events such as luminal protein secretion in some instances and initiates cell death in others. Until now, $[Ca^{2+}]_i$ increases were thought to represent physiological signals when they occurred as oscillations at the single cell level. In contrast, large and sustained $[Ca^{2+}]_i$ increases without oscillations were thought to initiate cell damage. This view was supported by the observation that supraphysiological CCK dose-dependently reduced the oscillatory nature of the $[Ca^{2+}]_i$ increase. Recent studies confirm the latter findings, but show in addition that exposure of acinar cells to free radicals causes not only a bulk increase in $[Ca^{2+}]_i$ but also calcium oscillations which had a lower frequency but a similar amplitude when compared with oscillations that followed physiological stimuli. In pancreatic acinar cells, the absolute degree of $[Ca^{2+}]_i$ increase does not definitely determine the cellular response. Instead, the duration of $[Ca^{2+}]_i$ increases may be more important, because under all experimental conditions of cell damage there was a sustained $[Ca^{2+}]_i$ increase. In contrast to recent suggestions of a direct relationship between $[Ca^{2+}]_i$ oscillations and subsequent exocytosis in pancreatic acinar cells, recent results show that free radicals can induce calcium oscillations which do not cause subsequent exocytosis but markedly inhibit the secretory response to various physiological stimuli [17]. Further experiments showed that the calcium release caused by free radicals originates mostly from thapsigargin-insensitive, ryanodine-sensitive stores. Thus, the origin and duration of increases in calcium, rather than its extent or oscillatory nature, determine whether the cell will secrete or die.

The abnormal type of $[Ca^{2+}]_i$ increase can trigger the activation of trypsin, acinar cell damage, and acute pancreatitis. This hypothesis is supported by studies which showed that calcium chelators inhibit the radical-induced activation of trypsin [17] as well as cell necrosis and apoptosis [18, 19]. It was also demonstrated that TAP generation, and thus trypsinogen activation under these conditions, depend on the availability of intracellular calcium. Thus, calcium may also play a major role in mediating the autodigestive process at this crucial step.

Calcium and Apoptosis of Pancreatic Acinar Cells

Free radicals, generated for example by menadione or peroxynitrite, may induce both necrosis and apoptosis [19, 20]. While a high concentration of menadione or peroxynitrite caused rapid cell necrosis, lower concentrations induced a DNA ladder in gel electrophoresis indicative of apoptosis [19, 20]. Similar results were obtained using a DNA fragmentation ELISA. The latter studies indicate that release of $[Ca^{2+}]_i$ may be involved in mediating both necrosis and apoptosis. It may depend on the type of the noxious factor and on the type of cell death in which calcium plays a predominant role. Binding and chelating of $[Ca^{2+}]_i$ inhibited both apoptosis and necrosis in vitro, suggesting that the $[Ca^{2+}]_i$ increases seen after various noxious factors are not merely a by-product but may directly mediate the cell damage [19, 20]. Therefore, blockade of the release of $[Ca^{2+}]_i$ may also have a clinical potential. As yet, however, most of the calcium chelators are nonspecific in also inhibiting the calcium responses to physiological stimuli and may thereby damage cells and tissues not involved in the primary disease.

Both menadione and peroxynitrite, as well as other mechanisms that release free radicals, also caused a rapid increase in $[Ca^{2+}]_i$, cell dehydration, and a secretory blockade [21]. It is noteworthy that release of $[Ca^{2+}]_i$ and cell shrinkage are early characteristics of the apoptotic process [19, 21]. Our studies also showed that free radicals can lead to activation of trypsinogen within 30 min. Therefore, recent observations link the early functional cell alterations of $[Ca^{2+}]_i$ increase, cell shrinkage, and secretory blockade to the consequences of trypsinogen activation and cell damage, in the form of both apoptosis and necrosis.

Oxidative Stress and Trypsinogen Activation

Our recent results show that oxidative stress causes a rapid activation of trypsin, which may be at least partly responsible for the resulting cell damage. In accordance with recent in vivo data, in vitro experiments showed that supramaximal concentrations of the CCK analogue cerulein also caused a rapid activation of trypsin, whereas "physiological" cerulein concentrations (i.e., concentrations which induce maximal amylase secretion) did not activate trypsin [9]. We have recently shown that trypsin activation due to supramaximal cerulein stimulation occurs inside the cell in the area which is covered by zymogen granules [10]. The present data suggest that zymogen granules are important targets of reactive oxygen species inside acinar cells. Since leakage of proteases from damaged cells accelerates xanthine oxidase-mediated injury, the enormous proteolytic potential of the pancreatic acinar cell makes it particularly susceptible to oxidative damage.

References

1. Chiari H (1896) Über Selbstverdauung des menschlichen Pancreas. Z Heilkunde 17:69–95
2. Niederau C, Schulz HU (1993) Current conservative treatment of acute pancreatitis: evidence of animal and human studies. Hepatogastroenterology 6:538–549
3. Niederau C, Frohnhoffs C, Schulz HU, Klonowski H (1995) Active pancreatic digestive enzymes show striking differences in their potential to damage isolated pancreatic acinar cells. J Lab Clin Invest 125:265–275
4. Niederau C, Liddle RA, Ferrell LD, Grendell JH (1986) Beneficial effects of cholecystokinin-receptor blockage and inhibition of proteolytic enzyme activity in experimental acute hemorrhagic pancreatitis in mice: evidence for cholecystokinin as a major factor in the development of acute pancreatitis. J Clin Invest 78:1056–1063
5. Lüthen R, Niederau C, Grendell JH (1995) Intrapancreatic activation of digestive enzymes during caerulein pancreatitis in rats: a possible role for changes in ATP and glutathione levels. Am J Physiol 268:G592–G604

6. Cavallini G, Tittobello A, Frulloni G, Masci E, Mariana A, DiFranesco V (1996) Gabexate for the prevention of pancreatic damage related to endoscopic retrograde cholangiopancreatography. N Engl J Med 335:919–923
7. Nagai H, Henrich H, Wünsch PH, Fischbach W, Mössner J (1989) Role of pancreatic enzymes and their substrates in autodigestion of the pancreas. Gastroenterology 96:838–847
8. Whitcomb DC, Gorry MC, Preston RA, Furey W, Sossenheimer MJ, Ulrich CD, Martin SP, Gates LK, Amann ST, Toskes PP, Liddle R, McGrath K jr, Uomo G, Post JC, Ehrlich G (1996) Hereditary pancreatitis is caused by a mutation in the cationic trypsinogen gen. Nat Genet 14:141–145
9. Niederau C, Klonowski H, Sarbia S, Lüthen R, Schulz HU, Häussinger D (1996) Oxidative injury to isolated rat pancreatic acinar cells versus isolated zymogen granules. Free Radic Biol Med 20:877–886
10. Lüthen R, Grendell JH, Häussinger D, Niederau C (1998) Trypsinogen activation occurs inside the acinar cell early in the course of acute cerulein-induced pancreatitis. Pancreas 17:38–43
11. Hurley PR, Cook A, Jehanli A, Austen BM, Hermon-Taylor J (1988) Development of radioimmunoassays for free tetra-L-aspartyl-lysine trypsinogen activation peptides (TAP). J Immunol Methods 111:195–203
12. Klonowski-Stumpe H, Han B, Lüthen R, Häussinger D, Niederau C (1998) Effects of cathepsin B inhibitors on trypsinogen activation in rat pancreas. Pancreas 16:96–101
13. Niederau C, Niederau M, Lüthen R, Strohmeyer G, Ferrell LD, Grendell JH (1990) Pancreatic exocrine secretion in acute experimental pancreatitis. Gastroenterology 99:1120–1127
14. Han B, Klonowski-Stumpe H, Sata N, Lüthen R, Schliess F, Häussinger D, Niederau C (1997) Cell volume changes modulate cholecystokinin and carbachol stimulated amylase release in isolated rat pancreatic acini. Gastroenterology 113:1756–1766
15. Häussinger D, Roth E, Lang F, Gerok W (1993) Cellular hydration state: an important determinant of protein catabolism in health and disease. Lancet 341:1330–1332
16. Niederau C, Crass RA, Silver G, Ferrell LD, Grendell JH (1988) Therapeutic regimens in acute experimental hemorrhagic pancreatitis. Effects of hydration, oxygenation, peritoneal lavage, and a potent protease inhibitor. Gastroenterology 95:1648–1657
17. Klonowski-Stumpe H, Schreiber R, Grolik M, Schulz HU, Häussinger D, Niederau C (1997) The effect of oxidative stress on cellular functions and cytosolic calcium of rat pancreatic acinar cells. Am J Physiol 272:G1489-G1498
18. Nicotera P, Bellomo G, Orrenius S (1992) Calcium-mediated mechanisms in chemically induced cell death. Annu Rev Pharmacol Toxicol 32:449–470
19. Sata N, Bin H, Klonowski H, Häusinger D, Niederau C (1997) Menadione exerts apoptosis and necrosis in pancreatic acinar cells. Free Radic Biol Med 3:844–850
20. Sata N, Bin H, Klonowski H, Häusinger D, Niederau C (1997) Peroxynitrite induces both apoptosis and necrosis in pancreatic acinar cells. Pancreas 15:278–284
21. Han B, Klonowski-Stumpe H, Lüthen R, Schreiber R, Häussinger D, Niederau C (1999) Menadione-induced oxidative stress inhibits cholecystokinin-stimulated secretion of pancreatic acini by cell dehydration. Am J Physiol (submitted for publication)

CHAPTER 3

Immunological Mechanisms in Acute Pancreatitis

J. Schölmerich

Introduction

In recent years it has become evident that both the intrapancreatic events and, even more, the extrapancreatic manifestations of severe acute pancreatitis (septic inflammatory response syndrome, whole-body inflammation) depend on immunological mechanisms. Thus far, this has not led to diagnostic or therapeutic consequences, with the exception of clinical trials with a PAF antagonist, lexipafant [1, 2]. In the following, the evidence for the importance of immunological mechanisms in the pathophysiology of severe acute pancreatitis will be presented. First the role of mediators in inflammation in general will be discussed, thereafter the role of cytokines in the pancreas itself during initial organ attack, then the role of cytokines as effectors in the systemic manifestations of acute pancreatitis, and finally possible consequences for diagnosis and treatment.

Role of Mediators in Inflammation

An abundance of cytokines and other mediators have been described which are involved mostly in local and systemic inflammatory responses. Most of these cytokines have a pluripotent action, as described, for example, for in-

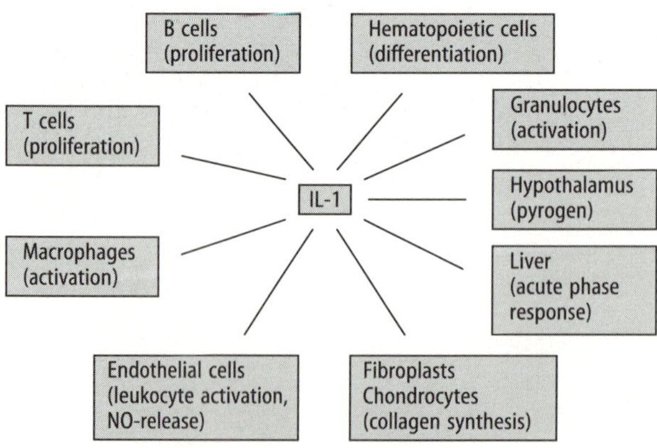

Fig. 1. Effects of interleukin-1 on different cell populations

terleukin-1 (Fig. 1). These mediators act on vast numbers of cells and induce most of the phenomena known to the clinician in all inflammatory disorders. Cytokines and other mediators are produced by an array of cells including monocytes/macrophages, fibroblasts, endothelial cells, lymphocytes, and epithelial cells. From studies of the small and large intestine it has become evident that epithelial cells are a major source of cytokines, and in particular chemokines, which attract inflammatory cells that in turn release cytokines [3]. It is therefore obvious to speculate that pancreatic acinar cells are able to do the same and could therefore be involved in immunological mechanisms in the pathogenesis of local and distant events in acute pancreatitis.

Cytokines and Chemokines in the Gland

The first suggestion that fatal pancreatitis is a consequence of excessive leukocyte stimulation came from H. Rinderknecht in 1988 [4]. At about the same time, our group described an early accumulation of leukocytes in the pancreas during attacks of acute pancreatitis as shown by leukocyte scintigraphy with technetium labeled leukocytes [5] (Fig. 2). Furthermore, the amount of leukocyte immigration was related to the outcome of the disease. Since it is obvious from the old quotation "cellulae non agent nisi fixatae" that chemokines (attracting leukocytes) and adhesion molecules must be involved in this process, we studied some cytokines and chemokines during the initial phase of acute pancreatitis. As expected, we found a significant level of interleukin-6 in the circulation of patients with later severe or fatal pancreatitis [6]. Furthermore, we detected a significant amount of circulating interleukin-8 in those patients with a fatal disease course (Fig. 3) [7]. These observations led to the concept that during the initial status of acute pan-

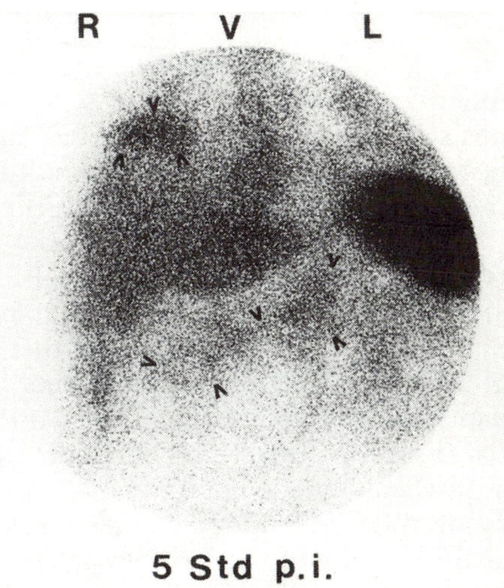

Fig. 2. Leukocyte scintigraphy in the early phase of severe acute pancreatitis

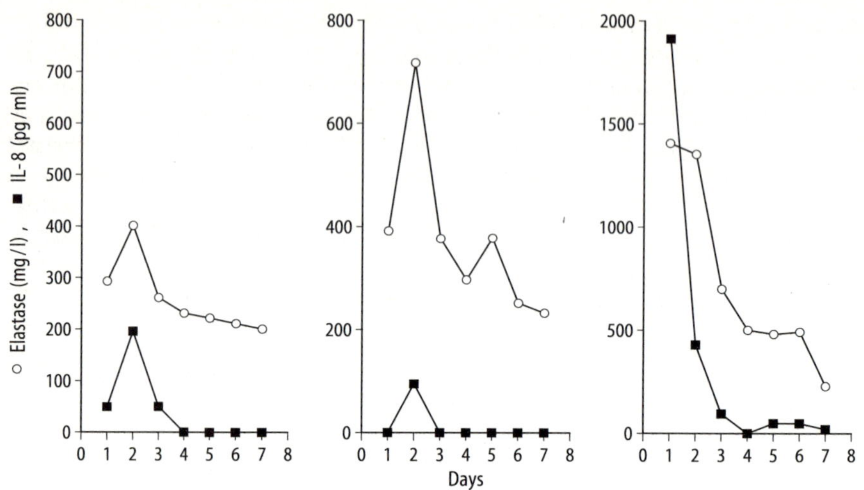

Fig. 3. Initial interleukin-8 serum concentrations in patients with different courses of acute pancreatitis

Table 1. IL-1 and TNFα have addictive effects in acute experimental pancreatitis (cerulein-induced) [10][a]

	Mortality (%)	Necrosis (0–4)	IL-6 (pg/ml)
Wild type	75**	3.6**	700**
IL-1-R$^{-/-}$	32	2.8	500
TNFα-R$^{-/-}$	30	2.7	450
IL-1-R and TNFα-R$^{-/-}$	15*	2.5	200*

[a] Effects were similar with interleukin-1 converting enzyme inhibitor/deletion.
* Significant vs wild type, IL-1-R$^{-/-}$, TNFα-R$^{-/-}$.
** Significant vs all knockouts.

creatitis highly elevated levels of circulating chemokines and cytokines are found in severe acute pancreatitis which seem to be correlated with prognosis [8, 9]. The fact that the half-life of interleukin-6 is about 5–10 min illustrates that there must be continuous production of the cytokine during the early phase of this disease.

Animal experiments with knockout models demonstrated that deletion of receptors for interleukin-1 or TNFα significantly reduced the mortality, the amount of necrosis, and the serum levels of interleukin-6; the combined knockout of both receptors further improved the outcome [10] (Table 1). Finally, other animal experiments showed that in two models of acute pancreatitis, the cerulein-induced and the bile acid-induced disease, differential display of messenger RNA detected two major rat chemokines (MOB-1, an α-chemokine and MCP-1 ($\alpha\,\beta$-chemokine) [11]. The inhibition of NF-κ-β by pyrrolidine dithiocarbamate resulted in reduction of the mRNA levels and of the severity of the induced pancreatitis. In vivo experiments and immunofluorescence localized the messenger RNA in acinar cells.

These findings, together with others, suggest that there is a local induction of messenger RNA for chemokines in the gland which, most likely by overflooding, releases chemokines, and probably cytokines as well, into the circulation. This has also been shown for TNF in experimental systems [12]. Thus, immune mechanisms are active inside the gland early in the disease and are responsible to some extent for the severity of the local events. A number of studies have added information about these effects, showing that local chemokine and cytokine production has to be included in the pathophysiological line of events in the pancreas.

Cytokines as Effectors of Systemic Inflammation in Severe Pancreatitis

Based on our earlier findings with regard to IL-6 and IL-8 [6–8], we more recently studied the only available human model of early pancreatitis, post-ERP pancreatitis, with regard to the time course of cytokine and chemokine release. By collecting blood samples from a significant number of patients undergoing ERP we were able to pick out those developing post-ERP pancreatitis and sequentially measure cytokines, anticytokines, CRP, and other parameters over the next 48 and in some instances 240 h [13, 14]. As expected from animal data, it turned out that IL-6 peaked 24 h earlier than C-reactive protein, which explains the better prognostic accuracy of the former for the later course of the disease. Furthermore, it was shown that IL-8 peaked significantly earlier than IL-6 and that the increase of IL-8 occurred almost immediately after ERP [14] (Fig. 4). At about the same time, the endogenous IL-1-receptor antagonist reached its peak, indicating an earlier release of IL-1, which induces this receptor antagonist (Fig. 5). From these and from the data of others it can be concluded that chemokines and cytokines, as well as their endogenous antagonists, are released into the systemic circulation early in the course of acute pancreatitis [8].

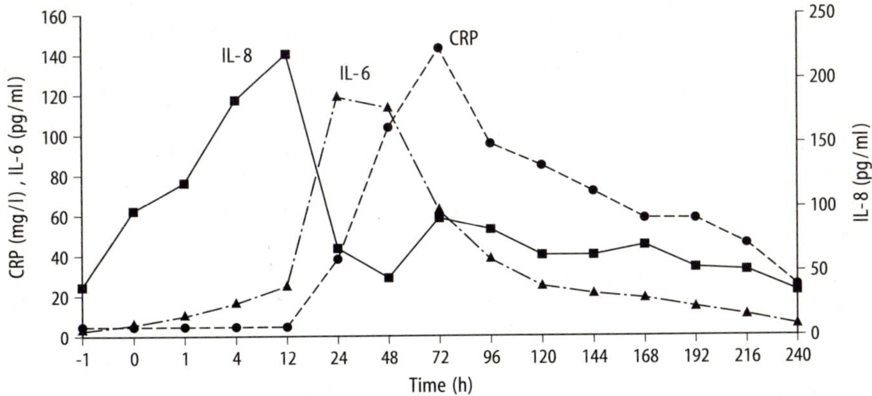

Fig. 4. Time course of serum interleukin-8 (*IL-8*), interleukin-6 (*IL-6*), and C-reactive protein (*CRP*) in post-ERP pancreatitis

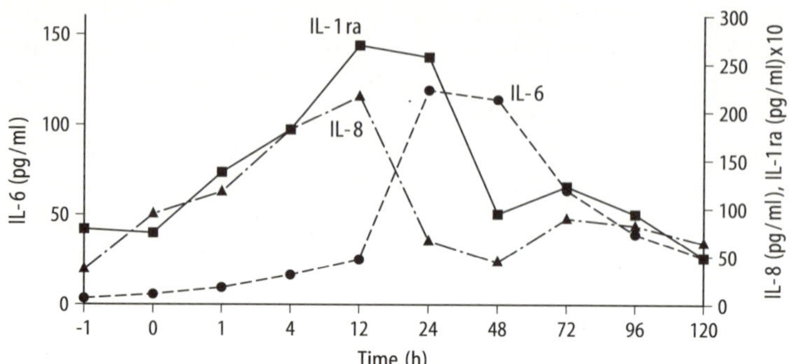

Fig. 5. Time course of serum interleukin-1 receptor antagonist (*IL-1ra*), interleukin-8 (*IL-8*), and interleukin-6 (*IL-6*) in post-ERP pancreatitis

Table 2. Levels of TNFα early in the course of human acute pancreatitis [15]

	Mild (n=59)	Severe (n=19)	Fatal (n=3)
TNFα (ng/ml)	9.6±7.9	11.0±9.0	Not detected
CRP (mg/l)	73 ±75	159 ±79	197±27
TNFα detected (%)	7	16	0

In contrast to others, we did not find TNFα during the course of post-ERP pancreatitis. This is in accordance with data from studies where the systemic levels of TNFα were not different between mild, severe, and fatal disease. In none of the patients with fatal disease was TNFα detected in the circulation (Table 2) [15]. However, in considering the ratio between TNF and its soluble receptors P55 and P75, which also represent an anti-inflammatory principle by binding TNF and preventing it from acting on its target cells, we demonstrated that there is a difference between mild and severe courses of the disease. In those patients with a severe course later, the ratio between the receptors and the proinflammatory cytokine decreased early, indicating consumption of these receptors, while this was not the case in patients with a mild disease course (Fig. 6) [16]. Similar findings have been obtained for interleukin-10 by others [17], who demonstrated that interleukin-10 levels initially were much higher in mild acute pancreatitis than in patients who later developed severe disease (424±364 vs. 15±6 pg/ml). All these data indicate that there is a significant release of proinflammatory cytokines and chemokines into the circulation during the initial phase of acute pancreatitis and a concordant decrease or loss of anti-inflammatory endogenous products in those patients developing severe disease.

This argument is further supported by the recent finding that animals that have a knockout for the β chemokine receptor CCR 1 have much less severe pulmonary damage in cerulein-induced acute pancreatitis as compared with animals that have the wild type (Table 3) [18]. Thus, it can be postulated that the systemic complications of acute pancreatitis are due mainly to the overflow of locally produced and later on distantly produced [19] chemokines

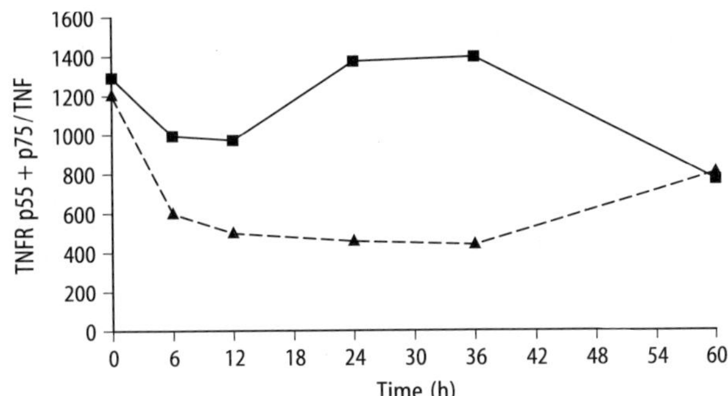

Fig. 6. Time course of the ratio of TNF receptors p55 and p75 to TNFα in serum in severe and mild acute pancreatitis

Table 3. Knockout of β-chemokine receptor CCR1 – prevention of lung failure in experimental pancreatitis [18][a] (MPO myeloperoxidase, BAL bronchoalveolar lavage)

	Wild type	$CCR1^{-/-}$	Wild-type cerulein	$CCR1^{-/-}$ cerulein
Capillary leak (%)	35	39	100	55
MPO (lung)	52	40	100	52
TNFα in BAL (pg/3 ml) after 12 h	–	–	400	0

[a] No change in pancreas itself except regarding MPO and TNF.

and cytokines which induce damage to distant organs such as lungs, kidneys, and the cardiovascular system (Fig. 7) [8].

Consequences for Diagnosis and Treatment

As expected on the basis of these experimental and human data, it turned out that interleukin-6, and probably even more interleukin-8, has a high predictive value for the later course of the disease (Tables 4, 5) [8, 9, 20–22]. It is obvious that the predicted value must be better than that of CRP, which is induced only by IL-6 in the liver and peaks at 48 or even 72 h. The biological correlation of IL-6 and CRP is delineated by the fact that there is a highly significant relationship between the peak levels of IL-6 and CRP in patients with post-ERP pancreatitis (Fig. 8) [13] as described earlier for patients with acute pancreatitis of different origin by our group [6]. The availability of early dipstick-like tests for these chemokines or cytokines will probably lead to the earlier recognition of patients with a higher risk of developing a severe or fatal course of the disease [8, 20, 23]. It may be anticipated that these tests will be able to pick up the right patients for early interventions using novel treatments such as PAF antagonists [1, 2].

In addition to these diagnostic consequences there are possible consequences for treatment. A number of anticytokine strategies exist and are used in other inflammatory disorders:

- Cytokine antibodies (TNF)
- Soluble cytokine receptors (TNF)
  Receptor antagonists (IL-1ra)
- Cytokine receptor antibodies
- Anti-inflammatory cytokines (IL-10)
- Anti-NF-κ-B principles
- Anti-adhesion principles (ICAM-1)

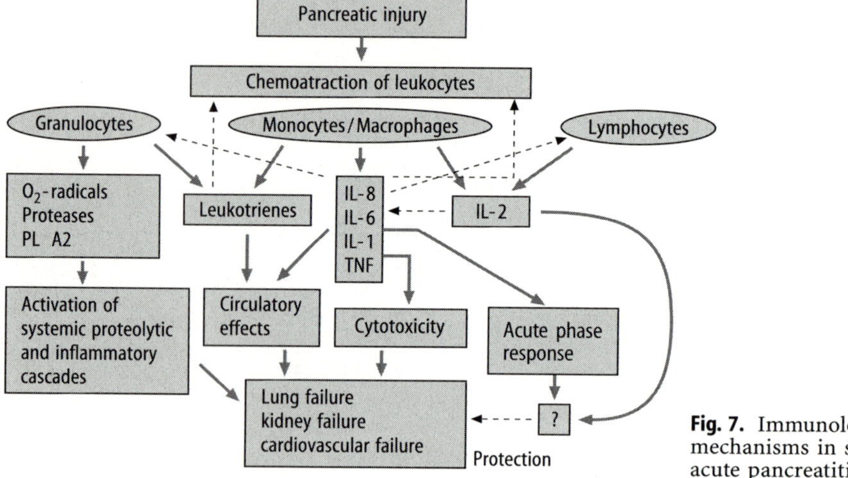

Fig. 7. Immunological mechanisms in severe acute pancreatitis

Table 4. Initial values predictive of a severe or fatal course of acute pancreatitis

	Positive predictive value (%)	Negative predictive value (%)	Cut-off
IL-6	91	82	>25 units/ml
Leukocyte elastase	86	79	>320 µg/l
α_2-macroglobulin	82	67	<1.5 g/l
CRP	73	73	>10 mg/dl
α_1-antitrypsin	59	50	>4 g/l
Clinical score	80	80	>3

Table 5. Use of cytokines in predicting severity of acute pancreatitis [21]

		Sensitivity (%)	Specificity (%)
Day 1	IL-6	**100**	**86**
	IL-8	100	81
	CRP	8	95
Day 2	IL-6	100	73
	IL-8	**100**	**91**
	CRP	57	86
Day 3	IL-6	86	91
	IL-8	**93**	**95**
	CRP	100	64

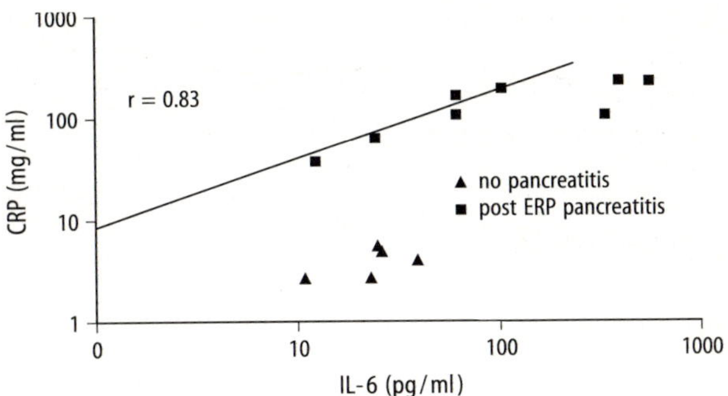

Fig. 8. Relationship between CRP and interleukin-6 (*IL-6*) peak levels in post-ERP pancreatitis; ■ patients with, ▲ patients without pancreatitis

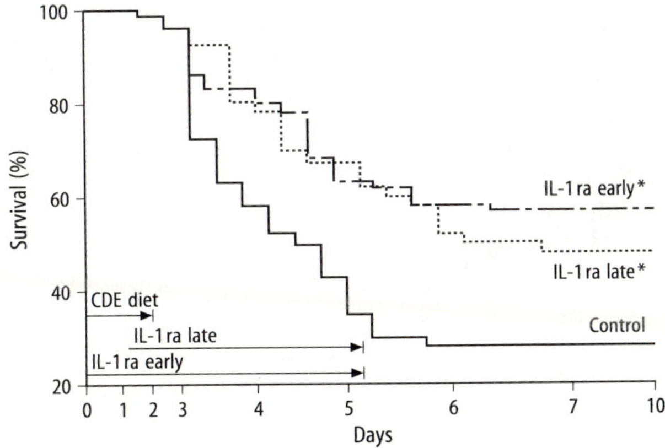

Fig. 9. Survival in experimental pancreatitis with and without administration of interleukin-1 receptor antagonist (*IL-1ra*) [24]

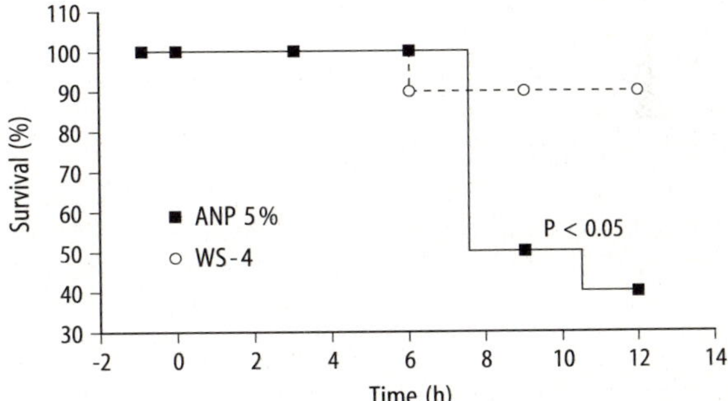

Fig. 10. Effect of an interleukin-8 antagonist (*WS-4*) on survival in bile salt-induced experimental pancreatitis (*ANP*) [25]

Most of those have not yet been used in human acute pancreatitis, but some have been studied in experimental systems. The endogenous receptor antagonist principle has been used for interleukin-1 in experimental pancreatitis [24]. It turned out that early (concomitant) as well as later (1 day) administration of this antagonist significantly reduced mortality in experimental pancreatitis (Fig. 9). Similar data have been found with an interleukin-8 antagonist in bile acid-induced rabbit pancreatitis [25] (Fig. 10). Furthermore,

Table 6. Effects of IL-10 after 10 h in experimental pancreatitis [26]

	TNFα (pg/ml)	Amylase (units/l)	Histology score (0–12)
Cerulein	120	3500	8
Plus IL-10 (1 h)[a]	**90***	**1300***	**5***
Plus IL-10 (4 h)	135	3400	7
Plus IL-10 (7 h)	142	3500	7

[a] After cerulein.
* Significant vs cerulein alone.

Table 7. Effects of anti-TNF in experimental acute pancreatitis [31]

	Bile-induced (fatal) pancreatitis	
	Pretreatment with TNF-antibody	No pretreatment
Survival (%)	77[a]	43
Survival (median, h)	72	33
Ascites (ml)	0.7	2.4
Lung congestion (n)	1.0	1.9

[a] All differences significant, 0.01–0.001.

the administration of interleukin-10, an anti-inflammatory cytokine which dampens most proinflammatory systems but does not completely abolish them, is helpful in experimental pancreatitis [26–28]. However, it is obvious from these data that only very early intervention may be helpful (Table 6). This system has been used in chronic inflammatory conditions such as inflammatory bowel disease (IBD) in human beings and has produced significant effects as well [29, 30].

Another principle, antibodies to TNFα, has been used in IBD as well and is meanwhile even licensed for this indication. This principle has been studied in experimental pancreatitis and has been found to improve survival and to decrease the number of complications [31] (Table 7). This has not been confirmed in all studies, however; local complications were mostly not affected [32]. This principle may even be damaging in certain situations. In the model of abdominal sepsis induced by cecal ligation and puncture [33] the simultaneous administration of anti TNF antibodies led to much earlier death as compared with later administration. Animals receiving the antibody 16 h after induction of abdominal sepsis survived 80 h and more (Fig. 11). In contrast, IL-10 actually improved survival and outcome in the same model [34].

Thus it can be stated that cytokines and other mediators are key players in inflammatory reactions. They are produced early in the pancreas and are released (and produced) in the systemic circulation. These cytokines and chemokines are responsible to a significant extent for systemic inflammatory reactions and distant organ complications, finally determining the prognosis for patients with severe acute pancreatitis. Serum levels are associated with

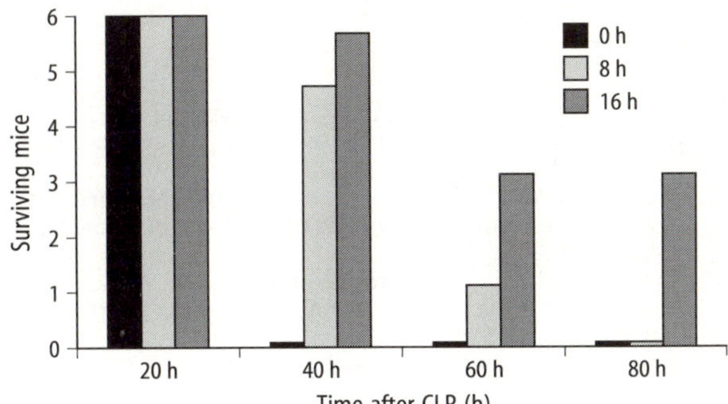

Fig. 11. Effects of anti-TNFα antibodies on survival given simultaneously (■), 8 h, or 16 h after cecal ligation and puncture (*CLP*) [33]

disease severity and can be used as prognostic parameters. An insufficient endogenous anticytokine response can lead to severe disease. Blockade or deletion of chemokine receptors and administration of antibodies and anti-inflammatory cytokines (mediators) prevent organ complications and may be used in clinical practice, even if given later with regard to distant organ complications.

Immunological mechanisms mediated by cytokines and other mediators are responsible for the systemic (whole-body) inflammation in acute pancreatitis and therefore for disease severity and probably mortality.

Outlook and Further Directions for Research

It is obvious from the data available at the moment that we need to learn more about the time course of mediator release, local and distant cellular reactions, and the impact of any of the cytokines known to be released during the initial attack. This may be best achieved using knockout models and the human model of post-ERP pancreatitis, where the patients can be studied during the initiation phase of the disease.

For diagnostic testing, studies should focus on the possibility of initial differentiation between patients with a severe and those with a less severe course of the disease. Therapeutic studies based on the principle of antimediators have been done with the PAF antagonist lexipafant, with positive results in early trials, but results of large-scale trials are lacking. From a biological point of view, studies with interleukin-10 and other pluripotent anti-inflammatory systems are warranted, since knockout of individual principles may be even deleterious. It is obvious that all proinflammatory cytokines are needed to some extent during different phases of the disease, as has been found differentially in inflammatory bowel disease for acute and chronic phases [35]. Therefore, clinical trials should be well designed and should consider the biological roles of the different pro- and anti-inflammatory mediators.

References

1. Kingsnorth AN, Galloway SW, Formela LJ (1995) Randomized, double-blind phase II trial of lexipafant, a platelet-activating factor antagonist, in human acute pancreatitis. Br J Surg 82:1414–1420
2. McKay CJ, Curran F, Sharples C, Baxter JN, Imrie CW (1997) Prospective placebo-controlled randomized trial of lexipafant in predicted severe acute pancreatitis. Br J Surg 84:1239–1243
3. Daig R, Andus T, Aschenbrenner E, Falk W, Schölmerich J, Gross V (1996) Increased interleukin 8 expression in the colon mucosa of patients with inflammatory bowel disease. Gut 38:216–222
4. Rinderknecht H (1988) Fatal pancreatitis, a consequence of excessive leukocyte stimulation. Intern J Pankreatol 3:105–112
5. Schölmerich J, Schümichen C, Lausen M, Gross V, Leser H-G, Lay L, Farthmann EH, Gerok W (1991) Scintigraphic assessment of leukocyte infiltration in acute pancreatitis using technetium 99m-hexamethyl propylene amine oxide as leukocyte label. Dig Dis Sci 36:65–70
6. Leser H-G, Gross V, Scheibenbogen C, Heinisch A, Salm R, Lausen M, Rückauer K, Andreesen R, Farthmann EH, Schölmerich J (1991) Elevation of serum interleukin-6 precedes acute-phase response and reflects severity in acute pancreatitis. Gastroenterology 101:782–785
7. Gross V, Andreesen R, Leser H-G, Lausen M, Farthmann EH, Gerok W, Schölmerich J (1992) Interleukin-8 and neutrophil activation in acute pancreatitis. Eur J Clin Invest 22:200–203
8. Schölmerich J (1996) Interleukins in acute pancreatitis. Scand J Gastroenterol 31 [Suppl 219]:37–42
9. Gross V, Leser H-G, Heinisch A, Schölmerich J (1993) Inflammatory mediators and cytokines – new aspects of the pathophysiology and assessment of severity of acute pancreatitis. Hepatogastroenterology 40:522–530
10. Denham W, Yang J, Fink G, Denham D, Carter G, Ward K, Norman J (1997) Gene targeting demonstrates additive detrimental effects of interleukin 1 and tumor necrosis factor during pancreatitis. Gastroenterology 113:1741–1746
11. Grady T, Liang P, Ernst SA, Logsdon CD (1997) Chemokine gene expression in rat pancreatic acinar cells is an early event associated with acute pancreatitis. Gastroenterology 113:1966–1975
12. Grewal HP, Mohey EDA, Gaber L, Kotb M, Gaber A (1994) Amelioration of the physiologic and biochemical changes of acute pancreatitis using an anti-TNF-alpha polyclonal antibody. Am J Surg 167:214–219
13. Meßmann H, Vogt W, Holstege A, Lock G, Heinisch A, Fürstenberg A, Leser H-G, Zirngibl H, Schölmerich J (1997) Post ERP pancreatitis as a model for cytokine induced acute phase response in acute pancreatitis. Gut 40:80–85
14. Meßmann H, Vogt W, Falk W, Vogl D, Zirngibl H, Leser HG, Schölmerich J (1998) Interleukins and their antagonists but not TNF and its receptors are released in post-ERP pancreatitis. Eur J Gastroenterol Hepatol 10:611–617
15. Paajanen H, Laat N, Jaakkola N, Pulkki K, Niinikoski J, Nordbach I (1995) Serum tumor necrosis factor compared with C-reactive protein in the early assessment of severity of acute pancreatitis. Br J Surg 82:271–273
16. Meßmann H, Grüne S, Sitter-Heinisch A, Agha A, Schmidt J, Mann S, Mann U, Holstege A, Zirngibl H. Schölmerich J (1997) TNF and TNF-receptors p55 and p75 in acute mild and severe pancreatitis. Gastroenterology 112:A464
17. Pezzilli R, Billi P, Miniero R, Barakat B (1997) Serum interleukin-10 in human acute pancreatitis. Dig Dis Sci 42:1469–1472
18. Gerard C, Frossard JL, Bhatia M, Sluja A, Gerard NP, Lu B, Steer M (1997) Targeted disruption of the β-chemokine receptor CCR1 protects against pancreatitis-associated lung injury. J Clin Invest 100:2022–2027
19. Norman J, Fink G, Franz M (1995) Acute pancreatitis induced intrapancreatic tumor necrosis factor gene expression. Arch Surg 131:966–970
20. Schölmerich J, Heinisch A, Leser H-G (1993) Diagnostic approach to acute pancreatitis: diagnosis, assessment of etiology and prognosis. Hepatogastroenterology 40:531–537
21. Pezzilli R, Billi P, Miniero R, Fiocchi M, Cappelletti O, Morselli-Labate AM, Barakat B, Sprovieri G, Miglioli M (1995) Serum interleukin-6, interleukin-8, and β_2-microglobulin in early assessment of severity of acute pancreatitis. Dig Dis Sci 40:2341–2348

22. Pezzilli R, Miniero R, Cappelletti O, Barakat B (1998) Serum interleukin 6 in the prognosis of acute biliary pancreatitis. Ital J Gastroenterol Hepatol 30:291–294
23. Rau B, Steinbach G, Gansauge F, Mayer JM, Grünert A, Beger HG (1997) The potential role of procalcitonin and interleukin-8 in the prediction of infected necrosis in acute pancreatitis. Gut 41:832–840
24. Norman J, Franz M, Messina J, Riker A, Fabri PJ, Rosemurgy AS, Gower WR (1994) Interleukin-1 receptor antagonist decreases severity of experimental acute pancreatitis. Surgery 117:648–655
25. Osman MO, Kristensen JU, Jacobsen NO, Lausten SB, Deleuran B, Deleuran M, Gesser B, Matsushima K, Larsen CG, Jensen SL (1998) A monoclonal anti-interleukin 8 antibody (WS-4) inhibits cytokine response and acute lung injury in experimental severe acute necrotising pancreatitis in rabbits. Gut 43:232–239
26. Lane JS, Todd KE, Mc Fadden DW, Reber HA, Ashley SW (1996) Interleukin-10 reduces severity early in the course of pancreatitis. Pancreas 13:445
27. Van Laethem JV, Marchant A, Delvaux A, Goldmann M, Robberecht P, Velu T, Deviere J (1995) Interleukin 10 prevents necrosis in murine experimental pancreatitis. Gastroenterology 108:1917–1922
28. Rongione AJ, Kusske AM, Kwan K, Ashley SW, Reber HA, McFadden DW (1997) Interleukin 10 reduces the severity of acute pancreatitis in rats. Gastroenterology 112:960–967
29. van Deventer SJ, Elson CO, Federak RN (1997) Multiple doses of intravenous interleukin 10 in steroid refractory Crohn's disease. Gastroenterology 113:283–289
30. Schreiber S (1997) Interleukin 10 in the intestine. Gut 41:274–275
31. Hughes CB, Grewal HP, Gaber LW, Kotb M, Mohey El-din AB, Mann L, Gaber AO (1996) Anti-TNF therapy improves survival and ameliorates the pathophysiologic sequelae in acute pancreatitis in the rat. Am J Surg 171:274–280
32. Guice KS, Oldham KT, Remick DG, Kunkel SL, Ward PA (1991) Anti-tumor necrosis factor antibody augments edema formation in cerulein-induced acute pancreatitis. J Surg Res 51:495–499
33. Echternacher B, Falk W, Maennel DN, Krammer PH (1990) Requirement of endogenous tumor necrosis factor/cachectin for recovery from experimental peritonitis. J Immunol 145:3762–3766
34. Rongione A, Kusske A, Kwan K, Ashley S, Reber H, McFadden D (1996) Interleukin 10 protects against lethality of intraabdominal infection and sepsis. Gastroenterology 110:A1104
35. Kojouharoff G, Hans W, Obermeier F, Männel DN, Andus T, Schölmerich J, Groß V, Falk W (1997) Neutralization of tumour necrosis factor (TNF) but not IL-1 reduces inflammation in chronic dextran sulphate sodium-induced colitis in mice. Clin Exp Immunol 107:353–358

CHAPTER 4

Mechanisms in Cellular Injury

Ch. Hanck and M.V. Singer

The exact mechanisms underlying the initiation and progression of acute pancreatitis remain unclear. Current research is concentrated on acinar cell events and the systemic complications of the early phase of acute pancreatitis (multiorgan failure, vascular leakage, excessive leukocyte activation, ARDS) (Rinderknecht et al. 1988).

Considerable progress has been made within the past few years in understanding the primary events leading to initiation of the disease. The dominant role of trypsin and trypsinogen activation in pancreatic autodigestion was underlined by the identification of mutations in the cationic trypsinogen gene of patients with hereditary pancreatitis (Whitcomb et al. 1996). Although the trypsin inhibitor gabexate mesilate did not show any benefit under clinical conditions when it was used (e.g., in established acute pancreatitis; Büchler et al. 1993) this might be a problem of timing, as trypsinogen inhibition has meanwhile been shown to prevent ERCP-induced pancreatitis (Cavallini et al. 1996).

The release of endogenous inflammatory mediators from the inflamed pancreas is not the initiating event in the evolution of acute pancreatitis (Denham et al. 1998b), but is supposed to be a determinant of the severity of the disease: Proinflammatory cytokines such as TNF-α and IL-1 were correlated with survival in severe experimental acute pancreatitis of transgenic mice (Denham et al. 1997). Other pathogenetic concepts besides the TNF-α pathway are the FAS pathway (both are involved in apoptosis) and the concept of T-cell-related cytotoxicity.

A synthetic interleukin-10 agonist was recently shown to diminish acute lung injury in rabbits with acute necrotizing pancreatitis (Osman et al. 1998). Transient transfection of a human interleukin-10 gene decreases the severity of pancreatitis (Denham et al. 1998a). Experimental models show that anti-IL-10 therapy given intravenously in cerulein-induced pancreatitis of female mice (Van Laethem et al. 1995) leads to reduced mortality; these findings were confirmed by Kusske et al. (Kusske et al. 1996) in a CDE model with intraperitoneal administration. The most noteworthy recent development regarding molecular mediators of acute pancreatitis has been the therapeutic use of antagonists of the platelet-activating factor (PAF) (McKay et al. 1996). Further candidates for clinical trials with potentially therapeutic implications are IL-1 RA and endothelin antagonists (Todd et al. 1997) and, in the context of immunoparalysis, the modulation of systemic complications (Hofheinz et al. 1997). Moreover, experimental research points to a disturbed microcirculation as a (co-)factor in the initiation of acute pancreatitis; hemodilution as a therapeutic option in human acute pancreatitis is currently under clinical investigation (Klar et al. 1993).

The relationship between acute and chronic pancreatitis has not yet been clarified. Recent research in hereditary pancreatitis (Whitcomb et al. 1996) speaks against a strict differentiation between "acute" and "chronic" pancreatitis. Activated cytokine mRNA expression for TNF-α in peripheral blood mononuclear cells of patients with late-stage alcoholic chronic pancreatitis demonstrates a systemic inflammatory response, suggesting that the same molecular mediators are operative in both "acute" and "chronic" pancreatitis (Hanck et al. 1998). Moreover, accumulating clinical and histomorphological evidence in the context of alcoholic pancreatitis (Ammann et al. 1996) suggests that chronic pancreatitis may result from recurrent acute pancreatitis. Further research is needed to understand the pathomechanisms which are supposed to be involved in the potential progression from acute to chronic pancreatitis (e.g., fibrogenesis and fibrolysis) (Riesle et al. 1997; Apte et al. 1998; Bachem et al. 1998).

References

Ammann RW, Heitz PhU, Klöppel G (1996) Course of alcoholic chronic pancreatitis: a prospective clinicomorphological long-term study. Gastroenterology 111:224–231

Apte MV, Haber PS, Applegate TL, Norton ID, McCaughan GW, Korsten MA, Pirola RC, Wilson JS (1998) Periacinar stellate shaped cells in rat pancreas: identification, isolation, and culture. Gut 43:128–133

Bachem MG, Schneider E, Gross H, Weidenbach H, Schmid RM, Menke A, Siech M, Beger H, Grunert A, Adler G (1998) Identification, culture, and characterization of pancreatic stellate cells in rats and humans. Gastroenterology 115:421–432

Büchler M, Malfertheiner P, Uhl W (1993) Gabexate mesilate in human acute pancreatitis. Gastroenterology 104:1165–1170

Cavallini G, Tittobello A, Frulloni L, Masci E, Mariani A, Di Francesco V, and the Italian Group (1996) Gabexate in digestive endoscopy. N Engl J Med 335:919–923

Denham W, Yang J, Fink G, Norman J (1997) Gene targeting demonstrates additive detrimental effects of IL-1 and TNF during pancreatitis. Gastroenterology 113:1741–1746

Denham W, Denham D, Yang J, Carter G, MacKay S, Moldawer LL, Carey LC, Norman J (1998a) Transient human gene therapy: a novel cytokine regulatory strategy for experimental pancreatitis. Ann Surg 227:812–820

Denham W, Yang J, Fink G, Denham D, Carter G, Bowers V, Norman J (1998b) TNF but not IL-1 decreases pancreatic acinar cell survival without affecting exocrine function: a study in the perfused human pancreas. J Surg Res 74:3–7

Hanck C, Hartmann A, Rossol S, Singer MV (1998) Cytokine gene expression in peripheral blood mononuclear cells suggests a systemic inflammatory response in alcoholic chronic pancreatitis. Abstract no 48, 8th meeting of the International Association of Pancreatology, Tokyo. Int J Pancreatol 23:224

Hofheinz H, Richter A, Nebe Th, Tsuji Y, Schmoll M, Fiedler F (1997) Immunomodulation with interferon-gamma in acute pancreatitis in rats. In: The immune consequences of trauma, shock and sepsis. Monduzzi, Bologna, pp 483–487

Klar E, Foitzik T, Buhr H, Messmer K, Herfarth C (1993) Isovolemic hemodilution with dextran 60 as treatment of pancreatic ischemia in acute pancreatitis. Clinical practicability of an experimental concept. Ann Surg 217:369–374

Kusske AM, Rongione AJ, Ashley SW, McFadden DW, Reber HA (1996) Interleukin-10 prevents death in lethal necrotizing pancreatitis in mice. Surgery 120:284–288

McKay C, Curran FJ, Sharples CE, Young CA, Baxter JN, Imrie CW (1996) The use of lexipafant in the treatment of acute pancreatitis. Adv Exp Med Biol 416:365–370

Osman MO, Jacobsen NO, Kristensen JU, Deleeuran B, Gesser B, Larsen CG, Jensen SL (1998) IT 9302, a synthetic interleukin-10 agonist, diminishes acute lung injury in rabbits with acute necrotizing pancreatitis. Surgery 124:584–592

Riesle E, Friess H, Zhao L, Wagner M, Uhl W, Baczako K (1997) Increased expression of transforming growth factor b after acute oedematous pancreatitis in rats suggests a role in pancreatic repair. Gut 40:73–79

Rinderknecht H (1988) Fatal pancreatitis, a consequence of excessive leucocyte stimulation? Int J Pancreatol 3:105–112

Todd KE, Lewis MP, Gloor B, Lane HS, Ashley SW, Reber HA (1997) An ETa/ETb endothelin antagonist ameliorates systemic inflammation in a murine model of acute hemorrhagic pancreatitis. Surgery 122:443–449

Van Laethem JL, Marchant A, Delvaux A, Goldman M, Robberecht P, Velu T, Devière J (1995) Interleukin 10 prevents necrosis in murine experimental acute pancreatitis. Gastroenterology 108:1917–1922

Whitcomb DC, Gorry MC, Preston RA, Furey W, Sossenheimer MJ, Ulrich CD, Martin SP, Gates LK Jr, Amann ST, Toskes PP, Liddle R, McGrath K, Uomo G, Post JC, Ehrlich GD (1996) Hereditary pancreatitis is caused by a mutation in the cationic trypsinogen gene. Nat Genet 14:141–145

CHAPTER 5

Acute Pancreatitis: Bacterial Translocation and Pancreatic Infections

St. W. Schmid, W. Uhl, and M. W. Büchler

Introduction

Acute pancreatitis ranges from a mild, transitory illness to a severe, rapidly fatal disease. While patients with mild acute pancreatitis can be treated on a regular ward, patients suffering from necrotizing pancreatitis (NP) should be treated in an intensive care unit. Improved intensive care therapy reduces early cardiorespiratory complications and mortality during the initial critical period dominated by severe inflammatory response syndrome (SIRS) [1]. However, during the course of the disease, infected pancreatic necrosis and septic complications are reported to develop in 40%–70% of patients with severe acute pancreatitis, which represents the major cause of morbidity and mortality [2–4]. Sepsis and related multiple organ failure are responsible for mortality in up to 80% of cases. The gut has been suggested as a possible origin of pancreatic infections in several experimental studies [5–10], but the exact route by which a sterile pancreatic necrosis becomes infected has not yet been clearly defined.

Possible Pathways for Pancreatic Infection

There are several hypothetical mechanisms by which bacteria may enter pancreatic and peripancreatic necrosis: (a) the hematogenous pathway via the circulation [5, 11], (b) transmural migration through the colon [9], (c) via colonic translocation of bacteria to the lymphatics [7, 8, 10], (d) via ascites [5, 7, 8], (e) via the biliary duct system [12, 13], and (f) from the duodenum via the main pancreatic duct [9, 14].

Since most pathogens in pancreatic infection are common gastrointestinal flora, the gut seems to be the principle source of pancreatitis-related infections and it is reasonable to postulate that bacterial translocation may be the mechanism of inoculation. Intestinal bacterial translocation may be defined as the passage of bacteria and bacterial products, such as exotoxins, endotoxins, and cell wall fragments, from the intestinal lumen to usually sterile extraintestinal sites. The intestinal mucosa normally provides a functional and anatomical barrier against intestinal organisms. However, this mucosal barrier is not complete and a minimal number of bacteria pass from the gastrointestinal tract through the mucosal lamina propria [15]. These contaminating organisms are usually cleared by immunocompetent cells in healthy individuals. In stress situations, however, this barrier fails, allowing these organisms to "translocate" to mesenteric lymph nodes, the portal venous circulation, the peritoneal cavity, and abdominal organs, with the resultant supervening sepsis and critical complications [16, 17]. This translocation is now recognized as a major cause of complicating infections in hospitalized patients, especially in immunocompromised individuals. Although the exact incidence of bacterial translocation in hospitalized patients is difficult to establish, many clinical studies indicate that systemic infections often originate from intestinal flora. Sedman et al. examined 267 general surgical patients by bacterial analysis of intestinal serosa and mesenteric lymph nodes taken at the time of surgery [18]. Excluding patients with distal intestinal obstruction and those with inflammatory bowel disease, in whom translocation was more common, the prevalence of bacterial translocation was 5%. Post-surgical complications were twice as prevalent in these patients.

It is of note that while the majority of complicating infections in animal studies and hospitalized patients is caused by a few species (*Escherichia coli*, other Enterobacteriaceae, and *Enterococcus* sp), the normal intestinal flora generally contains more than 400 species of bacteria [19]. In pancreatic infection, these germs also account for the majority of infections.

Numerous investigators have analyzed the clinical conditions which facilitate bacterial translocation, including enteric overgrowth, mesenteric ischemia, hemorrhagic shock, trauma, surgery, liquid alimentation, bowel stasis, and immunosuppression. Based on these animal studies, three potential mechanisms exist for the pathogenesis of bacterial translocation in acute pancreatitis:

1. Altered permeability of the intestinal mucosa: Acute pancreatitis causes severe volume depletion, with a reduction in cardiac output and intestinal blood flow [20, 21]. This probably leads to ischemic injury of the intestinal mucosa, with a consequent failure of mucosal barrier function.
2. Decreased host defense: Impaired phagocytic and reticuloendothelial function, demonstrated by a reduced clearance of *E. coli* from the circulation, has been noted by Widdison et al. [22], while Gianotti et al. have proven that local and systemic bacterial clearance is impaired in a rat model with acute pancreatitis [23].
3. Disruption of indigenous gut flora: Impairment of intestinal motility may play a pathophysiological role in the development of bacterial overgrowth, resulting in bacterial translocation to mesenteric lymph nodes [8, 24].

Ample animal studies exist to implicate enteric bacterial translocation in the pathogenesis of pancreatic infection. Wang et al. found a significant increase in bacterial translocation from the gut to mesenteric lymph nodes and lungs after 12 h and to the systemic circulation, ascites, and the pancreas at 24 h in rats [25]. These experiments demonstrated that translocation of enteric bacteria occurs during the early stage of acute pancreatitis and that the mesenteric lymph node-thoracic duct-circulation may be a major route for bacterial dissemination. But questions remain as to how pancreatic infection develops. Do bacteria translocate to mesenteric lymph nodes, from there to the blood circulation, and then to the pancreas, or do the organisms migrate transmurally through the colon, the ascites, and finally to the pancreas?

Experimental studies still provide equivocal results. Runkel et al. detected viable enteric bacteria in mesenteric lymph nodes of 100% of rats and in distant sites such as blood, liver, and spleen in 30% of rats with acute pancreatitis induced by biliopancreatic obstruction [10], and Isaji et al. found enteric pathogens in blood, ascites, and spleen in 12% of mice with diet-induced acute pancreatitis [26]. However, *less than 10%* of animals in both studies exhibited pancreatic infection, making it debatable whether the gut was really the origin- of the bacteria in these studies. Using the taurocholate model, however, Schwarz et al. showed bacterial infection of necrotic areas in more than 70% of the animals within 24 h [27]. In addition, Kazantsev et al. confirmed bacterial translocation to mesenteric lymph nodes and the pancreas in dogs with taurocholate/trypsin injection pancreatitis using plasmid-labeled *E. coli* [28]. They recovered labeled *E. coli* from mesenteric lymph nodes in 75% and from the pancreas in 63% of the dogs, proving the enteric origin of the bacteria in this study.

Medich et al. induced acute cerulein pancreatitis in rats in order to determine whether translocation of live bacteria to the pancreas, mesenteric lymph nodes, liver, and spleen occurred; they also measured the presence of orally fed fluorescent beads (sensitive inert markers of translocation) in the pancreas and mesenteric lymph nodes. Live bacteria were recovered from 33% of the pancreata of rats with acute pancreatitis but from none of the control rats. Beads were visualized in 91% of the pancreata of rats with acute pancreatitis but in none of the pancreata from control rats. Since beads were not visualized in the mesenteric lymph nodes of rats with acute pancreatitis, the authors concluded that acute pancreatitis promotes bacterial translocation, leading to transperitoneal infection of the pancreas [29]. A second, similar study by Arendt et al. indicated that bacteria do not spread from the peritoneal cavity in cerulein-induced acute pancreatitis in rats [30]. Additional experiments by Widdison et al., however, support the hypothesis that infection of pancreatic necrosis occurs transmurally from the colon. These authors showed that enclosing the colon in an impermeable bag prevented infection of pancreatic necrosis in a necrotizing model of acute pancreatitis [31].

Now that we have established a possible role for bacterial translocation, a number of therapeutic issues bear comment. Foitzik et al. demonstrated that early pancreatic infection following severe acute pancreatitis can be reduced with a full-gut decontamination regimen or with an antibiotic concentrated by the pancreas (imipenem), but not by unconcentrated antibiotics of similar spectrum (cefotaxime) or by oral antibiotics alone [32]. Their findings suggested, first, that both direct bacterial translocation from the gut and hematogenous spread interact in pancreatic infection with hematogenous seeding dominant at extrapancreatic sites and, second, that imipenem may be useful in clinical pancreatitis.

With regard to the clinical picture, the exact mechanism of bacterial translocation is also still a matter of considerable debate. However, a recent investigation demonstrated clinical evidence that aerobic gram-negative infections of pancreatic necrosis are of gut origin [33].

Thus, the question of how enteric bacteria enter pancreatic necrosis remains unanswered. The most probable pathways seem to be either transcolonic translocation or hematogenous spread. The answer is of utmost importance, however, since this will affect exactly how we administer prophylaxis to these patients in an attempt to prevent pancreatic infection.

Clinical Significance of Pancreatic Infection

According to the classification of the Atlanta symposium [34] acute severe pancreatitis is associated with organ failure and/or local complications, including necrosis, abscess, or pseudocyst. Pancreatic infection is generally associated with the development of pancreatic necrosis, which is defined as either diffuse or focal area(s) of nonviable pancreatic parenchyma, typically associated with peripancreatic fat necrosis. A pancreatic abscess is a circumscribed intra-abdominal collection of pus, usually in proximity to the pancreas, containing little or no pancreatic necrosis, which arises as a consequence of acute pancreatitis or pancreatic trauma. It is likely that pancreatic abscesses arise as a consequence of limited necrosis, with subsequent liquification and secondary infection later in the course of severe acute pancreatitis. A pseudocyst is defined as a collection of pancreatic juice enclosed by a wall of fibrous or granulation tissue which develops in acute pancreatitis, pancreatic trauma, or chronic pancreatitis. Bacteria may be present in a pseudocyst but often are of no clinical significance, since they represent contamination and not clinical infection. When pus is present, the lesion is more correctly termed a pancreatic abscess.

The frequency of bacterial infection of necrotic areas in the natural course of severe human acute pancreatitis (without antibiotics) has been examined in several studies [3, 4, 35]. Bacterial infection of pancreatic necrosis has been detected by fine-needle aspiration as early as the first week after onset of acute pancreatitis [4, 36]. In patients undergoing surgery for severe acute pancreatitis, Beger et al. demonstrated an overall contamination rate of 24% within the first week of the onset of acute pancreatitis, increasing to 46 and 71% in the second and third week, respectively [3]. Accordingly, patients with severe acute pancreatitis have the highest risk for pancreatic infection in the third week after onset of the disease. The overall infection rate in this series was 39%. Similar results were reported by Gerzof et al., who performed percutaneous CT-guided aspiration and gram staining, and by Bassi et al., who examined smears taken intraoperatively [4, 35]. However, the frequencies of (peri)pancreatic infections were higher at 60% and 63%, respectively.

Infection of pancreatic necrosis, however, develops later during the course of the disease and is dependent on the extent of intra- and extrapancreatic necrosis [3, 37, 38]. As shown by Beger et al., morphological analysis by contrast-enhanced CT scanning revealed a higher rate of infection in patients

Table 1. Correlation of extent of necrosis on contrast-enhanced CT scan and infection rate in patients with severe acute pancreatitis (from [83])

Extent of necrosis (%)	Sterile ($n=155$)	Infected ($n=71$)
<30	57	35
>30–<50	22	23
>50	21	42

with extensive necrosis: Two thirds of the patients with infected necrosis exhibited a total amount of necrosis of more than 30%, while 60% of patients with sterile necrosis revealed necrotic areas of less than 30% of the total pancreas [39] (Table 1). Therefore, the presence of a significant extent of necrosis (>30% in CT scan) is predictive for severe disease and identifies patients prone to develop (septic) complications [27, 36].

The important influence of bacterial infection on morbidity and mortality in severe acute pancreatitis has been analyzed in surgically treated patients suffering from infected pancreatic necrosis and in patients operated on with sterile necrosis [3]. Of 170 patients with severe acute pancreatitis, 42% had infected pancreatic necrosis and 58% had sterile necrosis. Preoperative morbidity was significantly higher in the group with infected pancreatic necrosis than in patients with sterile necrosis with respect to pulmonary (56% vs. 72%), renal (28% vs. 45%), and cardiocirculatory (13% vs. 30%) insufficiency. The hospital stay was significantly longer for patients with infected pancreatic necrosis than for those with sterile necrosis (64 vs. 45 days). The mortality was also significantly higher in the infected group, at 20% (14 of 71 patients), compared with 11% (ten of 99 patients) in the sterile group. Mortality in sterile necrosis is related to a systemic inflammatory response with consecutive multiple organ failure, most frequently occurring during the first 2 weeks after onset of the disease [40–43].

In summary, it has been demonstrated that infection of pancreatic necrosis is a significant prognostic factor in severe acute pancreatitis. Since infection is the leading cause of morbidity and mortality from acute pancreatitis, diagnosis and optimal treatment of infectious complications are the central challenge.

Bacteria

Cultures of infected pancreatic necrosis yielded a monomicrobial flora in 60%–87% of cases, whereas a polymicrobial flora was confirmed in only 13%–40% of cases (Table 2) [3, 4, 35]. There is usually a preponderance of gram-negative aerobic bacteria (*E. coli*, *Pseudomonas* spp, *Proteus*, *Klebsiella* spp), but gram-positive bacteria (*Staphylococcus aureus*, *Streptococcus faecalis*, *Enterococcus*), anaerobes, and rarely fungi have also been found [2–4, 35, 40, 44–47]. The incidence of fungi may increase in long-term disease but especially after prolonged antibiotic treatment [3, 35]. Luiten et al. differen-

Table 2. Frequency of bacteria in infected pancreatic necrosis among 77 patients (from [84])

Infection	Patients (%)
Monomicrobial	69
Escherichia coli	23
Staphylococcus aureus	14
Enterococcus	6
Klebsiella sp.	5
Polymicrobial	31
Escherichia coli	22
Enterococcus	16
Staphylococcus aureus	3
Klebsiella sp.	4
Pseudomonas	1
Proteus	4
Candida	5

tiated between gram-negative and gram-positive infection in patients with infected necrosis prospectively [48]. They found that gram-negative infection was associated with an increased mortality compared with gram-positive pancreatic infection.

Prevention of Infection of Pancreatic Necrosis

Given the poor prognosis for patients with severe acute pancreatitis and infection, the possibility of prevention and/or treatment of infection has received considerable attention. A summary of the options follows.

Intravenous Antibiotic Therapy

Early studies of prophylactic intravenous antibiotics failed to show any favorable effect on the outcome of patients suffering from acute pancreatitis [49–51]. However, most of the patients included in these studies suffered from mild acute pancreatitis. In addition, later studies focusing on pancreatic tissue concentrations following intravenous administration revealed that ampicillin, which has been used as antibiotic, failed to reach either therapeutic concentrations in the infected gland or the requisite bactericidal activity against the majority of organisms present in infected pancreatic necrosis [52, 53]. The basis for this altered pharmacokinetic behavior of antibiotics is the fact that the pancreas has a blood-pancreas barrier comparable to the blood-brain barrier [54]; this barrier is responsible for the selective uptake of antibiotic drugs into the pancreas. Bearing this in mind, Büchler et al. found chinolons (ciprofloxacin, ofloxacin) and imipenem to be substances with high pancreatic tissue levels as well as high bactericidal activity against most of the organisms present in pancreatic infection [52]. In contrast, aminoglycosides are unable to penetrate into human pancreatic tissue in bactericidal

Table 3. Efficacy factors (*EF*) for different bactericidal antibiotics in pancreatic tissue; i.e., an efficacy factor of 1.0 would indicate that the antibiotic inhibited all bacteria commonly found in pancreatic infection (from [52])

Antibiotic	EF
Aminoglycosides	
Netilmicin	0.14
Tobramycin	0.12
Acylureidopenicillins	
Mezlocillin	0.71
Piperacillin	0.72
Cephalosporins	
Cefotiam	0.75
Ceftizoxime	0.76
Cefotaxime	0.78
Ceftriaxone	0.79
Chinolons	
Ciprofloxacin	0.86
Ofloxacin	0.87
Carbapenem	
Imipenem	0.98

concentrations (Table 3) [52]. Bassi et al. studied the concentrations of several antibiotics by microbiological and high-performance liquid chromatography assays; they recommended pefloxacin and metronidazole and, to a variable extent, imipenem and mezlocillin as the first-choice antibiotics for preventing infected necrosis during severe acute pancreatitis [53].

The efficacy factors of several antibiotic classes are listed in Table 3. This factor includes the type and frequency of bacteria found in infected pancreatic necrosis, antibiotic tissue concentrations, and the percentage of inhibited bacterial strains according to the minimal antibiotic inhibitory concentration. Consequently, an ideal efficacy factor of 1 corresponds to complete inhibition of bacteria in infected pancreatic necrosis. Imipenem has an excellent efficacy factor of 0.98, whereas aminoglycosides have a very low factor. Metronidazole is exclusively active against anaerobes and should be used only in combination with non-anaerobic antibiotics.

Prophylactic use of imipenem in a controlled clinical trial was able to significantly reduce the incidence of pancreatic and nonpancreatic sepsis in patients with CT-proven severe acute pancreatitis, but the overall mortality, the rate of multiorgan failure, and the necessity for surgery were unaffected (Table 4) [55]. The possible weak points of this study are the relatively low numbers of patients (74 overall) and the fact that only two of 16 patients with >50% necrosis were randomized to the control group (with a consequent bias in "selection" for the control group). In addition, the antibiotic therapy may have been started too late after onset of the disease [36]. These results correspond to those of Foitzik et al. with an animal model of severe acute pancreatitis; they found a significantly reduced rate of pancreatic infection after the administration of imipenem, with unchanged mortality [32].

The combination of ceftazidime, amikacin, and metronidazole also decreased the incidence of sepsis in patients with severe alcoholic acute pan-

Table 4. Controlled randomized studies with respect to prophylactic antibiotic treatment in severe acute pancreatitis

Reference	Drug	Patients (n)		Rate of pancreatic infection (%)		Rate of MOF (%)		Mortality (%)	
		C	T	C	T	C	T	C	T
Pederzoli et al. [55]	Imipenem	33	41	30	12*	39	29	12	7
Sainio et al. [57]	Cefuroxime	30	30	40	30	–	–	23	3**
Schwarz et al. [58]	Ofloxacin/ metronida zole	13	13	53	61	–	–	15	0
Luiten et al. [40]	rectal SDD/ i.v. cefotaxime	52	50	38	18***	–	–	35	22

MOF, multiorgan failure; C, control; T, treatment group; SDD, rectal administration of colistin-sulphate, amphotericin, and norfloxacin.
$^{*}p<0.01$, $^{**}p=0.028$, $^{***}p=0.03$.

creatitis receiving antibiotic therapy, but no statistical difference was found with regard to mortality [56]. However, the number of patients (23) was also low. In contrast, Sainio et al. observed a significantly reduced mortality in patients with alcohol-induced severe acute pancreatitis treated with an early prophylactic antibiotic (cefuroxime), from 23% in the control group to 3% in the treatment group, which probably reflects a significantly decreased frequency of infectious complications [57]. Once again, the number of patients was low (30 vs. 30), the antibiotic treatment was changed after a mean of 9.2 days for 20 of the 30 patients in the antibiotic group, and antibiotics were started in 23 of 30 patients in the control group at a mean of 6.1 days.

In a clinical controlled study, Schwarz et al. reported that antibiotic prophylaxis with ofloxacin and metronidazole intravenously neither prevented nor delayed bacterial infection of pancreatic necrosis [58]. However, it significantly improved the clinical course if started before the onset of infection.

In summary, the clinical study of Sainio et al. using cefuroxime and the experimental study by Mithofer et al. using imipenem-cilastatin and ciprofloxacin are the only investigations which were able to demonstrate a reduced mortality following prophylactic treatment with antibiotics [57, 59].

Since patients with mild acute pancreatitis usually show an uneventful course with rapid recovery irrespective of the medical treatment they receive, antibiotic prophylaxis is not indicated in these cases. Based on the recent controlled studies, it seems possible, however, that morbidity and eventually mortality will be reduced in severe acute pancreatitis by early treatment with an antibiotic concentrated by the pancreas (e.g., imipenem), with a resultant decrease in the need for surgical intervention. Ideally, therefore, patients with pancreatic necrosis and/or signs of septic complications should be treated with a prophylactic antibiotic that has the appropriate pharmacokinetic properties. There is an enormous need for more adequate clinical studies to assess the effect of prophylactic antibiotic treatment in severe or necrotizing acute pancreatitis.

Selective Bowel Decontamination (SDD)

The elimination of intestinal bacteria may be a possible way to reduce or eliminate infection of pancreatic necrosis. Stoutenbeek et al. reported in 1984 that the selective decontamination of the digestive tract with nonabsorbable antibiotics, administered through the gastric tube, reduced the aerobic gram-negative intestinal flora in multiple trauma patients [60]. In combination with systemic cefotaxime, directed against early endogenous infection, the total infection rate decreased from 81% to 16%. Several other studies revealed that selective decontamination eliminates gram-negative bacteria from the intestinal tract and sometimes reduces gram-negative septic complications in intensive care patients. However, the results with regard to reduction of mortality are conflicting [61–65].

Since the risk of infection of pancreatic necrosis increases with gram-negative intestinal colonization, the elimination of gram-negative pathogens by prophylactic selective decontamination with enteral administered antibiotics appears to be an effective method to prevent pancreatic necrosis from becoming infected. As a consequence, several experimental investigations have examined the use of selective decontamination in severe acute pancreatitis [5, 7, 32, 66].

Based on the fact that colectomy and intestinal lavage combined with kanamycin instillation proved effective in reducing mortality from sodium taurocholate-induced acute hemorrhagic pancreatitis in the rat, translocation of intestinal flora has to be regarded as a major factor influencing mortality in experimental severe pancreatitis [5]. However, in the colectomized rats, gram-negative bacteremia was not prevented, suggesting incomplete reduction of intestinal flora; this was comparable to lavaged rats with an absence of gram-negative micro-organisms in the blood as well as in ascites. Isaji et al. also demonstrated that reduction of intestinal flora inhibits secondary infection caused by bacterial translocation and improves survival in diet-induced hemorrhagic pancreatitis in mice [26].

In an uncontrolled clinical study, SDD reduced the infection rate and sepsis in patients with acute pancreatitis complicated by acute respiratory failure, but mortality remained unaffected [62]. A previously published paper analyzed SDD in patients with severe acute pancreatitis in a randomized prospective trial [40]. Fifty of 102 patients were treated by oral and rectal administration of colistin-sulphate, amphotericin, and norfloxacin combined with short-term systemic prophylaxis with cefotaxime until oral and rectal cultures became sterile. In patients treated with SDD the overall incidence of infected necrosis (18% vs. 38% in control group, $p=0.03$) and the rate of relaparotomies (3.1 in the control group vs. 0.9 in the SDD group, $p<0.05$) were significantly reduced, probably due to a marked reduction in gram-negative infected necrosis from 33% in the control group to only 8% in the SDD group ($p=0.003$). However, overall mortality in patients treated with selective decontamination was not significantly reduced compared with the control group (22% vs. 35%). This study failed to prove an overgrowth and translocation of gram-positive bacteria (enterococci, staphylococci), as shown in other studies [67, 68]. The authors concluded, however, that SDD reduces mortality in patients with severe acute pancreatitis owing to a significant reduction in the development of gram-negative infection of pancreatic necrosis. Consequently, SDD should be started before secondary infection has occurred. However, no influence on early mortality (<2 weeks) was observed, considering that the follow-up was longer in this study than in other trials (40 days). In addition, the concept of surgical treatment differed from other trials. But the most important question remains unanswered: whether the positive results in the treatment group were achieved by the topical treatment with SDD or by the short-term administration of i.v. antibiotics.

Enteral Nutrition

To avoid meal-stimulated pancreatic secretion, patients with acute pancreatitis are withdrawn from enteral feeding and even receive total parenteral nutrition. This may have an adverse effect, since enteral mucosal atrophy in critically ill patients may promote bacterial translocation from the gut and therefore increase the risk for infection of the pancreas. In a recent study, McClave et al. investigated early total enteral nutrition (via a nasojejunal feeding tube placed endoscopically) versus total parenteral nutrition (via a central or peripheral line) in acute pancreatitis, started within 48 h of admission. Enteral nutrition has been found to be safe and effective, but significantly less costly than total parenteral nutrition [69]. Thus, early enteral feeding seems possible, and the clinical implication of enteral nutrition in acute NP and its impact on infection of pancreatic necrosis should be evaluated in further studies.

Treatment of Infected Pancreatic Necrosis

Local infection of necrotic areas of the pancreas influences the course of the disease, the prognosis, and the clinical management. Bacterial infection of pancreatic necrosis is generally suspected in patients who develop signs of sepsis on the basis of a bacteriologically positive fine-needle aspiration biopsy. Conservative treatment will lead to 100% mortality in patients with signs of local and systemic septic complications [2, 70–72]. While infected pancreatic necrosis is a clear indication for surgery, the management of sterile necrosis is a matter of controversy. Most surgical centers have adopted a very aggressive surgical approach to severe acute pancreatitis during the past two decades, but there is now a growing trend toward treating patients with sterile severe acute pancreatitis conservatively. However, a severe deteriorating clinical course in patients who do not respond to maximal ICU therapy is still regarded as an indication for surgical therapy [2, 73–76]. Thus, the valid criteria for operative interventions in patients with sterile necrosis are still undetermined and remain a matter of debate.

There is general agreement that surgical treatment of severe acute pancreatitis should be postponed as long as possible, until a certain demarcation of necrosis occurs. The second or third week seems to guarantee optimal operative conditions for necrosectomy. Surgical methods for the treatment of necrosis are varied and it is debatable which is the best. The recommended and currently accepted technique of surgical management is an organ-preserving approach which involves débridement or a necrosectomy combined with a management concept that maximizes postoperative evacuation of retroperitoneal debris and exudate. Three comparable techniques are available: (a) closed continuous lavage, utilizing open débridement with local continuous high-volume lavage [77, 78]; (b) management by planned, staged relaparotomies [79]; and (c) open packing with frequent planned reoperations [80]. In experienced hands, these approaches have reduced the mortality of severe acute pancreatitis to <15%.

Still unproven strategies are percutaneous CT-guided catheter drainage, recently described by Freeny et al. [81], and transoral endoscopic drainage and irrigation lavage by means of a nasobiliary tube, reported by Baron et al. [82]. Further evaluation of these techniques is needed before they can be adopted into clinical practice.

Our Approach to Necrotizing Pancreatitis

After pancreatic necrosis has been confirmed by a contrast-enhanced CT scan, patients with NP are treated in the ICU and receive imipenem/cilastatin 3–4×0.5 g/day intravenously for at least 14 days. When clinical signs of sepsis are present, patients undergo fine-needle aspiration with Gram's staining and culture. This procedure is repeated if necessary. Surgical intervention is initiated as soon as infected pancreatic necrosis is verified. At laparotomy the gastrocolic and duodenocolic ligaments are divided and the pancreas is exposed. Débridement or necrosectomy, either digital or with the careful use of instruments, permits the exclusive removal of all demarcated devitalized tissue, preserving the vital pancreatic parenchymal tissue. After surgical débridement, thorough hemostasis with transfixion stitches using monofilament suture material is mandatory. In our experience, necrosectomy must not be done aggressively and it is not necessary to meticulously remove all the devitalized tissue, because any necrotizing tissue left behind will be washed out by the lavage fluid later on. Extensive intraoperative lavage follows. For closed postoperative continuous local lavage, at least two double-lumen Salem tubes (20–24 Ch) and single-lumen silicone rubber tubes (28–32 Ch) are inserted and the gastrocolic and duodenocolic ligaments are sutured to create a closed retroperitoneal lesser sac compartment. During the first 7 days, 40 l of peritoneal dialysis solution are used daily for lavage. The amount of fluid is rapidly reduced over the following days, depending on the

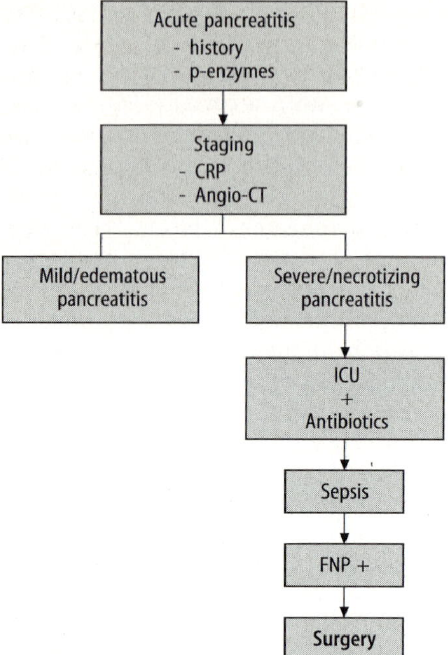

Fig. 1. Algorithm for clinical decision-making in acute pancreatitis (CRP C-reactive protein, FNP fine-needle puncture)

clinical course of the patient and the appearance of the outflowing fluid. The drainage tubes are removed successively within 2–3 weeks.

From November 1993 to September 1996, a total of 95 patients with acute pancreatitis were admitted to the Department of Visceral and Transplantation Surgery of the University Hospital of Bern. Figure 1 illustrates the decision-making steps followed. Contrast-enhanced CT established the diagnosis of NP in 44 patients (46%). Mean Ranson and APACHE II scores were 4.7 (range 2–8) and 9.9 (range 1–19), respectively. Patients with NP received antibiotic therapy for at least 14 days and were treated in the ICU with maximum conservative measures. Only one patient with a fulminant disease course and sterile pancreatic necrosis was operated on in the first week due to the lack of a recognizable response to ICU therapy. The other 43 patients (98%) responded initially to ICU treatment. Patients developing clinical signs of sepsis underwent fine-needle aspiration of the (peri)pancreatic area with Gram's staining and culture. In 14/44 patients (32%) infection of (peri)pancreatic necrosis was confirmed 21±3.3 days after onset of the disease. The surgical group ($n=15$) was managed by necrosectomy and closed retroperitoneal lavage over a mean of 22 days (range 12–36 days). In the postoperative period one patient had to be reoperated due to hemorrhage, and two other patients developed abscesses which were successfully treated by an interventional approach. The mean length of hospital stay for the group with sterile pancreatic necrosis was 21 days (range 14–28) and for those with infected pancreatic necrosis 64 days (range 29–90). Two patients in the surgical group died of septic multiple organ failure.

Acknowledgements. The authors wish to acknowledge Mark Kidd for his critical evaluation of and commentary on this manuscript.

References

1. Uhl W, Schrag HJ, Schmitter N, Nevalainen TJ, et al (1997) Pathophysiological role of secretory type I and II phospholipase A_2 in acute pancreatitis: an experimental study in rats. Gut 40:386–392
2. Widdison AL, Karanjia ND (1993) Pancreatic infection complicating acute pancreatitis. Br J Surg 80:148–154
3. Beger HG, Bittner R, Block S, Büchler M (1986) Bacterial contamination of pancreatic necrosis. A prospective clinical study. Gastroenterology 91:433–438
4. Gerzof SG, Banks PA, Robbins AH, Johnson WC, et al (1987) Early diagnosis of pancreatic infection by computed tomography-guided aspiration. Gastroenterology 93:1315–1320
5. Lange JF, van Gool J, Tytgat GN (1987) The protective effect of a reduction in intestinal flora on mortality of acute haemorrhagic pancreatitis in the rat. Hepatogastroenterology 34:28–30
6. Gianotti L, Munda R, Alexander JW, Tchervenkov JI, Babcock GF (1993) Bacterial translocation: a potential source for infection in acute pancreatitis. Pancreas 8:551–558
7. Marotta F, Geng TC, Wu CC, Barbi G (1996) Bacterial translocation in the course of acute pancreatitis: beneficial role of nonabsorbable antibiotics and lactitol enemas. Digestion 57:446–452
8. Tarpila E, Nystrom PO, Franzen L, Ihse I (1993) Bacterial translocation during acute pancreatitis in rats. Eur J Surg 159:109–113
9. Widdison AL, Karanjia ND, Reber HA (1994) Routes of spread of pathogens into the pancreas in a feline model of acute pancreatitis. Gut 35:1306–1310
10. Runkel NS, Moody FG, Smith GS, Rodriguez LF, et al (1991) The role of the gut in the development of sepsis in acute pancreatitis. J Surg Res 51:18–23
11. Webster MW, Pasculle AW, Myerowitz RL, Rao KN, Lombardi B (1979) Postinduction bacteremia in experimental acute pancreatitis. Am J Surg 138:418–420
12. Konok GP, Thompson AG (1969) Pancreatic ductal mucosa as a protective barrier in the pathogenesis of pancreatitis. Am J Surg 117:18–23
13. Runkel NS, Rodriguez LF, Moody FG (1995) Mechanisms of sepsis in acute pancreatitis in opossums. Am J Surg 169:227–232
14. Byrne JJ, Joison J (1964) Bacterial regurgitation in experimental pancreatitis. Am J Surg 107:18–23
15. Wells CL, Jechorek RP, Erlandsen SL (1990) Evidence for the translocation of Enterococcus faecalis across the mouse intestinal tract. J Infect Dis 162:82–90
16. Deitch EA (1990) The role of intestinal barrier failure and bacterial translocation in the development of systemic infection and multiple organ failure. Arch Surg 125:403–404
17. Border JR, Hassett J, LaDuca J, Seibel R, et al (1987) The gut origin of septic states in blunt multiple trauma (ISS=40) in the ICU. Ann Surg 206:427–448
18. Sedman PC, Macfie J, Sagar P, Mitchell CJ, et al (1994) The prevalence of gut translocation in humans. Gastroenterology 107:643–649
19. Wells CL (1996) Colonization and translocation of intestinal bacterial flora. Transplant Proc 28:2653–2656
20. Trapnell JE (1981) Pathophysiology of acute pancreatitis. World J Surg 5:319–327
21. Wulff K, Sjostrom B (1974) Influence of acute pancreatitis on central hemodynamic, regional blood flow distribution and arteriovenous shunting in the dog. Eur Surg Res 6:354–363
22. Widdison AL, Karanjia ND, Alvarez C, Reber HA (1992) Influence of levamisole on pancreatic infection in acute pancreatitis. Am J Surg 163:100–103; discussion pp 103–104
23. Gianotti L, Solomkin JS, Munda R, Alexander JW (1995) Failure of local and systemic bacterial clearance in rats with acute pancreatitis. Pancreas 10:78–84
24. Leveau P, Wang X, Soltesz V, Ihse I, Andersson R (1996) Alterations in intestinal motility and microflora in experimental acute pancreatitis. Int J Pancreatol 20:119–125

25. Wang X, Andersson R, Soltesz V, Leveau P, Ihse I (1996) Gut origin sepsis, macrophage function, and oxygen extraction associated with acute pancreatitis in the rat. World J Surg 20:299–307
26. Isaji S, Suzuki M, Frey CF, Ruebner B, Carlson J (1992) Role of bacterial infection in diet-induced acute pancreatitis in mice. Int J Pancreatol 11:49–57
27. Schwarz M, Büchler M, Thomsen J, Friess H, et al (1993) Pancreatic infection in experimental acute pancreatitis: a frequent finding. Digestion 54:A119
28. Kazantsev GB, Hecht DW, Rao R, Fedorak IJ, et al (1994) Plasmid labeling confirms bacterial translocation in pancreatitis. Am J Surg 167:201–206; discussion pp 206–207
29. Medich DS, Lee TK, Melhem MF, Rowe MI, et al (1993) Pathogenesis of pancreatic sepsis. Am J Surg 165:46–50
30. Arendt T, Wendt M, Olszewski M, Falkenhagen U, et al (1997) Cerulein-induced acute pancreatitis in rats – does bacterial translocation occur via a transperitoneal pathway? Pancreas 15:291–296
31. Widdison AL, Karanjia ND, Reber HA (1990) Route(s) of spread of bacteria to the pancreas in acute necrotizing pancreatitis. Pancreas 5:736
32. Foitzik T, Fernandez-del Castillo C, Ferraro MJ, Mithofer K, et al (1995) Pathogenesis and prevention of early pancreatic infection in experimental acute necrotizing pancreatitis. Ann Surg 222:179–185
33. Luiten EJ, Hop WC, Endtz HP, Bruining HA (1998) Prognostic importance of gram-negative intestinal colonization preceding pancreatic infection in severe acute pancreatitis. Results of a controlled clinical trial of selective decontamination. Intensive Care Med 24:438–445
34. Bradley ELD (1993) A clinically based classification system for acute pancreatitis. Summary of the international symposium on acute pancreatitis, Atlanta, Ga., September 11–13, 1992. Arch Surg 128:586–590
35. Bassi C, Falconi M, Girelli R, Nifosi F, et al (1989) Microbiological findings in severe acute pancreatitis. Surg Res Commun 5:1–4
36. Isenmann R, Buchler M, Uhl W, Malfertheiner P, et al (1993) Pancreatic necrosis: an early finding in severe acute pancreatitis. Pancreas 8:358–361
37. Ranson JH, Balthazar E, Caccavale R, Cooper M (1985) Computed tomography and the prediction of pancreatic abscess in acute pancreatitis. Ann Surg 201:656–665
38. Banks PA (1991) Infected necrosis: morbidity and therapeutic consequences. Hepatogastroenterology 38:116–119
39. Beger HG, Buchler M, Bittner R, Block S, et al (1988) Necrosectomy and postoperative local lavage in necrotizing pancreatitis. Br J Surg 75:207–212
40. Luiten EJ, Hop WC, Lange JF, Bruining HA (1995) Controlled clinical trial of selective decontamination for the treatment of severe acute pancreatitis. Ann Surg 222:57–65
41. Blamey SL, Imrie CW, J ON, Gilmour WH, Carter DC (1984) Prognostic factors in acute pancreatitis. Gut 25:1340–1346
42. Karimgani I, Porter KA, Langevin RE, Banks PA (1992) Prognostic factors in sterile pancreatic necrosis. Gastroenterology 103:1636–1640
43. Steinberg W, Tenner S (1994) Acute pancreatitis. N Engl J Med 330: 1198–1210
44. Bittner R, Block S, Büchler M, Beger HG (1987) Pancreatic abscess and infected pancreatic necrosis. Different local septic complications in acute pancreatitis. Dig Dis Sci 32:1082–1087
45. Bradley ELD (1991) Operative management of acute pancreatitis: ventral open packing. Hepatogastroenterology 38:134–138
46. Pederzoli P, Bassi C, Vesentini S, Girelli R, et al (1990) Retroperitoneal and peritoneal drainage and lavage in the treatment of severe necrotizing pancreatitis. Surg Gynecol Obstet 170:197–203
47. Banks PA, Gerzof SG, Langevin RE, Silverman SG, et al (1995) CT-guided aspiration of suspected pancreatic infection: bacteriology and clinical outcome. Int J Pancreatol 18:265–270
48. Luiten EJ, Hop WC, Lange JF, Bruining HA (1997) Differential prognosis of gram-negative versus gram-positive infected and sterile pancreatic necrosis: results of a randomized trial in patients with severe acute pancreatitis treated with adjuvant selective decontamination. Clin Infect Dis 25:811–816
49. Craig RM, Dordal E, Myles L (1975) The use of ampicillin in acute pancreatitis (letter). Ann Intern Med 83:831–832
50. Howes R, Zuidema GD, Cameron JL (1975) Evaluation of prophylactic antibiotics in acute pancreatitis. J Surg Res 18:197–200

51. Finch WT, Sawyers JL, Schenker S (1976) A prospective study to determine the efficacy of antibiotics in acute pancreatitis. Ann Surg 183:667–671
52. Büchler M, Malfertheiner P, Friess H, Isenmann R, et al (1992) Human pancreatic tissue concentration of bactericidal antibiotics. Gastroenterology 103:1902–1908
53. Bassi C, Pederzoli P, Vesentini S, Falconi M, et al (1994) Behavior of antibiotics during human necrotizing pancreatitis. Antimicrob Agents Chemother 38:830
54. Burns GP, Stein TA, Kabnick LS (1986) Blood-pancreatic juice barrier to antibiotic excretion. Am J Surg 151:205–208
55. Pederzoli P, Bassi C, Vesentini S, Campedelli A (1993) A randomized multicenter clinical trial of antibiotic prophylaxis of septic complications in acute necrotizing pancreatitis with imipenem. Surg Gynecol Obstet 176:480–483
56. Delcenserie R, Yzet T, Ducroix JP (1996) Prophylactic antibiotics in treatment of severe acute alcoholic pancreatitis. Pancreas 13:198–201
57. Sainio V, Kemppainen E, Puolakkainen P, Taavitsainen M, et al (1995) Early antibiotic treatment in acute necrotising pancreatitis. Lancet 346:663–667
58. Schwarz M, Isenmann R, Meyer H, Beger HG (1997) Antibiotic use in necrotizing pancreatitis. Results of a controlled study. Dtsch Med Wochenschr 122:356–361
59. Mithofer K, Fernandez-del Castillo C, Ferraro MJ, Lewandrowski K, et al (1996) Antibiotic treatment improves survival in experimental acute necrotizing pancreatitis. Gastroenterology 110: 32–240
60. Stoutenbeek CP, van Saene HK, Miranda DR, Zandstra DF (1984) The effect of selective decontamination of the digestive tract on colonisation and infection rate in multiple trauma patients. Intensive Care Med 10:185–192
61. Tetteroo GW, Wagenvoort JH, Ince C, Bruining HA (1990) Effects of selective decontamination on gram-negative colonisation, infections and development of bacterial resistance in esophageal resection. Intensive Care Med 16:S224–228
62. McClelland P, Murray A, Yaqoob M, Van Saene HK, et al (1992) Prevention of bacterial infection and sepsis in acute severe pancreatitis. Ann R Coll Surg Engl 74:329–334
63. Rocha LA, Martin MJ, Pita S, Paz J, et al (1992) Prevention of nosocomial infection in critically ill patients by selective decontamination of the digestive tract. A randomized, double blind, placebo-controlled study. Intensive Care Med 18:398–404
64. Gastinne H, Wolff M, Delatour F, Faurisson F, Chevret S (1992) A controlled trial in intensive care units of selective decontamination of the digestive tract with nonabsorbable antibiotics. The French Study Group on Selective Decontamination of the Digestive Tract. N Engl J Med 326:594–599
65. Cerra FB, Maddaus MA, Dunn DL, Wells CL, et al (1992) Selective gut decontamination reduces nosocomial infections and length of stay but not mortality or organ failure in surgical intensive care unit patients. Arch Surg 127:163–167
66. Gianotti L, Munda R, Gennari R, Pyles R, Alexander JW (1995) Effect of different regimens of gut decontamination on bacterial translocation and mortality in experimental acute pancreatitis. Eur J Surg 161:85–92
67. Jackson RJ, Smith SD, Rowe MI (1990) Selective bowel decontamination results in gram-positive translocation. J Surg Res 48: 444–447
68. Webb CH (1992) Antibiotic resistance associated with selective decontamination of the digestive tract. J Hosp Infect 22:1–5
69. McClave SA, Greene LM, Snider HL, Makk LJ, et al (1997) Comparison of the safety of early enteral vs parenteral nutrition in mild acute pancreatitis. JPEN J Parenter Enteral Nutr 21:14–20
70. Becker JM, Pemberton JH, DiMagno EP, Ilstrup DM, et al (1984) Prognostic factors in pancreatic abscess. Surgery 96:455–461
71. Beger HG, Büchler M (1986) Decision-making in surgical treatment of acute pancreatitis: operative or conservative management of necrotizing pancreatitis? Theor Surg 1:61–68
72. Bradley ELD (1989) Antibiotics in acute pancreatitis. Current status and future directions. Am J Surg 158:472–477
73. Isenmann R, Buchler MW (1994) Infection and acute pancreatitis. Br J Surg 81:1707–1708
74. Bradley EL III, Allen K (1991) A prospective longitudinal study of observation versus surgical intervention in the management of necrotizing pancreatitis. Am J Surg 161:19–24; 24–25 (discussion)
75. Büchler M, Malfertheiner P, Uhl W, Beger HG (1988) Conservative treatment of necrotizing pancreatitis in patients with minor pancreatic necrosis. Pancreas 3:592

76. Büchler M, Uhl W, Beger HG (1993) Surgical strategies in acute pancreatitis. Hepatogastroenterology 40:563–568
77. Büchler M, Uhl W, Isenmann R, Bittner R, Beger HG (1993) Necrotizing pancreatitis: necrosectomy and closed continuous lavage of the lesser sac. The Ulm experience. In: Beger HG, Büchler M, Malfertheiner P (eds) Standards in pancreatic surgery. Springer, Berlin Heidelberg New York
78. Larvin M, Chalmers AG, Robinson PJ, McMahon MJ (1989) Débridement and closed cavity irrigation for the treatment of pancreatic necrosis. Br J Surg 76:465–471
79. Sarr MG, Nagorney DM, Mucha P Jr, Farnell MB, Johnson CD (1991) Acute necrotizing pancreatitis: management by planned, staged pancreatic necrosectomy/débridement and delayed primary wound closure over drains. Br J Surg 78:576–581
80. Bradley ELD (1993) A fifteen year experience with open drainage for infected pancreatic necrosis. Surg Gynecol Obstet 177:215–222
81. Freeny PC, Hauptmann E, Althaus SJ, Traverso LW, Sinanan M (1998) Percutaneous CT-guided catheter drainage of infected acute necrotizing pancreatitis: techniques and results. AJR Am J Roentgenol 170:969–975
82. Baron TH, Thaggard WG, Morgan DE, Stanley RJ (1996) Endoscopic therapy for organized pancreatic necrosis. Gastroenterology 111:755–764
83. Uhl W, Schrag HJ, Wheatley AM, Büchler MW (1994) The role of infection in acute pancreatitis. Dig Surg 11:214–219
84. Beger HG, Rau B, Isenmann R (1998) Bacterial infection of pancreatic necrosis. In: Büchler MW, Uhl W (eds) Acute pancreatitis: novel concepts in biology and therapy. Blackwell, Berlin

CHAPTER 6

Staging and Early Nasoenteral Feeding in Acute Pancreatitis

C. W. IMRIE

This article on acute pancreatitis (AP) is about staging (mild and severe forms of the disease) and early nasoenteral feeding. The potential impact this is having at present (and probably will have in the future) on the way we are thinking about and managing patients with acute pancreatitis is considerable.

Identifying the group of patients with severe acute pancreatitis is very important. About 20%–25% of patients have the severe form of the disease. This is the group of interest in terms of newer therapies, because patients with mild disease do not need any new therapy. All patients with gallstones should undergo cholecystectomy or endoscopic sphincterotomy at first admission.

Patients with severe disease are optimally managed in a high-dependency setup or in an intensive care unit. The early identification of these high-risk patients is not easy. It has been the subject of a great deal of communications and papers over many years. Patients with severe disease according to the Atlanta criteria are those who have developed organ failure or later local complications [1]. All the multifactorial systems and other methods of grading severity were initially geared to identifying the systemic inflammatory response syndrome in patients who were likely to present major therapeutic problems in the first week of illness [2–5].

Acute Pancreatitis
- Amylase >3 ULN (upper limit of normal) or blood lipase >2 ULN
- Consistent clinical picture and ultrasound

Severe Acute Pancreatitis
- Organ failure ± local complications

Atlanta criteria (Bradley 1992)

In our own algorithm with regard to the management of severe acute pancreatitis our purpose is to try to identify objectively this group with severe disease as soon as possible. The object is obviously to allocate them to a bed in an appropriate part of the hospital, but before that they undergo an ultrasound examination. If there is any evidence clinically that they belong in the severe group or that they have objective markers of severity, if there is clear evidence on ultrasonography of stones, or if they have an abnormal liver

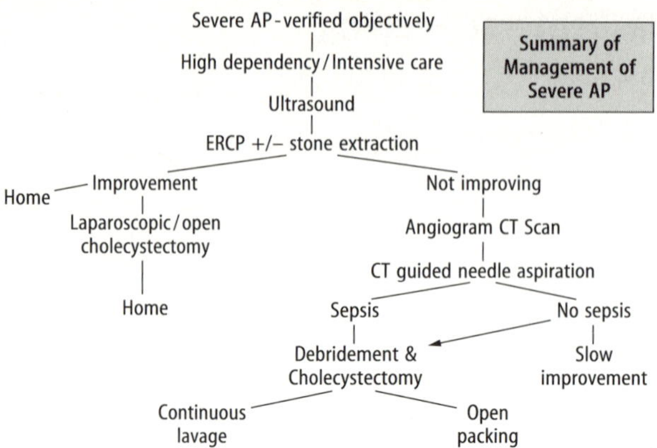

Fig. 1. Summary of management of severe acute pancreatitis

function test, they then go within the shortest possible time for ERCP and stone extraction. This is difficult on a Sunday, but Monday to Saturday this can usually be done within 18 h and often much sooner (Fig. 1).

The problem is *early accurate grading*. The systems which John Ranson and I were involved in developing are really too slow, as is C-reactive protein [6–8] with regard to therapeutic assessment of any new agent. What can be done for early grading is careful clinical assessment, and this tends to have been ignored in much of the literature. This is understandable, in that clinical assessments cannot be compared between one center and another. However, clinical assessment is very important, and chest X-ray, body mass index, and the Acute Physiology and Chronic Health Evaluation II (APACHE II) [9] plus CT can all be done quite rapidly.

Body Mass Index (BMI) is something that costs very little to measure and is a useful index of severity. Paul Lankisch was really the first who drew attention to the importance of obesity [10]. Morbid obesity is defined as a BMI of greater than 40 kg/m^2, but any patient with a BMI over 30 tends to be in the severe group. Of the multifactorial grading systems, *APACHE II* [9] is really the only one that can be used immediately, and it has therefore been employed in many of the studies of octreotide and of lexipafant in the past 8 or 10 years. *Contrast-enhanced CT scanning* [11–14] has been used to grade patients in antibiotic studies in the first few hours after admission [15–17], but most experts are concerned that a CT scan performed too early would miss the exact volume of poorly perfused or nonperfused pancreas. There is considerable debate over whether CT can really be used as an early grading approach. The only other system that can be examined is the *respiratory system*, to see if there are any radiological abnormalities. A patient with an early pleural effusion tends to be in the severe group.

Accurate Early Grading of Severe AP

1. Clinical assessment
2. Body Mass Index (BMI >30 kg/m^2)

Table 1. Clinical assessment at admission and 48 h later in AP [20]

	At admission	At 48 h
Sensitivity (%)	44	66
PPV (%)	69	77

PPV, Positive Predictive Value

Table 2. Clinical assessment of severity of AP [21]

	Assessment of an experienced clinician	
	Sensitivity (%)	Specificity (%)
At admission	68	87
At 48 h	82	96

3. APACHE II (immediate score >5)
4. Contrast-enhanced CT scan (with Balthazar score of 1–10)

In 1985, as part of a study of peritoneal lavage to see whether this was of any value in severe acute pancreatitis, objective grading of severity was looked at. It was found that the initial clinical assessment by clinicians was very poor for both gallstones and alcohol-related disease [18]. Fewer than 40% of the patients who developed clinically severe pancreatitis were identified in the emergency room. Peritoneal aspiration identified 90% with an alcohol etiology, but only 25% with gallstones accurately, while the Glasgow prognostic score identified 65%–70% of these etiologies well [18, 19].

Four years later, the Leeds group assessed a group of 290 consecutive patients and found that clinical grading of severity was fairly poor at admission but improved to almost 80% accuracy after 48 h (Table 1) [20]. We looked at a smaller group of patients in Glasgow and found that with only one clinician examining all the patients we were able to achieve a high sensitivity and specificity at 48 h (Table 2).

However, we know that the APACHE II score can be quite good for grouping patients. Those patients who have an uncomplicated course usually have an APACHE II score of under 6; those with a complicated course tend to fall within a higher range, whereas those with a fatal outcome have much higher levels (Fig. 2). The major drawback of the APACHE II score is that patients in the Western world are living longer nowadays and are fitter at the age of 70 than they were when the scheme was drawn up in 1984. The chronic health evaluation aspect of the APACHE system probably needs to be changed now, 15 years after the original publication appeared. If we are really going to make this a good system we should probably change and modify it for use in assessing acute pancreatitis in 1999.

Obesity, which was already mentioned, relates to outcome, and in a study in Capetown it was shown that in a group of 19 patients with BMI greater than 30 there were seven deaths (compared with only four deaths in a group

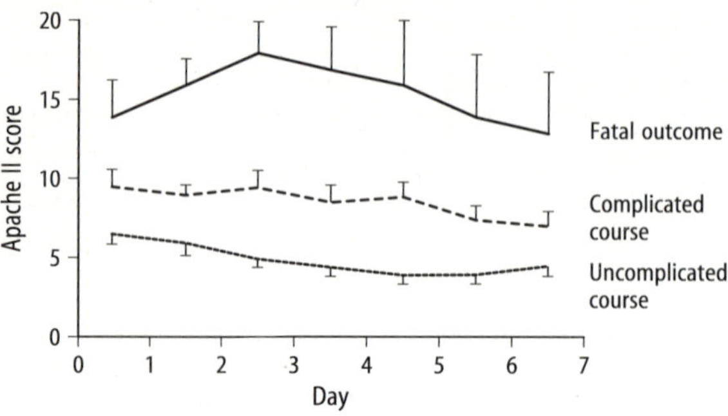

Fig. 2. APACHE II score

Table 3. Body Mass Index Score [23]

Body Mass Index[a]	Score
≤25	0
25<–<30	1
≥30	2

[a] Body Mass Index = weight (kg)/height (m^2).

of 80 lighter persons) and, for the obese, higher complication rates were recorded [22]. The suggestion was that obesity did predict severity, and it also tends to predict respiratory failure.

Johnson, in Southampton, has suggested that we combine the APACHE II score with BMI (APACHE 0). In a prospective study of 184 patients he has utilized this system by giving 1 point for a patient with a BMI between 25 and 30 and 2 points for a patient with a BMI over 30 [23] (Table 3). When the patients were grouped according to BMI less than 25, 25–30, and greater than 30 there was a corresponding pattern in their disease course, local complications increasing with the heavier patients, organ failure increasing, severity of disease increasing, there was little difference in mortality between the first and the second groups but a significant difference in the third group (Fig. 3). A simple thing such as BMI confers considerable advantage in grading severity and confirms what has been the subjective experience for many years.

In the same study, Johnson showed that he could improve the accuracy of an APACHE II score greater than 8 from 77% to 82% by adding in the obesity factor. If he moved the cut-off of the APACHE to 9 or greater he also found an improvement in accuracy. This indicates that APACHE 0 is better than APACHE II alone (Table 4).

If CT is to be applied for grading severity, it is important that some form of objective scoring system is used. The original alphabetical scoring system (A–E) which Balthazar described in an earlier paper [11] is very poor; it failed in the Rotterdam study of Luiten very badly [24]. It is better to use the later Balthazar grading system, which is numerical (1–10) [12], i.e., for less than 30% necrosis, between 30% and 50%, or greater than 50%, 2, 4, or 6

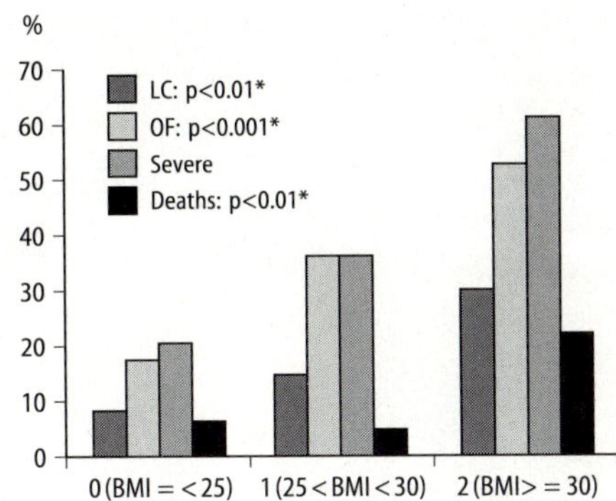

Fig. 3. BMI score and severity: local complication and organ failure rates [23]

Table 4. APACHE II vs APACHE 0 [23]

Cut-off	PPV	NPV	Accuracy
>8			
APACHE II	63	84	77
APACHE 0	67	94	82
>9			
APACHE II	71	84	80
APACHE 0	74	91	85

NPV; PPV, Negative and Positive Predictive Values

Table 5. CT grading of acute pancreatitis [12]

Grade	Description	Score[a]		Necrosis	Score
A	Normal	0	–	–	–
B	Focal, diffuse enlargement; contour irregularity; inhomogeneous attenuation	1	–	<30%	2
C	B + peripancreatic haziness/streaky densities	2	+	50%	4
D	B, C +I III defined peripancreatic fluid collection	3	–	>50%	6
E	B, C + ≥2 III defined peripancreatic fluid collections	4	–	–	–

[a] Score range: 0–10.

points, respectively, are added to the 0, 1, 2, 3, 4 points from the original assessment of the CT scan (Table 5).

Thus, to predict severity at admission we really only have the presence of obesity or pleural effusions, combined with the clinical status of the patient. While it takes a little longer, the APACHE II and APACHE 0 score can be used at admission. Biochemical markers at 48 h and also blood CRP are very

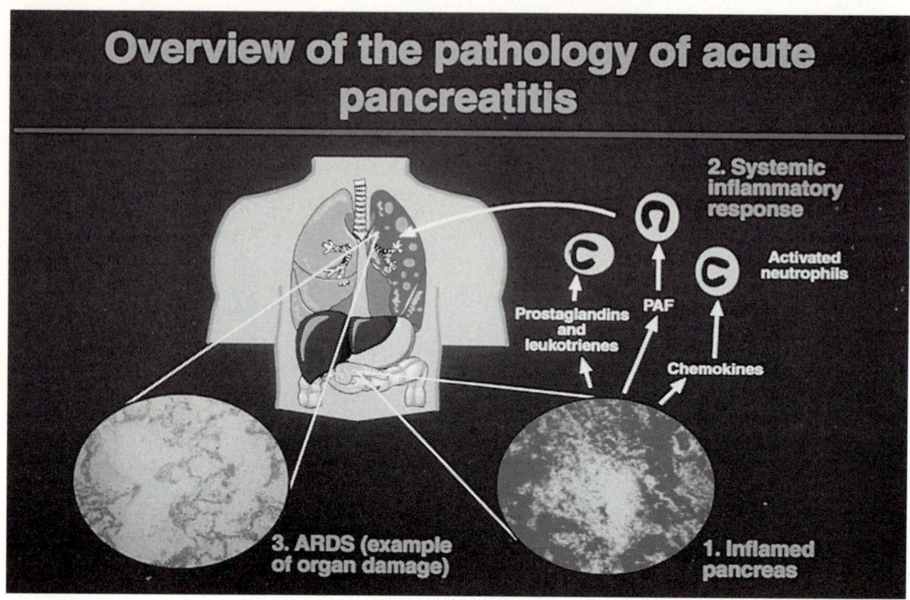

Fig. 4. Overview of the pathology of acute pancreatitis (with permission of British Biotech Pharmaceuticals)

useful – the higher the level, the poorer the prognosis – although there is a very big skew of results, which makes it too unreliable for exclusive use in individual patients [6–8].

The alternative grading systems have drawbacks. The Ranson Score is used almost invariably in its original 1974 version [2], even with populations predominantly comprising a gallstone etiology. The second system, described for gallstone patients in 1981 [3], really should be the one used. The Glasgow score in its 8-factor format is reasonably consistent for both gallstone AP and alcohol AP patients, but both of these systems take too long to apply, as does C-reactive protein in the assessment of any new therapy for early use in patients with severe AP.

Patients become very ill largely because their lungs, hearts, and kidneys become compromised. The degree of injury within the pancreas is obviously enormously important, but the reason for death tends to be multiorgan failure, and the predominant damage is to the respiratory system (Fig. 4).

One hypothesis as to why the patients become ill is related to the systemic inflammatory response syndrome. A patient with mild pancreatitis following original trauma to the pancreas develops a normal inflammatory response, which tends to resolve spontaneously with adequate fluid replacement and analgesia. The patient who has a more severe inflammatory response may progress to early multiorgan dysfunction syndrome. However, all of these things are considered reversible. The problem is that a second hit, e.g., another stone passing through the ampulla of Vater or an infection, results in late multiorgan dysfunction syndrome (MODS), and this group has the highest mortality (Fig. 5).

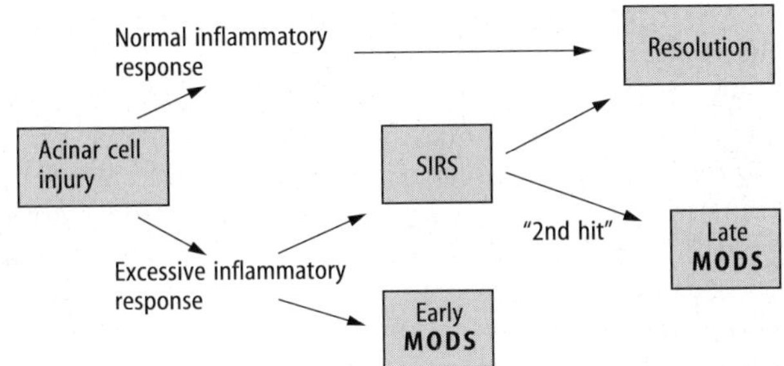

Fig. 5. Pathogenesis of organ failure and acute pancreatitis

Several changes are possible in the therapeutic approach to severe acute pancreatitis:

- Early endoscopic sphincterotomy by an expert should always be considered (especially where an indication of gallstones and/or cholangitis is present)
- I.v. antibiotic therapy may be helpful
- Early nasoenteral feeding
- Early i.v. lexipafant may significantly lower mortality

I want to consider here early nasoenteral feeding and review the current evidence. Andersson and co-workers (Lund, Sweden) published a study on giving lexipafant, a platelet activating factor antagonist, prior to the insult of acute pancreatitis [24]. They had shown in earlier control studies that jejunal permeability increases just a few hours after the onset of experimental pancreatitis. They were able to reverse this change by giving lexipafant beforehand. Obviously, this is not a potential clinical situation, except in the case of ERCP-induced pancreatitis. Thus, our focus has moved somewhat from the pancreas to the potential effects, predominantly on the jejunum and less so on the ileum (Fig. 6). Bowel mucosal permeability changes may be minimized by the provision of small volumes of enteric feeding.

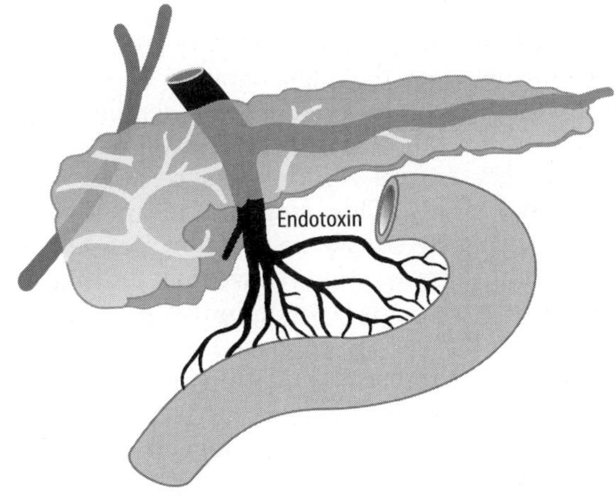

Fig. 6. Gut permeability changes occur early in severe AP

An intriguing study of taurocholate-induced AP in rats was presented at the Tokyo meeting of the International Association of Pancreatology in July 1998. In this study from the Barcelona group, a standard group of rats were subjected to taurocholate-induced pancreatitis, but in one of the four groups, a preliminary portocaval shunt was made immediately before the insult of the taurocholate-induced AP [25]. These rats were excluded if they lost more than 2 ml of blood in the portocaval shunt, so it was a very tricky piece of surgery. Bronchoalveolar lavage analysis was performed in all the groups, and macrophage activation was shown by measuring NO, TNF, and MIP 2 release. The intriguing point in this paper was that this macrophage activation in the lungs was not shown at all in the group of animals with the preliminary portocaval shunt. The surprising finding is that whatever toxins pass into the portal circulation seem to require the liver to modify them before the lungs are adversely affected.

The study implies that portocaval shunt confers a benefit in this situation, but obviously we are not going to perform prophylactic portocaval shunts in patients. The passage of the inflammatory mediators through the liver appears to be vital for their activation [25]. This work will surely stimulate a number of other research groups to investigate what happens in the liver.

Returning to the use of enteral feeding, we should examine a 34-patient study published by Windsor and colleagues, in which 13 patients had objective evidence of severe AP [26]. They randomized 16 of these 34 patients to enteral feeding and 18 to intravenous feeding. There were six cases of severe AP and no deaths in the enterally fed group compared with seven cases of severe AP and two deaths in the intravenously fed group. This is obviously a very small study with a restricted number of patients, and there were only 13 with severe pancreatitis, but it did show some interesting results. Of the 11 enterally fed patients with profound systemic inflammatory response syndrome at the beginning of the first week there were only two with the syndrome at the end of the week. None of this group developed major sepsis or multiorgan failure, or died, whereas in the intravenously fed group there were still ten with profound SIRS at the end of 1 week; three had major sepsis, five developed multiorgan failure, and two died [26].

In the same study they found that the markers of SIRS, namely CRP, and APACHE II, were reduced in the group of patients who were enterally fed, and furthermore that IgM anticore endotoxin antibodies rose in the intravenously fed group but not in the enterally fed one, and the antioxidant capacity fell in the intravenously fed group but rose in the enterally fed group, implying that enteral feeding was certainly better than parenteral feeding in this small study. This may not mean that enteral feeding is tremendously valuable; it may simply be that intravenous feeding is of limited value. What we should do is to stop intravenous feeding unless there is no alternative. At this stage we do not have definitive proof that enteral feeding is beneficial.

Kalfarentzos et al. published a paper claiming that enteral nutrition was superior to parenteral nutrition in severe AP [27]. All 38 patients in their study had objective evidence of severe pancreatitis; 18 patients were fed nasojejunally, 20 intravenously, and all of the patients had at least three Glasgow criteria as markers of severity. There were fewer complications with en-

Table 6. The Kalfarentzos study [27]

Characteristics	Enteral feeding ($n=18$)	Parenteral feeding ($n=20$)
Sex (M:F)	8:10	7:13
Age (years)	63.0	67.2
Etiology (n)		
Gallstones	14	16
Alcohol	3	2
Other	1	2
Glasgow criteria	4.2	4.6
APACHE II	12.7	11.8
CRP	290	335
Catheter sepsis	0	2
Glucose >200 mg	4	9
Infected necrosis	1	4
Abscess	1	0
Fistula	0	2
Pseudocyst	0	1
Major sepsis	5	10
Cost/day (UK£)	30	100

teral feeding than with intravenous feeding, and there was a lower risk of sepsis (see also Table 6).

They found no difference in the total days of stay in respiratory intensive care or in total hospital stay between the two groups. There were approximately 12 days in RICU and 40 days in hospital. The implications of this study are that enteral feeding did not made any difference in hospital stay but that it is cheaper and somewhat safer in terms of infection [27].

There is also further data from a group in Belgium covering a pilot study in which they used early enteral nutrition by nasojejunal feeding in both moderate and severe AP [28]. They were successful with this in 20 of 21 patients at an average of 36 h following admission. They utilized a 2-lumen nasogastrojejunal tube placed after endoscopic location of a jejunal guidewire. They did not routinely give antibiotics in the latter part of the study but they did in the early part, and they questioned whether antibiotics should be withheld if early enteral feeding is used.

We have taken this one stage further in Glasgow by looking at a pilot study of nasogastric feeding [29]. Everyone else has looked only at nasojejunal feeding and all the theories say that this is the only form we should consider. In our pilot study we put the question: "Can nasogastric feeding be practical and safe?" The study material was as follows:

- 26 consecutive patients with severe disease
- three or more positive Glasgow prognostic criteria
- APACHE II of 6 or greater
- Balthazar CT severity index of at least 5

There is no question that this was a group of severely ill patients. Feeding commenced within 48 h of admission to our unit. Just over half the patients came to us primarily and some of them were being fed within 8 h. Initially, we were using a commercial feed, at a rate of 20 ml/h, but we found – to our surprise, considering the recommendations in the textbooks – that for many of the patients this could be moved up fairly quickly. We used this low-fat semi-elemental peptide feed (Nutricia), commencing at full strength at a rate of 20–30 ml/h and gradually increasing to 100 ml/h.

In this group of 26 patients the time to target rate of administration was a median of 36 h. The median hospital stay for the group was 17 days, and the span in intensive care was 7 days. There were four deaths, all of them associated with multiorgan system failure [29].

We thus have a situation where early enteral feeding has been used in severe AP in several publications and presentations within the last 12 months: Windsor and colleagues in Leeds [26], the Kalfarentzos-headed group in Greece [27], and Nakad and coworkers in Brussels [28] all used the nasojejunal route, and Eatock and colleagues in Glasgow [29] examined the nasogastric route.

We are currently randomizing patients into a study comparing nasojejunal and nasogastric feeding. Of the initial 26 patients we treated with nasogastric feeding there were four who did not tolerate it at different stages. One of them was an elderly woman who kept pulling the tube out; after seven placements we decided that was enough. There were two others who had large nasogastric aspirates, and in these cases we relocated the tube into the jejunum. Thus we conclude that nasoenteric feeding appears both practical and safer than intravenous feeding in cases of severe AP.

References

1. Bradley EL III (1993) A clinically based classification system for acute pancreatitis. Summary of the International Symposium on Acute Pancreatitis, Atlanta, Ga., September 11–13, 1992. Arch Surg 128:586–590
2. Ranson JHC, Rifkind KM, Roses DF, Fink SD, Eng K, Spencer FC (1974) Prognostic signs and the role of operative management in acute pancreatitis. Surg Gynecol Obstet 139:69–81
3. Ranson JHC (1979) The timing of biliary surgery in acute pancreatitis. Ann Surg. 189:654–663
4. Imrie CW, Benjamin IS, Ferguson JC, McKay AJ, Mackenzie I, O'Neill J, Blumgart LH (1978) A single-centre double-blind trial of Trasylol therapy in primary acute pancreatitis. Br J Surg 65:337–341
5. Blamey SL, Imrie CW, O'Neill J, Gilmour WH, Carter DC (1984) Prognostic factors in acute pancreatitis. Gut 25:1340–1346
6. Wilson C, Heads A, Shenkin A, Imrie CW (1989) C-reactive protein, antiproteases and complement factors as objective markers of severity in acute pancreatitis. Br J Surg 76:177–181
7. Buchler M, Malfertheiner P, Beger HG (1986) Correlation of imaging procedures, biochemical parameters and clinical stage in acute pancreatitis. In: Malfertheiner P, Ditschuneit H (eds) Diagnostic procedures in pancreatic disease. Springer, Berlin Heidelberg New York, pp. 123–129
8. Puolakkainen P, Valtonen V, Paananen A, Schroder T (1987) C-reactive protein (CRP) and serum phospholipase A2 in the assessment of the severity of acute pancreatitis. Gut 28:764–771
9. Knaus WA, Wagner DP, Draper EA, Zimmerman JE. APACHE II final form and national validation results of a severity of disease classification system. Crit Care Med 12:213–229
10. Lankisch PG, Schirren CA (1990) Increased body weight as a prognostic parameter for complications in the course of acute pancreatitis. Pancreas 5:626–629

11. Balthazar EJ, Ranson JH, Naidich DP, Megibow AJ, Caccavale R, Cooper MM (1985) Acute pancreatitis: prognostic value of CT. Radiology 156:767–772
12. Balthazar EJ, Robinson DL, Megibow AJ, Ranson JH (1990) Acute pancreatitis: value of CT in establishing prognosis. Radiology 174:331–336
13. Kivisaari L, Schroder T, Sainio V, Somer K, Standertskjold-Nordenstam CG (1991) CT evaluation of acute pancreatitis: 8 years clinical experience and experimental evidence. Acta Radiol Suppl [Stockh] 377:20–24
14. Beger HG (1989) Surgical management of necrotising pancreatitis. Surg Clin North Am 69:529–549
15. Pederzoli P, Bassi C, Vesentini S, Campedelli A (1993) A randomized multicenter clinical trial of antibiotic prophylaxis of septic complications in acute necrotizing pancreatitis with imipenem. Surg Gynecol Obstet 176:480–483
16. Sainio V, Kemppainen E, Puolakkainen P, Taavitsainen M, Kivisaari L, Valtonen V, Haapiainen R, Schroder T, Kivilaakso E (1995) Early antibiotic treatment in acute necrotising pancreatitis. Lancet 346:663–667
17. Schwarz M, Isenmann R, Meyer H, Beger HG. Antibiotika bei nekrotisierender Pankreatitis. Dtsch Med Wochenschr 122:356–361
18. Corfield AP, Cooper MJ, Williamson RC, Mayer AD, McMahon MJ, Dickson AP, Shearer MG, Imrie CW (1985) Prediction of severity in acute pancreatitis: prospective comparison of three prognostic indices. Lancet 2(8452):403–407
19. Mayer AD, McMahon MJ, Corfield AP, Cooper MJ, et al (1985) Controlled clinical trial of peritoneal lavage for the treatment of severe acute pancreatitis. N Engl J Med 312:403–404
20. Larvin M, McMahon MJ (1989) APACHE-II score for assessment and monitoring of acute pancreatitis. Lancet 2:201–205
21. Heath DI, Imrie CW (1994) The Hong Kong criteria and severity prediction in acute pancreatitis. Int J Pancreatol 15:179–185
22. Funnell IC, Bornman PC, Weakley SP, et al (1993) Obesity: an important prognostic factor in acute pancreatitis. Brit J Surg 80:484–486
23. Johnson CJ, Toh SKC (1998) The APACHE II prognostic system combined with obesity, an improved method of grading severity of acute pancreatitis. Churchill Livingstone, Edinburgh (Recent advances in surgery, vol. 21)
24. Andersson R, Wang X, Sun Z, Deng X, Soltesz V, Ihse I (1998) Effect of a platelet-activating factor antagonist on pancreatitis-associated gut barrier dysfunction in rats. Pancreas 17:107–119
25. Sabater L, Closa D, Fernandez-Cruz L, et al (1998) Liver mediates the activation of alveolar macrophages during acute pancreatitis. Proceedings of Eighth International Association of Pancreatology, Tokyo
26. Windsor AC, Kanwar S, Li AG, Barnes E, Guthrie JA, Spark JI, Welsh F, Guillou PJ, Reynolds JV (1998) Compared with parenteral nutrition, enteral feeding attenuates the acute phase response and improves disease severity in acute pancreatitis. Gut 42:431–435
27. Kalfarentzos F, Kehagias J, Mead N, Kokkinis K, Gogos CA (1997) Enteral nutrition is superior to parenteral nutrition in severe acute pancreatitis: results of a randomized prospective trial. Br J Surg 84:1665–1669
28. Nakad A, Piessevaux H, Marot JC, Hoang P, Geubel A, Van Steenbergen W, Reynaert M (1998) Is early enteral nutrition in acute pancreatitis dangerous? About 20 patients fed by an endoscopically placed nasogastrojejunal tube. Pancreas 17:187–193
29. Eatock FC, Brombacher GD, Steven A, Imrie CW, Carter CR (submitted) Nasogastric feeding in severe acute pancreatitis may be practical and safe. Gut 1999

CHAPTER 7

Acute Pancreatitis: Medical and Endoscopic Treatment

CH. LÖSER and U.R. FÖLSCH

Introduction

Acute pancreatitis is a common disorder with an incidence that has increased significantly within the past few decades [1–3]. Although the reasons for this obvious increase in incidence are not fully understood, they may be related in part to the general increase in alcohol consumption and abuse, as well as to the improved ability to diagnose an acute pancreatitis by laboratory and morphological procedures. Despite significant improvement of our knowledge in recent years, there is still a great deal of uncertainty and controversial discussion with regard to the role and importance of the various etiological and pathophysiological mechanisms, the relevance of prognostic scores, the clinical assessment of the natural course of the disease, or recent therapeutic concepts for patients with acute pancreatitis [3–9]. Deciding what constitutes an adequate therapeutic approach for patients with acute pancreatitis is still a major clinical problem, especially in cases of acute necrotizing pancreatitis.

The clinical severity of this disease varies widely, from a mild, self-limiting form with interstitial edema to severe, necrotizing pancreatitis with still a high mortality. While acute interstitial edematous pancreatitis is rather frequent (80%–90%) but mild (mortality 0%–3%), acute necrotizing pancreatitis is less frequent (10%–20%) but is still burdened by a high mortality (up to 50%) and therefore remains a difficult clinical problem with regard to prognostic assessment and adequate therapeutic approaches [3, 4, 7]. Major causes of acute pancreatitis are gallstones (40%–50%) and alcoholism (30%–40%), and 10%–30% are idiopathic cases of unknown origin [3, 10].

Principles of Basic Treatment

The basic principles of therapy and supportive care in patients with acute pancreatitis are as follows:

1. Immediate hospitalization
2. Oral food and fluid restriction
3. Nasogastric suction (symptoms of subileus)

4. Adequate parenteral fluid and electrolyte replacement
5. Control of central venous pressure, fluid balance
6. Adequate pain relief
7. Prophylaxis of stress ulcer disease
8. Adequate parenteral high-caloric substitution in severe cases
9. Repeated assessment and continuous monitoring of clinical status
10. Prophylactic antibiotics in severe cases and biliary pancreatitis

It is absolutely mandatory to admit patients with suspected acute pancreatitis to a hospital immediately for further diagnostic and close-meshed clinical observation [3, 4, 7, 11, 12]. Once the diagnosis has been established, continuous observation and monitoring of the patient is the most important initial measure. In cases of moderate to severe forms of acute pancreatitis it is established practice to admit the patient to an intensive care unit for close-meshed clinical observation under maximal supportive care conditions. In cases of severe, acute pancreatitis the patient should be transferred early to a specialized medical center. Today, conservative intensive care is widely accepted as the most important initial therapeutic measure [3–16]. Oral food and fluid restriction, adequate parenteral fluid and electrolyte replacement according to the central venous pressure and urinary excretion, and adequate relief of pain are the major initial goals. Though nasogastric suction and therapy with H_2-receptor antagonists have not been found to have any influence on the course of acute pancreatitis, the former will help to relieve subjective discomfort caused by meteorism and subileus, while H_2-inhibitors are useful in the prophylaxis of stress-induced ulcerations [4, 7, 17, 18]. Since acute pancreatitis may cause significant formation of retroperitoneal fluid, adequate initial, CVP-guided parenteral substitution of volume (up to 10 l/day) is important to prevent or correct hemodynamic deterioration.

Initial conservative intensive care is well established as the first stage of treatment in patients with acute pancreatitis and has contributed significantly to lowering the mortality and morbidity of this disease in recent years. Close-meshed evaluation of the clinical status by physical examination, abdominal palpation, monitoring of blood pressure and heart rate, fluid balance, central venous pressure and urinary excretion, accompanied by frequent laboratory evaluations (electrolytes, WBC and RBC, arterial pO_2, acid-based homeostasis, creatinine, urea, blood sugar, calcium, total protein, albumin, blood coagulation, etc.) is important for early assessment of complications and prediction of clinical course and outcome. Besides local complications (peripancreatic necrosis or inflammation, abscess, bleeding, ascites, pseudocysts, fistulae, etc.) primarily systemic complications such as shock due to circulatory failure, respiratory or renal insufficiency, coagulation disorders, and sepsis may threaten the life of the patient [19, 20]. Problem-oriented treatment of patients with acute pancreatitis is summarized in Table 1.

Table 1. Problem-oriented treatment in acute pancreatitis

Problem	Treatment
Impacted biliary stone	ERC, endoscopic papillotomy
Shock	Substitution of fluid and albumin, catecholamines (dopamine)
Respiratory failure	Assisted ventilation with positive end-space expiratory pressure (PEEP)
Renal failure	Diuretics, dopamine, hemodialysis
Sepsis	Percutaneous fine-needle puncture, antibiotics, surgery
Hyperglycemia	Insulin in low doses
Coagulopathy	Heparin, fresh-frozen plasma
Hypocalcemia	Infusion of calcium plus albumin
Necrosis	
Sterile	Antibiotics, observation
Infected	Antibiotics, débridement
Pseudocysts	Observation, drainage
Abscess	Drainage, surgery

Assessment of Severity

A major initial goal in cases of acute pancreatitis is the early discrimination between a mild edematous and a severe necrotizing course of the disease associated with an evaluation of the individual prognosis of the patient. A number of initial prognostic scoring systems (Ranson, Glasgow, Banks, Agarwal-Pitchumony, etc.) and parameters for follow-up monitoring (APACHE II-score, C-reactive protein, LDH, alpha$_2$-macroglobulin, alpha$_1$-antitrypsin, PMN-elastase, phospholipase A_2, trypsinogen activation peptide, interleukin 6, etc.) have been established (for reviews see [13, 21–25]). For clinical practice, C-reactive protein and LDH were established in many studies as easy to determine and ubiquitously available laboratory parameters for the evaluation of the prognosis and appearance of necrosis in individual patients. PMN-elastase [26], trypsinogen activation peptide (TAP) [27], and interleukin 6 [28] are the most interesting new parameters which still need more detailed evaluation. Intravenous contrast-enhanced computer tomography has become the gold standard for the sensitive detection and adequate follow-up of pancreatic necrosis [3, 21, 22].

Conservative Treatment

Despite some progress that has been made in recent years, little is known with regard to the complex pathophysiological factors and mechanisms involved in the initiation and further development of an acute pancreatitis in human beings. It is generally accepted that "autodigestion", caused by a premature intrapancreatic activation of digestive enzymes, is the pathophysiological end-stage of the disease; however, little has been discovered about the

Table 2. Conservative, causally oriented concepts in the treatment of acute pancreatitis that failed to exert a positive effect in controlled or open clinical studies

Treatment concept	Reference(s)
Inhibition of pancreatic secretion	
Atropine	[30]
Calcitonin	[31]
Somatostatin/octreotide	[32–34]
Glucagon	[35, 36]
Fluorouracil	[37]
H_2-receptor antagonists	[18, 38, 39]
Inhibition of autodigestive enzymes	
Aprotinin	[41–43]
Gabexate-mesilate/camostate	[44–46]
Phospholipase A_2-inhibitors	[47]
Fresh-frozen plasma	[48]
Reduction of inflammation	
Indomethacin	[49]
Prostaglandins	
Removal of toxic substances	
Peritoneal lavage[a]	[52–56]
Sump drainage	[51]
Hemofiltration[a]	[57]
Inactivation of oxygen-free radicals	[50]

[a] At present under further investigation.

early stages of pathogenesis, and therefore advances in conservative therapeutic concepts have remained scarce over the past few years. Many drugs and procedures have been intensively investigated in various animal models of acute pancreatitis and many studies showed successful amelioration of the induced disease; nevertheless, when the same substances and procedures were investigated in human trials, a vast majority of the studies ended up with negative results [29]. Table 2 summarizes the conservative attempts of treatments based on causally oriented concepts in patients with acute pancreatitis which failed to have beneficial effects in controlled or open clinical trials (for review see [3–9, 13]).

Several attempts were made to inhibit pancreatic secretion by pharmacological means in order to put the pancreas at rest. Nevertheless, these studies using atropine [30], calcitonin [31], somatostatin or octreotide [32–34], glucagon [35, 36], fluorouracil [37], or H_2-receptor antagonists [18, 38, 39] were generally disappointing, and the agents proved to have no significant effect on the course and the mortality of acute pancreatitis. It now appears doubtful whether decreasing pancreatic secretion makes any sense in the treatment of acute pancreatitis, since several authors were able to show in experimental animal models that exocrine pancreatic secretion is strongly inhibited during acute pancreatitis [40].

The concept of inhibiting autodigestive pancreatic enzymes by the administration of protease or phospholipase inhibitors such as aprotinin [41–43], camostate, or gabexate-mesilate [44–46], phospholipase A_2 inhibitors [47], or fresh-frozen plasma [48] failed to show significant benefits in the treatment of patients with acute pancreatitis. A further promising possibility was the use of peritoneal lavage for diagnostic-prognostic [52] as well as therapeutic [53–55] reasons. Although these studies provided conflicting results, most failed to find any positive effect [53, 55]. In a recently published study, long-term peritoneal lavage has been shown to exert a beneficial effect on complications and mortality [56], but further clinical studies are needed before it can be decided whether or not peritoneal lavage should be recommended in the treatment of patients with acute pancreatitis. A further clinically interesting attempt is to remove toxic substances from patients with acute pancreatitis by means of early hemofiltration [57]. The clinical effects of early hemofiltration as well as hemodilution are presently under investigation in clinical trials.

Ongoing Clinical Studies

As indicated above in detail, the advances in conservative therapeutic concepts based on our understanding of the different underlying pathophysiological mechanisms have remained small over the past decades. Nevertheless, there are some highly interesting new concepts with promising initial results that merit further clinical evaluation. Candidates presently under investigation are, for example, prolonged peritoneal lavage, hemofiltration, plasma exchange and isovolemic hemodilution, e.g., with dextran, systemic administration of novel antibiotics, bacterial decontamination of the gut in order to prevent bacterial infection of pancreatic necrosis, and recently developed anti-inflammatory drugs, such as the platelet-activating factor (PAF) antagonists. None of these therapeutic options can be recommended for clinical use unless their clinical value is established in the various ongoing studies.

The most promising new drug at present is the PAF antagonist lexipafant. PAF is a proinflammatory lipid mediator which plays a significant role in a variety of pathophysiological conditions, and experimental data reveal a central role for PAF as a mediator in acute pancreatitis [58, 59]. Kingsnorth and co-workers [60] demonstrated in a double-blind, placebo-controlled study that administration of the PAF antagonist lexipafant (60 mg i.v. for 3 days) significantly reduced the incidence of organ failure and was associated with a reduced ICU and hospital stay and with a nonsignificant reduction in the number of deaths in the treatment group compared with the placebo group. These data were extended in a British multicenter trial which found a significant reduction in mortality, local complications, and septic complications in lexipafant-treated patients with acute pancreatitis [61]. A worldwide multicenter trial on the clinical effects of lexipafant in patients with different forms of acute pancreatitis was recently closed after the inclusion of 1500 patients. When the various results and details of this large and well-performed study are presented, the question of whether lexipafant exerts any clinical benefit in any subgroup of patients with acute pancreatitis might be answered.

Antibiotics in Acute Pancreatitis

About 40%–60% of necroses in patients with necrotizing pancreatitis are infected within 1–3 weeks after onset of the disease, and about 75% of the pathogenes involved are gram-negative bacteria, while 10% are anaerobics [62]. In the presence of a reasonable suspicion of infected pancreatic necrosis, US- or CT-guided fine-needle aspiration should be done, and antibiotic treatment initiated in accordance with the antibiogram [63–65]. Our knowledge of the role and effects of the various antibiotics in patients with acute pancreatitis is still incomplete and needs further intensive clinical evaluation. At present, a general prophylactic antibiotic therapy for all patients with acute pancreatitis is not reasonable, though it is generally accepted that early administration of antibiotics is indicated for patients with severe or complicated courses of the disease or those with an acute pancreatitis of biliary origin [3, 4, 63–65]. While earlier studies failed to show significant benefits of prophylactic antibiotic treatment, recently published studies in patients with necrotizing pancreatitis were able to prove a beneficial effect of early prophylactic treatment with antibiotics, and imipenem, cephalosporines, chinolons, and metronidazole seem to be the first-line drugs [66–68]. Further details on bacterial translocation and pancreatic infections are given in Chap. 5.

Nutritional Support

It is generally accepted that patients with acute pancreatitis should fast until the clinical conditions have improved, in order to put the pancreas to rest. However, it is a matter of controversy and not well documented whether total parenteral nutrition or enteral nutrition via jejunal feeding are the preferential routes for adequate caloric supplementation [69, 70]. Patients with severe cases of acute pancreatitis require adequately high caloric substitution of nutrients. Recently published data from animal studies and early controlled clinical trials in human subjects suggest that enteral nutrition via jejunal feeding might be superior to the established route of parenteral alimentation, though further comparative prospective studies are needed before recommendations for clinical practice can be given [70, 71]. Nevertheless, it is well known that total parenteral nutrition results in a highly significant early atrophy of gut mucosa, which significantly supports the transmigration of luminal bacteria. Therefore, it is evident that the maintenance of structural and functional integrity of the gut mucosa is a reasonable goal in patients with acute pancreatitis in order to avoid the infection of pancreatic necrosis by transmigrated bacteria from the gut lumen. Further studies are warranted to prove the clinical benefits of early enteral nutrition via jejunal tubes in comparison to the established total parenteral nutrition, before general recommendations can be made.

Management of Pain

Patients with acute pancreatitis generally suffer severe abdominal pain and therefore, a major goal of initial treatment is the achievement of early, potent pain relief. As with patients who have had cardiac infarction, it is most important to put the patient at rest by adequately relieving pain and further symptoms. Potent analgesics such as buprenorphine, pentazocine, or procaine hydrochloride (2 g/24 h i.v.) are commonly used. Though it is known from experimental data that morphine is able to increase the pressure of Oddi's sphincter, there is no clinical evidence that this is of relevance in clinical practice.

Treatment of Biliary Pancreatitis

In 35%–50% of cases gallstones are the cause of an acute pancreatitis. In clinical practice persistent incarceration of gallstones is a rare event [72, 73], and smaller stones that become impacted intermittently are obviously more frequent [74, 75]. It is generally accepted that patients with signs of persistently impacted gallstones benefit from early ERC/EPT treatment [76].

Whether or not patients with biliary pancreatitis will benefit from early ERC/EPT has been under discussion for some time and was the subject of five studies which are briefly summarized here: Neoptolemos and co-workers [77] were the first to investigate early ERC in a prospectively controlled study of 121 patients with suspected biliary pancreatitis. This study, which was carried out by one highly skilled endoscopist, reveals no significant differences in mortality and overall complications between conventional management and urgent ERCP; however, among patients with predicted severe cases overall complications were significantly lower in the invasive compared with the conventional subgroup [77]. Leser et al. [78] did not show a benefit of early ERC in a prospectively controlled study of patients with severe nonbiliary pancreatitis. Fan et al. [79] investigated a heterogeneous group of patients with different underlying origins of pancreatitis and found no significant difference in the rate of either local or systemic complications between the invasive and conventionally treated groups. However, biliary sepsis was observed only in the conventionally treated group, and the authors feel that emergency ERCP is generally indicated for all patients with acute pancreatitis, irrespective of the cause of the disease and irrespective of the predicted severity of pancreatitis. There are a variety of flaws in the design of this study, and this general conclusion is not substantiated by the results it presents.

Nowak et al. [80] carried out diagnostic ERCP in 280 patients with suspected acute biliary pancreatitis within 24 h of admission. Seventy-five patients with impacted stones were treated by immediate sphincterotomy (group I). Two hundred and five patients with a normal papilla were randomly assigned to treatment with immediate sphincterotomy (group II,

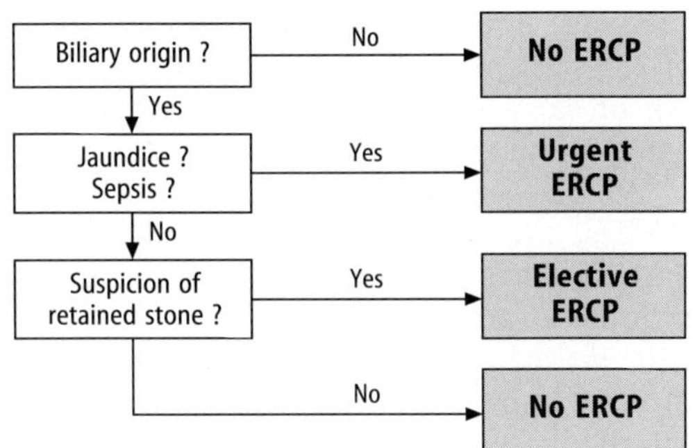

Fig. 1. Differential indications for ERCP in patients with acute pancreatitis

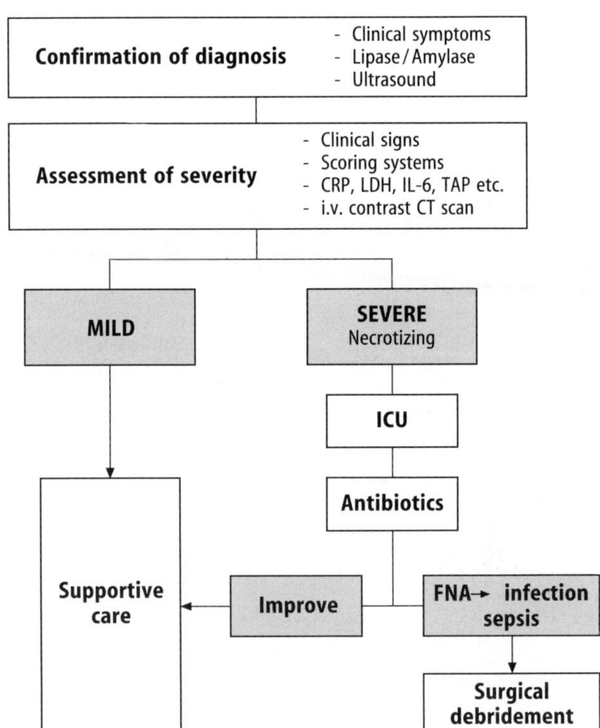

Fig. 2. Algorithm of decision-making and therapeutic strategies in cases of acute pancreatitis. The differential use of endoscopy (ERCP) is given in Fig. 1

n=103) or to conventional management (group III, *n*=102). The authors observed significantly fewer complications in the sphincterotomy groups (I and II) compared with group III. However, the benefit of sphincterotomy in group I is debatable, since a control group was not included. Groups I and II cannot be compared with group III in a prospective randomized trial, because group I was constructed by selecting patients with impacted gallstones. So far, this study has been published only in abstract form. Essential details such as the characteristics of the patients before treatment (for example, whether there was any fever or jaundice) and an analysis of the complications are not available. In a recently published randomized multicenter trial of 238 patients, Fölsch et al. [81] were not able to demonstrate a clinical benefit of early ERCP in patients with suspected biliary pancreatitis but no evidence of an impacted gallstone or biliary complications.

With regard to the clinical conclusions which can be drawn from these studies, the situation is hampered by the fact that there are many and, in part, important differences between them concerning inclusion criteria, definitions, and study design. Figure 1 summarizes the clinical decision-making with regard to the necessity for endoscopic interventions on the basis of our present knowledge. Early ERCP is indicated only when impacted gallstones (markedly elevated bilirubin) or cholangitis (septic fever) are assumed. The indication for ERCP is not dependent on the severity of pancreatitis but rather on the biliary complications of the disease. ERCP is definitely not recommended when nonobstructive pancreatitis is obvious after clinical evaluation or on laboratory findings and ultrasound examination. In patients with biliary pancreatitis but no signs of biliary complications, elective ERCP is sufficient and appropriate [82, 83]. Figure 2 summarizes the route of clinical decision-making and recommended therapeutic strategies for patients with acute pancreatitis.

References

1. Lankisch PG, Schirren C, Schmidt H, Schönfelder G, Creutzfeldt W (1989) Etiology and incidence of acute pancreatitis: a 20-year study in a single institution. Digestion 44:20–25
2. Corfield AP, Cooper MJ, Williamson RCN (1985) Acute pancreatitis: a lethal disease of increasing incidence. Gut 26:724–729
3. Steinberg W, Tenner S (1994) Acute pancreatitis. N Engl J Med 330:1198–1210
4. Löser Chr, Fölsch UR (1993) A concept of treatment in acute pancreatitis – results of controlled trials, and future developments. Hepatogastroenterology 40:569–573
5. Berk JE (1995) The management of acute pancreatitis: a critical assessment as Dr. Bockus would have wished. Am J Gastroenterol 90:696–703
6. Banks P (1997) Practice guidelines in acute pancreatitis. Am J Gastroenterol 92:377–386
7. Niederau C, Schulz H-U (1993) Current conservative treatment of acute pancreatitis: evidence from animal and human studies. Hepatogastroenterology 40:538–549
8. Forsmark CF, Toskes PP (1995) Acute pancreatitis. Medical management. Crit Care Clin 11:295–322
9. Ranson JHC (1995) The current management of acute pancreatitis. Adv Surg 28:3–112
10. Mössner J (1989) Pathogenese und Pathophysiologie der akuten Pankreatitis. Internist 30:705–717
11. Fölsch UR, Löser C (1992) Aktuelle Trends bei der Behandlung der akuten Pankreatitis. Dtsch Arztebl 89:B-2459–B-2468
12. Fölsch UR (1987) Principles of intensive care of patients with acute pancreatitis. In: Beger HG, Büchler M (eds) Acute pancreatitis. Springer-Verlag, Berlin Heidelberg New York, pp 289–292
13. Reynaert MS, Dugernier T, Kestens PJ (1990) Current therapeutic strategies in severe acute pancreatitis. Intensive Care Med 16:352–362
14. Gebhardt C, Bödeker H, Blinzler L, Kraus D, Hergdt G (1994) Wandel in der Therapie der schweren akuten Pankreatitis. Chirurg 65:33–41
15. Banks PA (1994) Acute pancreatitis: conservative management. Dig Surg 11:220–225
16. Sigurdsson GH (1994) Intensive care management of acute pancreatitis. Dig Surg 11:231–241

17. Navarro S, Ros E, Aused R, Garcia Puges AM, Pique JM, Bonet JV (1984) Comparison of fasting, nasogastric suction and cimetidine in the treatment of acute pancreatitis. Digestion 30:224–230
18. Loiudice TA, Lang J, Mehta H, Banta L (1984) Treatment of acute alcoholic pancreatitis: the roles of cimetidine and nasogastric suction. Am J Gastroenterol 79:553–558
19. Pitchumoni CS, Agarwal N, Jain NK (1988) Systemic complications of acute pancreatitis. Am J Gastroenterol 83:5 97–606
20. Renner IG, Savage WT, Pantoja JL, Renner VJ (1985) Death due to acute pancreatitis. A retrospective analysis of 405 autopsy cases. Dig Dis Sci 30:1005–1018
21. Büchler M (1991) Objectification of the severity of acute pancreatitis. Hepatogastroenterology 38:101–108
22. Freeny PC (1991) Diagnosis and detection of complications of acute pancreatitis. Hepatogastroenterology 38:109–115
23. Banks PA (1991) Predictors of severity in acute pancreatitis. Pancreas 6 [Suppl 1]:7–12
24. Demmy TL, Burch JJ, Feliciano DV, Mattox KL, Jordan GL (1988) Comparison of multiple-parameter prognostic systems in acute pancreatitis. Am J Surg 156:492–496
25. Malfertheiner P, Dominguez-Munoz JE (1993) Prognostic factors in acute pancreatitis. Int J Pancreatol 14:1–8
26. Malfertheiner P, Kemmer TP (1991) Clinical picture and diagnosis of acute pancreatitis. Hepatogastroenterology 38:97–100
27. Wilson AS, Austen BM, Imrie CW, Herman-Taylor J (1990) Trypsinogen activation peptides assay in the early prediction of severity of acute pancreatitis. Lancet 335:4–8
28. Leser H-G, Gross V, Scheibenbogen C, Heinisch A, Salm R, Lausen M, Rückauer K, Andreesen R, Farthmann EH, Schölmerich J (1991) Elevation of serum interleukin-6 concentration precedes acute-phase response and reflects severity in acute pancreatitis. Gastroenterology 101:782–785
29. Steinberg W, Schlesselman SE (1987) Treatment of acute pancreatitis. Gastroenterology 93:1420–1427
30. Cameron JL, Mekiyan D, Zuidema GD (1979) Evaluation of atropine in acute pancreatitis. Surg Gynecol Obstet 148:206–208
31. Goebell H, Ammann R, Herfarth C, Horn J, Hotz J, et al (1979) A double-blind trial of synthetic salmon calcitonin in the treatment of acute pancreatitis. Scand J Gastroenterol 14:881–889
32. Usadel KH, Überla KK, Leuschner U (1985) Treatment of acute pancreatitis with somatostatin – results of the multicenter double-blind trial. Dig Dis Sci 30:992
33. Choi TK, Mok F, Zhan WG, Fan ST, Lai ECS, Wong J (1989) Somatostatin in the treatment of acute pancreatitis: a prospective randomized controlled trial. Gut 30:223–227
34. Uhl W, Malfertheiner P, Adler G, Bruch HP, Lankisch PG, Lorenz D, Gaus W, Beger HG, Büchler MW (1999) A randomized controlled multicentric trial on the role of octreotide in human acute pancreatitis. Gut (in press)
35. Kronberg U, Bülow S, Joergensen PM, Svendsen LB (1980) A randomized double-blind trial of glucagon in the treatment of biliary disease. Am J Gastroenterol 73:423
36. Waterworth MW, Barbezat GO, Bank S (1974) Glucagon in treatment of acute pancreatitis. Lancet 1:1231
37. Saario IA (1983) 5-Fluorouracil in the treatment of acute pancreatitis. Am J Surg 145:349–352
38. Broe PJ, Zinner MJ, Cameron JL (1982) A clinical trial of cimetidine in acute pancreatitis. Surg Gynecol Obstet 154:13–16
39. Meshkinpour H, Molinari MD, Gardner L, Berk JE, Hoehler FK (1979) Cimetidine in the treatment of acute alcoholic pancreatitis: a randomized, double-blind study. Gastroenterology 77:687–690
40 Niederau C, Niederau M, Lüthen R, Strohmeyer G, Ferrell LD, Grendell JH (1990) Pancreatic exocrine secretion in acute experimental pancreatitis. Gastroenterology 99:1120–1127
41. Skyring A, Singer A, Tornya P (1965) Treatment of acute pancreatitis with Trasylol: report of a controlled therapeutic trial. Br Med J 2:627–629
42. Trapnell JE, Rigby CC, Talbot CH, Duncan EHL (1974) A controlled trial of Trasylol in the treatment of acute pancreatitis. Br J Surg 61:177–182
43. Imrie CW, Benjamin IS, Ferguson JC, McKay AJ, Mackenzie I, O'Neill J, Blumgart LH (1978) A single centre double blind trial of Trasylol therapy in primary acute pancreatitis. Br J Surg 65:337–341

44. Freise J, Meker P, Schmidt FW, Horbach L (1986) Gabexat mesilat in der Behandlung der akuten Pankreatitis. Ergebnisse der hannoverschen multizentrischen Doppelblindstudie mit 50 Patienten. Z Gastroenterol 24:200–211
45. Goebell H und die Deutsche Pankreas-Studiengruppe (1988) Multizenter-Doppelblindstudie mit dem Proteinasen-Inhibitor Gabexat-Mesilat (FOY) bei akuter Pankreatitis in niedriger Dosierung. Z Gastroenterol 26:477
46. Büchler M, Malfertheiner P, Uhl W, Stöckmann F, Schölmerich J, Adler G, Rolle K, Ditschuneit H, Beger HG (1990) The German multicenter double-blind randomised study of gabexate-mesilate (4 g/day i.v.) in acute pancreatitis. Gastroenterology 98:A214
47. Tykkä HT, Vaittinen EJ, Mahlberg KL, Railo JE, Pantzar PJ, Sarna S, Tallberg T (1985) A randomized double-blind study using $CaNA_2$ EDTA, a phospholipase A_2 inhibitor, in the management of human acute pancreatitis. Scand J Gastroenterol 20:5–12
48. Leese T, Holliday M, Heath D, Hall AW, Bell PRF (1987) Multicentre clinical trial of low volume fresh frozen plasma therapy in acute pancreatitis. Br J Surg 74:907–911
49. Ebbehoj N, Fries J, Svendsen JLB, Bülow S, Madsen P (1985) Indomethacin treatment of acute pancreatitis. A controlled double-blind trial. Scand J Gastroenterol 20:778–800
50. Uden S, Bilton D, Guyon PM, Kay PM, Braganza JM (1990) Rationale for antioxidant therapy in pancreatitis and cystic fibrosis. Adv Exp Med Biol 264:555–572
51. Ranson JHC, Rifkind KM, Roses DF, Fink SD, Eng K, Spencer FC (1974) Prognostic signs and the role of operative management in acute pancreatitis. Surg Gynecol Obstet 139:69–81
52. Pickford IR, Blackett RL, McMahon MJ (1977) Early assessment of severity of acute pancreatitis using peritoneal lavage. Br Med J 2:1377–1379
53. Mayer AD, McMahon MJ, Corfield AP, Cooper MJ, Williams CN, Chir M et al (1985) Controlled clinical trial of peritoneal lavage for the treatment of severe acute pancreatitis. N Engl J Med 312:399–404
54. Ranson JHC, Spencer FC (1978) The role of peritoneal lavage in severe acute pancreatitis. Ann Surg 187:565–575
55. Ihse I, Evander A, Holmberg JT, Gustafson I (1986) Influence of peritoneal lavage on objective prognostic signs in acute pancreatitis. Ann Surg 204:122–127
56. Ranson JHC, Berman RS (1990) Long peritoneal lavage decreases pancreatic sepsis in acute pancreatitis. Ann Surg 211:708–718
57. Blinzler L, Haußer J, Bödeker H, Zaune U, Martin E, Gebhardt C (1991) Conservative treatment of severe necrotizing pancreatitis using early continuous venovenous hemofiltration. Contrib Nephrol 93
58. Dabrowski A, Gabrylelewicz A, Chyczewski L (1991) Effect of platelet activating factor antagonist (BN 52021) on caerulein-induced acute pancreatitis with reference to oxygen radicals. Int J Pancreatol 8:1–11
59. Fujuimura K, Kubota Y, Ogura M et al (1992) Role of endogenous platelet-activating factor in caerulein-induced pancreatitis in rats: protective effects of PAF-antagonist. J Gastroenterol Hepatol 7:199–202
60. Kingsnorth AN, Galloway SW, Formela LJ (1995) Randomized, double-blind phase II trial of lexipafant, a platelet-activating factor antagonist, in human acute pancreatitis. Br J Surg 82:1414–1420
61. Kingsnorth AN (1997) Early treatment with lexipafant, a platelet activating factor antagonist, reduces mortality in acute pancreatitis: a double blind randomized, placebo controlled study. Gastroenterology 112:A453
62. Beger HG, Bittner R, Block S, Büchler M (1986) Bacterial contamination of pancreatic necrosis. A prospective clinical study. Gastroenterology 91:433–438
63. Byrne JJ, Treadwell TL (1989) Treatment of pancreatitis – when do antibiotics have a role? Postgrad Med 85:333–339
64. Bradley EL (1989) Antibiotics in acute pancreatitis – current status and future directions. Am J Surg 158:472–477
65. Barie PS (1996) A critical review of antibiotic prophylaxis in severe acute pancreatitis. Am J Surg 172 [Suppl 6A]:38S-43S
66. Pederzoli P, Bassi C, Vesentini S, Campedelli A (1993) A randomized multicenter clinical trial of antibiotic prophylaxis of septic complications in acute necrotizing pancreatitis with imipenem. Surg Gynecol Obstet 176:480–483
67. Sainio V, Kemppainen E, Puolakkainen P, Taavitsainen M, Kivisaari L, Valtonen V, Haapiainen R, Schröder T, Kivilaakso E (1995) Early antibiotic treatment in acute necrotising pancreatitis. Lancet 346:663–667
68. Delcenserie R, Yzet T, Ducroix JP (1996) Prophylactic antibiotics in treatment of severe acute alcoholic pancreatitis. Pancreas 13:198–201

69. Havala T, Shronts E, Cerra F (1989) Nutritional support in acute pancreatitis. Gastroenterol Clin North Am 18:525–542
70. McClave SA, Snider H, Owens N, Sexton LK (1997) Clinical nutrition in pancreatitis. Dig Dis Sci 42:2035–2044
71. McClave SA, Greene LM, Snider HL, Makk LJK, Cheadle WG, Owens NA, Dukes LG, Goldsmith LJ (1997) Comparison of the safety of early enteral vs parenteral nutrition in mild acute pancreatitis. JPEN 21:014–020
72. Acosta JM, Pellegrini CA, Skinner DB (1980) Etiology and pathogenesis of acute biliary pancreatitis. Surgery 88:118–125
73. Kim U, Shen HY, Bodner B (1988) Timing of surgery for acute gallstone pancreatitis. Am J Surg 156:393–396
74. Houssin D, Castaing D, Lemoine J, Bismuth H (1983) Microlithiasis of the gallbladder. Surg Gynecol Obstet 157:20–24
75. Farinon AM, Ricci GL, Sianesi M, Percudani M, Zanella E (1987) Physiopathologic role of microlithiasis in gallstone pancreatitis. Surg Gynecol Obstet 164:252–256
76. Fölsch UR (1988) Endoskopische Papillotomie bei akuter biliärer Pankreatitis: gesicherte oder experimentelle Therapie? Endoskopie heute 2:30–32
77. Neoptolemos JP, Carr-Locke DL, London NJ, Bailey IA, James D, Fossard DP (1988) Controlled trial of urgent endoscopic retrograde cholangiopancreatography and endoscopic sphincterotomy versus conservative treatment for acute pancreatitis due to gallstones. Lancet 2:979–983
78. Leser HG, Gross V, Heinisch A, Schölmerich J (1993) Frühpapillotomie bei schwerer akuter Pankreatitis ohne Choledocholithiasis: Ergebnisse einer Multicenter-Studie. Z Gastroenterol 31:544 (abstract)
79. Fan S-T, Lai ECS, Mok FPT, et al (1993) Early treatment of acute biliary pancreatitis by endoscopic papillotomy. N Engl J Med 328:228–232
80. Nowak A, Nowakowska-Dulawa E, Marek TA, Rybicka J (1995) Final results of the prospective, randomized, controlled study on endoscopic sphincterotomy versus conventional management in acute biliary pancreatitis. Gastroenterology 108 [Suppl]:A380 (abstract)
81. Fölsch UR, Nitsche R, Lüdtke R, Hilgers RA, Creutzfeldt W, and the German Study Group on Acute Biliary Pancreatitis (1997) Early ERCP and papillotomy compared with conservative treatment for acute biliary pancreatitis. N Engl J Med 336:237–242
82. Nitsche R, Fölsch UR (1999) Role of ERCP and sphincterotomy in acute pancreatitis. Baillieres Clin Gastroenterol (in press)
83. Fölsch UR, Nitsche R, Hilgers RA, Lüdtke R, Creutzfeldt W (1992) Papillotomie bei akuter Pankreatitis – mehr Nutzen als Risiken? Bildgebung 19 [Suppl 1]:25–27

CHAPTER 8

Surgical Treatment of Acute Pancreatitis

H. G. BEGER, B. RAU, J. MAYER, and R. ISENMANN

Classification of Acute Pancreatitis

Former classifications of acute pancreatitis have been based on the etiology of the disease. This has led to great confusion, as comparison of the patients with regard to course and severity of the disease and outcome has been hampered. During the past decades, the definition of acute pancreatitis has undergone considerable modifications. The current classification has been defined by the Atlanta consensus conference. It is based on the clinical picture of the disease and distinguishes between mild and severe courses [1, 2].

The overwhelming majority of patients with acute pancreatitis suffer from mild disease which responds to conservative treatment. Fatalities and complications are rare. The pathomorphological picture is characterized by interstitial edema, and complete functional and morphological restitution of the gland is the rule. In mild acute pancreatitis, surgical treatment is contraindicated.

In contrast, 10%–20% of the patients develop severe disease, which in pathomorphological terms is characterized by the development of intra- or peripancreatic necrosis. Severe acute pancreatitis is associated with a considerable rate of organ failure and local complications. The majority of deaths due to the disease are observed in patients with pancreatic necrosis.

From the clinical point of view, it is of importance to distinguish between sterile and infected pancreatic necrosis. Infected pancreatic necrosis is defined as the presence of bacteria in diffuse or focal areas of nonviable pancreatic parenchyma. Bacterial infection of pancreatic necrosis commonly occurs during the second week after onset of the disease.

The term pancreatic abscess describes a localized collection of purulent material with little or no necrosis in the pancreas or peripancreatic region, surrounded by a wall of fibrotic tissue. In contrast, infected pancreatic pseudocysts are defined as localized and encapsulated collections of infected pancreatic juice, not containing pus or necrotic material. Both pancreatic abscess and infected pseudocysts are local complications of severe acute pancreatitis. In comparison to infected necrosis, they are characterized by a mild to moderate clinical picture with significantly lower APACHE II and Ranson scores. Systemic complications and fatal courses are less frequent in these patients [3].

Indications for Surgical Treatment

The indications for surgical treatment in severe acute pancreatitis have undergone considerable changes during the past few years and still are under discussion. Today, there is general agreement that only patients with pancreatic necrosis are candidates for surgical treatment. Formerly, early surgical intervention was advocated [4–6]. Disappointing results led to a more restrictive approach, and our current principles of management are based on the observation that 30%–40% of patients with sterile pancreatic necrosis do not require surgery and can be managed by conservative treatment [7–9]. Thus, the initial treatment of severe acute pancreatitis should be conservative management in the ICU as long as the patient responds to it. There are, however a number of clear-cut indications for which surgery should be performed:

- There is general agreement that surgery is mandatory for infected necrosis and should be performed soon after bacterial infection has been diagnosed [7, 10–13].
- Ongoing multiorgan failure despite maximum intensive medical therapy over a period of 48–72 h is accepted as an indication for surgery regardless of whether there is evidence of pancreatic infection [7, 8, 12, 13].
- Abdominal complications (persistent ileus, intra-abdominal bleeding, suspected GI-tract perforation) pose additional indications for surgical treatment.

Rationales for surgery in necrotizing pancreatitis are numerous: First, bacteria and their toxic compounds are released into the circulation and are responsible for remote organ failure. Thus, the removal of infected necrotic material is a therapeutic necessity. Second, the formation of late complications such as pancreatic abscesses can be prevented by removing the infected debris. Third, preservation of still viable pancreatic tissue will achieve good long-term results with respect to pancreatic exocrine and endocrine function.

Relevance of Pancreatic Infection

Infected pancreatic necrosis is found in 1%–10% of all patients suffering from acute pancreatitis and in 40%–70% of all patients with necrotizing pancreatitis [3, 12, 14, 15]. Data from our institution indicate the significance of infectious complications in acute pancreatitis (Table 1). It is the most common complication of severe acute pancreatitis and has a tremendous clinical impact. There are significant differences in morbidity and mortality between patients with infected and those with sterile necrosis. Systemic complications such as pulmonary insufficiency, renal failure, shock, sepsis, and sepsis-like syndrome as well as coagulopathy are more frequent in patients with infected pancreatic necrosis [16, 17]. As in other series, systemic complications are more frequent in our patients with pancreatic infection (Table 2), and the hospital stay of this subgroup as well as their time in the ICU is considerably longer.

Table 1. Incidence of severe acute pancreatitis in 1442 patients

	Patients	% of NP	% of AP
Interstitial pancreatitis	1015		70.4
Necrotizing pancreatitis	300		20.8
Sterile necrosis	201	67.0	13.9
Infected necrosis	99	33.0	6.8
Pancreatic abscess	40		2.8
Pseudocysts	87		6.0

Table 2. Clinical relevance of infected necrosis in 300 patients with severe acute pancreatitis, Department of General Surgery, University of Ulm, May 1982–December 1996

	Systemic complications	
	In sterile necrosis (201 patients)	In infected necrosis (99 patients)
Pulmonary insufficiency (%)[a]	58.7	74.7
Sepsis/sepsis syndrome (%)[b]	36.3	54.5
Coagulopathy (%)[c]	42.8	54.5
Renal insufficiency (%)[d]	21.4	21.2
Hospitalization (days)[e]	45 (2–209)	62 (1–238)
ICU duration (days)[e]	21 (1–184)	27 (1–238)
Mortality	26 patients (12.9%)	94 patients (25.2%)

[a] pO_2<60 mmHg
[b] *Sepsis*: T>38.5°C/Leu >16 giga/l/BE – 4 mmol/l for >48 h and positive blood culture/aspirate. *Sepsis syndrome*: Sepsis: T>38.5°C/Leu >12 giga/l /BE – 2.5 mmol/l and negative blood culture/aspirate.
[c] Prothrombin time <70% and/or activated partial thromboplastin time >45 s.
[d] Serum creatinine >180 pmol/l.
[e] Patients (n=221) undergoing surgical treatment.

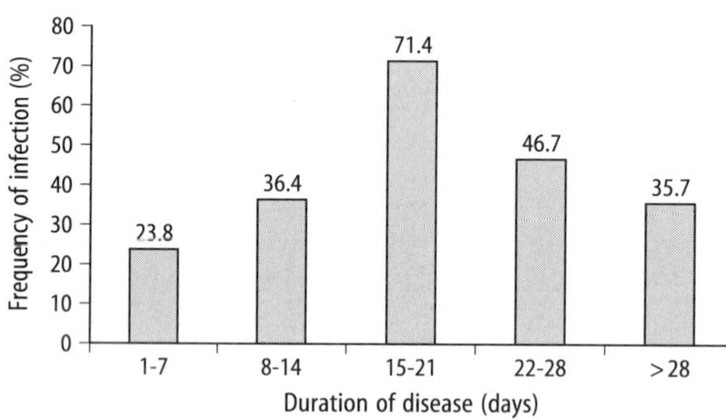

Fig. 1. Incidence of infected necrosis in patients undergoing surgery. Time of appearance of bacteria in intraoperative smears

Bacterial infection of pancreatic necrosis correlates with the duration of the disease. A time-dependent increase in its incidence has been shown (Fig. 1). Using fine-needle aspiration, bacteria can be detected a median of 6 days after onset of acute pancreatitis [18, 19]. A second factor determining the incidence of bacterial infection is the extent of necrosis. It increases with the amount of necrotic intrapancreatic tissue (Fig. 2).

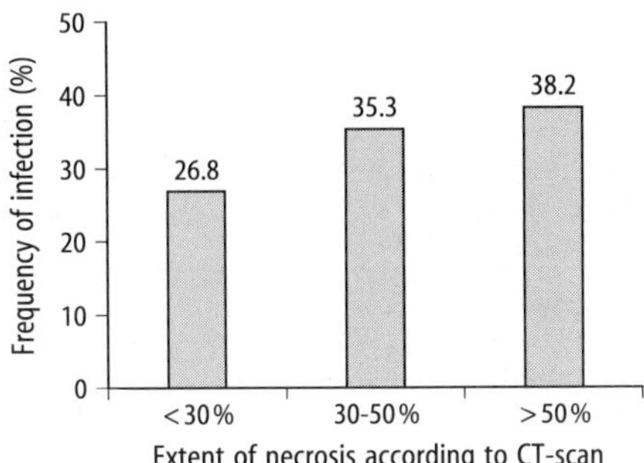

Fig. 2. Relation between the extent of pancreatic necrosis found on contrast-enhanced CT scanning and incidence of infection in 225 patients with necrotizing pancreatitis, University of Ulm, May 1982–December 1996

Bacterial Spectrum of Infected Pancreatic Necrosis

The bacterial spectrum of infected pancreatic necrosis is well defined. Data have been obtained from smears obtained either during surgical necrosectomy [20, 21] or by computer-tomography guided fine-needle aspiration [18]. In general, infected pancreatic necrosis is a monomicrobial infection, dominated by gram-negative germs. *Escherichia coli* is the strain commonly found in infected necrosis, but it also harbors gram-positive bacteria such as enterococci and *Staphylococcusaureus* as well as anaerobes and fungi (Table 3).

As especially the colon contains the greatest variety and number of germs anywhere in the body, it is assumed that the bacteria found in pancreatic infection originate from the gastrointestinal tract. The routes by which the organisms might reach the necrotic areas remain unclear. Direct translocation, hematogenous or lymphatic spread, or infection via the pancreatic duct and the common bile duct all have been supposed as pathways of infection [22–24]. The exact mechanisms are still a matter of experimental investigation, and to date, none of them has consistently been confirmed or ruled out.

Table 3. Spectrum of bacteria and frequency in infected pancreatic necrosis among 105 patients, Department of General Surgery, University of Ulm May 1982–December 1993

Type of infection	Frequency (%)
Monomicrobial	69
Escherichia coli	23
Staphylococcus aureus	14
Enterococcus	6
Klebsiella	5
Polymicrobial	31
E. coli	22
Enterococcus	16
Staph. aureus	3
Klebsiella	4
Pseudomonas	1
Proteus	4
Candida	5

Table 4. Value of ultrasound-guided fine-needle aspiration for predicting infected pancreatic necrosis in a prospective series of 88 patients, Department of General Surgery, University of Ulm, January 1988–February 1996

Fine-needle aspiration	Confirmed	
	Positive (*n*=31)	Negative (*n*=102)
Positive (*n*=36)	31	5
Negative (*n*=107)	5	102
Sensitivity (%)	86	
Specificity (%)		95
Diagnostic accuracy (%)	93	

Diagnosis of Infected Pancreatic Necrosis

In the absence of reliable imaging and laboratory markers that indicate infected pancreatic necrosis, diagnosis of bacterial infection is best made by fine-needle aspiration (FNA) under the guidance of either CT or ultrasound, with Gram staining and culture of the aspirate. FNA has been introduced into the diagnostic algorithm of necrotizing pancreatitis a decade ago and has proven its reliability and safety in several studies. Sensitivity for prediction of infected necrosis is reported to range from 90 to 100%, with specificity ranging from 96% to 100% [18, 25–28]. At our institution, ultrasound-guided FNA is performed as a standard procedure in patients with CT-proven pancreatic necrosis and persisting systemic complications or with a newly developed or persisting septic clinical picture [25]. In a prospective series of 88 patients, this procedure was found to have a sensitivity of 86% and a specificity of 95% for prediction of infected pancreatic necrosis (Table 4). Its high diagnostic accuracy enables early detection and timely surgical intervention and thus provides a chance to prevent further local and systemic complications caused by bacterial infection.

Indications for Surgical Management in Sterile Necrosis

The management of patients with sterile necrosis is controversial. Experience has shown that 30%–40% of these patients can be treated sucessfully without operating. Surgery in this situation is aimed at preventing the systemic release of a number of vasoactive and toxic substances that lead to remote organ failure. Exudation of fluid containing activated pancreatic enzymes and biologically active mediators to the peripancreatic region and the abdominal cavity is one of the characteristics of severe acute pancreatitis [29]. Systemic delivery of these substances takes place via the portal circulation, and there is strong evidence that the systemic release of these substances correlates with an increased incidence of organ failure. Our present strategy in sterile necrosis is based on the observation that successful conservative management is characterized by response to extended ICU treatment. This is de-

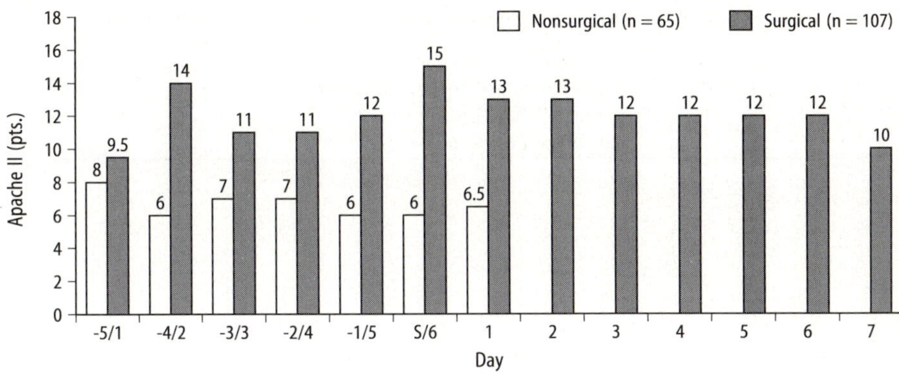

Fig. 3. APACHE II scores in 172 patients with sterile pancreatic necrosis. Comparison of surgical patients (days 5–1 preoperative and days 1–7 postoperative) to nonsurgical patients (days 1–7 after admission)

monstrated by a decrease in the APACHE II scores of these patients (Fig. 3). As long as the patient responds to conservative treatment alone, surgical intervention is not necessary [8]. It is accepted that surgery is indicated for patients who do not respond to maximum conservative treatment over a period of more than 72 h. The question of whether or not sterile necrosis should be operated on at all is currently under discussion. However, there is no contolled series comparing operative and observational treatment for this group of patients.

Timing of Surgical Treatment in Necrotizing Pancreatitis

The timing of operative intervention in necrotizing pancreatitis is still a matter of controversy. The intervention can be performed early, within the first 7 days, or late, after the postacute phase during or after the second week. There is no doubt that initial management should be conservative. Experience shows that even in the presence of organ dysfunction, maximum intensive support should be provided for at least 3 days. We advocate operative intervention for patients who do not respond to this supportive regimen by about the second week of the disease. The rationale for this delayed concept is to wait until demarcation of necrosis has occurred. Early intervention during days 1–7 (in the acute phase) should be applied only in rare cases with a fulminant course or if infection of necrosis has been confirmed objectively.

Techniques of Surgical Treatment

Numerous approaches have been advocated in the surgical management of necrotizing pancreatitis during the past decades, ranging from nonresective methods to extensive resections. Owing to disappointing results, nonresective

Table 5. Surgical treatment of necrotizing pancreatitis – results of different surgical techniques

Reference	Mortality		Pancreatic fistulas	Small-bowel fistulas	Colonic fistulas	Hemorrhage
	Patients	%				
Conventional						
39	6/12	50.0				
40	16/38	42.1	5/38		3/38	4/38
8	5/29	17.2				
41	14/17	82.4				
42	4/14	28.6	3/14	0/14	1/14	1/14
43	2/12	16.7	2/12	0/12	0/12	0/12
44	1/36	2.8				2/36
45	4/18	22.2	0/18	1/18	4/18	1/18
Total	52/176	29.5	10/82 (12%)		9/82 (11%)	8/118 (7%)
Open/semiopen						
46	2/10	20	0/10	4/10	0/10	2/10
47	6/28	21.4	0/28	0/28	0/28	1/28
15	4/23	17.4	6/23	3/23	5/23	6/23
48	7/43	16.2	3/43		5/43	
49	3/15	20.0	1/15		4/15	4/15
50	10/71	14.1	33/71		5/71	5/71
51	40/125	32.0	0/125	15/125	17/125	24/125
Total	72/315	22.9	43/315 (14%)		58/315 (18%)	42/315 (13%)
Closed						
52	9/27	33.3				
53	3/14	21.4	0/14	6/14	2/14	1/14
54	40/191	17.9	16/191		21/191	18/191
55	18/140[a]	12.9	10/95		9/95	3/95
Total	70/372	18.8	26/300 (9%)		38/300 (13%)	22/300 (7%)

[a] Primary admissions and early referrals only.

procedures and extensive resections have been abandoned. Today, the benefit of surgical necrosectomy is unquestioned, but subsequent management remains a matter of considerable discussion (Table 5).

Conventional Drainage

Conventional débridement and Penrose/sump drainage has been the classic approach in necrotizing pancreatitis. It is associated with persistent intra-abdominal infections and a high rate of reoperations. Recently, the success rate was shown to depend on the extent and completeness of débridement. The use of wider drainages and the insertion of multiple sump and rubber drains in combination with aggressive débridement have led to acceptable results at a few centers which still favor this method.

Open and Semiopen Management

Based on the observation that recurrent pancreatic sepsis is a common sequel of conventional drainage, some surgeons pursue aggressive operative approaches involving open packing and frequent and planned reoperations. Following necrosectomy, the affected area is packed with nonadherent gauze. The abdomen is left open and the package is changed every 24–48 h under sedation in the ICU. The technique has been modified at other centers by insertion of a synthetic mesh or zipper in the abdominal fascia to allow easy reentry for planned relavage.

Although these methods have provided favorable results when used in experienced hands, repeated intra-abdominal manipulations increase the risk of intra-abdominal hemorrhage, bowel or pancreatic fistulas, and bowel obstruction with subsequent ileus. Consequently, ICU therapy is often mandatory for several weeeks.

Necrosectomy and Closed Lavage of the Lesser Sac (Closed Management)

In contrast to open and semiopen techniques, closed management combines surgical débridement of necrotic areas and extensive postoperative lavage of the retroperitoneum. The method was introduced in the early 1980s and is currently applied at several centers. It avoids repeated intra-abdominal manipulation with the risk of a prolonged stay in intensive care, local bleeding, intestinal fistula, mechanical ileus, and incisional hernias.

After opening of the lesser sac, careful surgical débridement with removal of necrotic material is done mainly digitally, in order to preserve still vital pancreatic parenchyma. This is followed by extensive intraoperative lavage with 6–12 l isotonic saline in order to clear the pancreatic bed. Large single-lumen catheters (Charr. 24–28), as well as double-lumen catheters (Charr. 16–18), are placed in the lesser sac for postoperative lavage (Fig. 4). Following this procedure, the gastrocolic and duodenocolic ligaments are sutured, creating a closed compartment which is rinsed postoperatively with 24 l of commercial hyperosmolar potassium-free dialysis fluid per day. In cases where the peritoneal cavity is additionally affected, local lavage of the lesser sac is combined with a short-term peritoneal lavage. Remaining necrotic material and biochemically active compounds are eliminated from the pancreatic region, and the drains can be removed after stepwise reduction of the daily lavage quantity.

In our experience, this procedure has proven to be safe and effective (Table 6). From May 1982 until December 1996, 140 patients with necrotizing pancreatitis underwent necrosectomy and local lavage of the lesser sac. The patients suffered from severe pancreatitis and had a median APACHE II score of 9 points and a median Ranson core of 4 points. Postoperative lavage was carried out over a median of 22 days with an initial fluid amount of 24 l/day. Reoperation was necessary in 51 patients (36.4%); 18 (12.9%) of our patients died. According to our experience, the concept of necrosectomy and

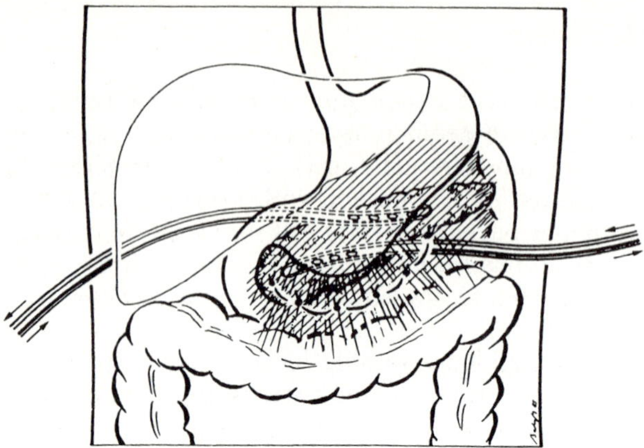

Fig. 4. Continuous lavage of the lesser sac after necrosectomy for necrotizing pancreatitis. Lavage is carried out with double-lumen catheters for a median of 3 weeks

Table 6. Results of necrosectomy and local lavage for necrotizing pancreatitis in 140 patients, University of Ulm, Department of General Surgery, 1982–1996

Parameter	Mean	Range
Preoperative		
Ranson points	4	0–9
APACHE II points	9.0	0–28
Postoperative		
Hospitalization (days)	53	7–192
ICU (days)	22	1–184
Lavage duration (days)	22	1–109
Lavage fluid (l/h)	24/24	2–36
Frequency of reoperation (%)	36.4	
Mortality (%)	12.9	

postoperative continuous lavage of the lesser sac is safe and successful for the surgical management of patients with necrotizing pancreatitis. In comparision to the results of other surgical approaches in necrotizing pancreatitis, such as the open or semiopen technique, it provides similar results with respect to clinical outcome and is superior in terms of the lower demand for technical expenditures, ICU therapy, and cost.

None of the three different approaches is superior to the others with regard to the basic principle of necrosectomy. In experienced hands, favorable results can be achieved with any of them, provided that all necrotic material and septic collections are thoroughly removed and that reoperation is performed promptly if there is evidence of ongoing sepsis (Table 5).

Surgical Treatment – Future Trends

Today, there is little discussion about the techniques of surgical treatment of severe acute pancreatitis. The current surgical standards are all comparable with regard to mortality and postoperative complications. Nevertheless, even at specialized centers, the mortality of severe acute pancreatitis is 15%–20% after surgical treatment. These figures appear to be improvable. Based on the observation that patients treated conservatively seem to have a better prognosis than those who have to undergo surgery, discussion is now centered on modification of our current indications for surgery. This has led to trends of prolonged conservative treatment even in patients with infected pancreatic necrosis, irrespective of persistent or ongoing organ failure and sepsis [30, 31]. To date, only selected groups of patients have been treated according to these protocols. As long as controlled clinical studies are lacking, results of prolongation of conservative management of these severely ill patients are difficult to interpret and future investigations will have to show the value of this approach.

There have been other approaches to reducing the complications of acute pancreatitis. Early use of antibiotic drugs in patients with pancreatic necrosis has been shown to reduce the incidence of pancreatic infection [32], mortality [33], or both [34]. The results are promising, but due to drawbacks in the design of the studies, a conclusive statement about the value of early antibiotics cannot yet be made [35, 36].

Other therapeutic concepts focus on the reduction of the systemic release of activated inflammatory mediators as well as chemotactic substances, which have been suggested to play a role in the pathogenesis of organ failure during severe acute pancreatitis. Although a number of different substances including calcitonin, somatostatin and its analogues, or protease inhibitors have failed to reduce the systemic complications of severe acute pancreatitis [37], further research is necessary in this field. Lexipafant, a platelet-activating factor antagonist, is currently under clinical investigation [38].

The concept of reducing the infectious complications of severe acute pancreatitis and/or the incidence of systemic failure is a promising approach to improving the prognosis, and further research seems to be justified in this field.

References

1. Bradley EL III (1993) A clinically based classification system for acute pancreatitis. Arch Surg 128:586–590
2. Frey C, Reber HA (1993) Clinically based classification system for acute pancreatitis. Pancreas 8:738–741
3. Bittner R, Block S, Büchler M, Beger HG (1987) Pancreatic abscess and infected pancreatic necrosis. Different local septic complications in acute pancreatitis. Dig Dis Sci 32:1082–1087
4. Nordback IH, Auvinen OA (1985) Long-term results after pancreas resection for acute necrotizing pancreatitis. Br J Surg 72:687–689
5. Ranson JC, Rifkind KM, Roses DF, Fink SD, Eng K, Spencer FC (1974) Prognostic signs and the role of operative management in acute pancreatitis. Surg Gynecol Obstet 139:69

6. Acosta JM, Rossi RR, Galli OM, Pellegini CA, Skinner DB (1978) Early surgery for gallstone pancreatitis: evaluation of a systemic approach. Surgery 83:367–370
7. Bradley EL, Allen K (1991) A prospective longitudinal study of observation versus surgical intervention in the management of necrotizing pancreatitis. Am J Surg 161:19–25
8. Rau B, Pralle U, Uhl W, Schoenberg MH, Beger HG (1995) Management of sterile necrosis in instances of severe acute pancreatitis. J Am Coll Surg 181:279–288
9. Karimgani I, Porter KA, Langevin RE, Banks PA (1992) Prognostic factors in sterile pancreatic necrosis. Gastroenterology 103:1636–1640
10. Bradley EL (1987) Management of infected pancreatic necrosis by open drainage. Ann Surg 206:542–550
11. Sarr MG, Nagorney DM, Much P jr, Farnell MB, Johnson CD (1991) Acute necrotizing pancreatitis: management by planned, staged pancreatic necrosectomy/débridement and delayed primary wound closure over drains. Br J Surg 78:576–581
12. Beger HG, Bittner R, Büchler M, Block S, Nevalainen TJ, Roscher R (1988) Necrosectomy and postoperative local lavage in necrotizing pancreatitis. Br J Surg 75:207–212
13. Isenmann R, Büchler MW (1994) Infection and acute pancreatitis. Br J Surg 81:1707–1708
14. Fedorak IJ, Ko TC, Djuricin G, McMahon M, Thompson KR, Prinz A (1991) Secondary pancreatic infections: are they distinct clinical entities? Surgery 161:19
15. Widdison AL, Karanjia ND (1993) Pancreatic infection complicating acute pancreatitis. Br J Surg 80:148–154
16. Isenmann R, Rau B, Schoenberg MH, Beger HG(1998) Determinants of organ failure (OF) in patients with necrotizing pancreatitis (NP). Gastroenterology 114:A470
17. de Beaux AC, Palmer KR, Carter DC (1995) Factors influencing morbidity and mortality in acute pancreatitis; an analysis of 279 cases. Gut 37:121–126
18. Gerzof SG, Banks PA, Robbins AH, Johnson WC, Spechler SJ, Wetzner SM, Snider JM, Langevin RE, Jay ME (1987) Early diagnosis of pancreatic infection by computed tomography-guided aspiration. Gastroenterology 93:1315–1320
19. Isenmann R, Büchler M, Uhl W, Pralle U, Malfertheiner P, Bialas C, Meyer H, Beger HG (1992) When does infection of pancreatic necrosis happen? Pancreas 7:A742
20. Beger HG, Bittner R, Block S, Büchler M (1986) Bacterial contamination of pancreatic necrosis – a prospective clinical study. Gastroenterology 91:433–438
21. Bassi C, Falconi M, Girelli R, Nifosi F, Elio A, Martini N, Pederzoli P (1989) Microbiological findings in severe pancreatitis. Surg Res Comm 5:1–4
22. Wells CL, Rotstein OD, Pruett TL, Simmons RL (1986) Intestinal bacteria translocate into experimental intra-abdominal abscesses. Arch Surg 121:102–107
23. Widdison AL, Karanjia ND, Reber HA (1994) Routes of spread of pathogens into the pancreas in a feline model of acute pancreatitis. Gut 35:1306–1310
24. Medich DS, Lee TK, Melhem MF, Rowe MI, Schraut WH, Lee KW (1993) Pathogenesis of pancreatic sepsis. Am J Surg 165:46–52
25. Rau B, Pralle U, Mayer JM, Beger HG (1998) Role of ultrasonographically guided fine-needle aspiration cytology in the diagnosis of infected pancreatic necrosis. Br J Surg 85:179–184
26. Stiles GM, Berne TV, Thommen VD, Molgaard CP, Boswell WD (1990) Fine needle aspiration of pancreatic fluid collections. Am Surg 56:764–768
27. Hiatt JR, Fink AS, King W II, Pitt HA (1987) Percutaneous aspiration of peripancreatic fluid collections: a safe method to detect infection. Surgery 101:523–530
28. Barkin JS, Pereiras R, Hill M, Levi J, Isikoff M, Rogers AI (1982) Diagnosis of pancreatic abscess via percutaneous aspiration. Dig Dis Sci 27:1011–1014
29. Chikh-Torab F, Berger D, Buttenschön K, Pralle U, Beger HG (1996) Inflammatory mediators in acute pancreatitis: high concentrations in the peripancreatic fluid. Digestion 57:156A
30. Rünzi M, Layer P, Niebel W, Eigler FW, Goebell H (1996) Infected necrosis in severe acute pancreatitis: an indication for immediate surgery? Pancreas 13:455
31. Dubner H, Steinberg W, Hill M, Bassi C, Chardavoyne R, Bank S (1996) Infected pancreatic necrosis and peripancreatic fluid collections: serendipitous response to antibiotic and medical therapy in three patients. Pancreas 12:298
32. Pederzoli P, Bassi C, Vesentini A, Campedelli A (1993) A randomized multicenter clinical trial of antibiotic prophylaxis of septic complications in acute necrotizing pancreatitis with imipenem. Surg Gynecol Obstet 176:480–483
33. Sainio V, Kemppainen E, Puolakkainen P, Taavitsainen M, Kivisaari L, Valtonen V, Haapiainen R, Schröder T, Kivilaakso E (1995) Early antibiotic treatment in acute necrotising pancreatitis. Lancet 346:663–667

34. Luiten EJT, Hop WCJ, Lange JF, Bruining HA (1995) Controlled clinical trial of selective decontamination for the treatment of severe acute pancreatitis. Ann Surg 222:57–65
35. Powell JJ, Miles R, Siriwardena AK (1998) Antibiotic prophylaxis in the initial management of severe acute pancreatitis. Br J Surg 85:582–587
36. Ho SH, Frey CF (1997) The role of antibiotic prophylaxis in severe acute pancreatitis. Arch Surg 132:487–493
37. Steinberg WM, Schlesselmann SE (1987) Treatment of acute pancreatitis. Gastroenterology 93:1420–1427
38. Kingsnorth AN, Galloway SW, Formela LJ (1995) Randomized, double-blind phase II trial of lexipafant, a platelet-activating factor antagonist, in human acute pancreatitis. Br J Surg 82:1414–1420
39. Alexandre JH, Guerrieri MT (1981) Role of total pancreatectomy in the treatment of necrotizing pancreatitis. World J Surg 5:369–377
40. Smadja C, Bismuth H (1986) Pancreatic débridement in acute necrotizing pancreatitis: an obsolete procedure. Br J Surg 73:408–410
41. Allardyce DB (1987) Incidence of necrotizing pancreatitis and factors related to mortality. Am J Surg 154:295–299
42. Wilson C, McArdle CS, Carter DC, Imrie CW (1988) Surgical treatment of acute necrotizing pancreatitis. Br J Surg 75:119–123
43. Teerenhovi O, Nordback I, Eskola J (1989) High volume lesser sac lavage in acute necrotizing pancreatitis. Br J Surg 76:370–373
44. Howard JM (1989) Delayed débridement and external drainage of massive pancreatic or peripancreatic necrosis. Surg Gynecol Obstet 168:25–29
45. Villazon A, Villazon O, Terrazas F, Rana R (1991) Retroperitoneal drainage in the management of the septic phase of severe acute pancreatitis. World J Surg 15:103–108
46. Wertheimer MD, Norris CS (1986) Surgical management of necrotizing pancreatitis. Arch Surg 121:484–487
47. Garcia-Sabrido JL, Tallado J, Christou NV, Polo JR, Valdecanatos E (1988) Treatment of severe intra-abdominal sepsis and/or necrotic foci by open-abdomen approach. Arch Surg 123:152–156
48. Waclawiczek HW, Chmelizek F, Heinerman M (1992) Das Laparostoma (open packing) im Behandlungskonzept infizierter Pankreasnekrosen. Wien Klin Wochenschr 104:443–447
49. Orlando R III, Welch JP, Akbari CM, Bloom GP, Macaulay WP (1993) Techniques and complications in open drainage for infected pancreatic necrosis. Surg Gynecol Obstet 177:65–71
50. Bradley EL III (1993) A fifteen-year experience with open drainage for infected pancreatic necrosis. Surg Gynecol Obstet 177:215–222
51. Függer R, Götzinger P, Sautner T (1995) Necrosectomy and laparostomy – a combined therapeutic concept in acute necrotizing pancreatitis. Eur J Surg 161:103–107
52. Gebhardt C, Gall FP (1981) Importance of peritoneal irrigation after surgical treatment of hemorrhagic, necrotizing pancreatitis. World J Surg 5:379–385
53. Larvin M, Chalmers AG, Robinson PJ, MacMahon MJ (1989) Débridement and closed cavity irrigation for the treatment of pancreatic necrosis. Br J Surg 76:465–471
54. Pederzoli P, Bassi C, Vesentini S, et al (1990) Retroperitoneal and peritoneal drainage and lavage in the treatment of severe necrotizing pancreatitis. Surg Gynecol Obstet 170:197–203
55. Beger HG, Krautzberger W, Bittner R, Block S, Büchler M (1985) Results of surgical treatment of necrotizing pancreatitis. World J Surg 9:972–979

Part II
Chronic Pancreatis

Chronic Pancreatitis: Do Different Etiologies (Alcohol, Obstruction) Invoke Different Mechanisms?

J. Mössner

Introduction

The pathogenesis of chronic pancreatitis is still poorly understood (Adler and Schmid 1997). Alcohol is the leading risk factor and most common etiology. In the industrialized countries at least 80% of all cases of chronic pancreatitis are due to alcohol abuse. At present, there are four competing hypotheses concerning the pathogenesis of this disease: (a) ethanol-induced fatty degeneration of acini, (b) damage to acini by oxygen-derived free radicals, (c) destruction of acini due to ductal hypertension resulting from obstruction by protein precipitates, (c) fibrosis as a consequence of repeated episodes of acute necrotizing pancreatitis.

According to the second Marseille classification of pancreatitis (Sarles 1986), besides alcohol-induced obstruction by pancreatic protein precipitates obstruction per se may cause chronic pancreatitis. This rather rare form of so-called obstructive chronic pancreatitis may be caused by scars after acute pancreatitis, tumor invasion, trauma, or anatomical variations such as pancreas divisum (Bradley 1991). Besides the leading etiology, i.e. alcohol, and the rare cause of non-alcohol-related obstruction, there are other rare causes of the disease: tropical chronic pancreatitis, hereditary chronic pancreatitis, autoimmune pancreatitis, hypercalcemia, and idiopathic forms. Irrespective of the various etiologies and possible different pathogenetic steps at the beginning of the disease, advanced chronic pancreatitis is characterized by irreversible degeneration of acinar cells, which are displaced by fibrous tissue.

Our limited knowledge about the pathogenesis of chronic pancreatitis is certainly due to the lack of appropriate animal models. Pancreatic fibrosis was induced in rats by dibutyltin dichloride (Sparmann et al. 1997). Thus, one may speculate that this animal model may help us to increase our understanding about the pathomechanism of this disease.

Alcohol-induced Chronic Pancreatitis

The pathogenesis of alcohol-induced chronic pancreatitis is poorly understood. According to the concept of Bordalo et al., ethanol induces *fatty degeneration* of acinar cells, similar to its effect on the liver (Bordalo et al.

1977). Braganza presents the concept of the deleterious effect of *oxygen-derived free radicals.* Alcohol, nicotine, and industrial pollutants overwhelm the detoxification capacity of the cytochrome-P-450 system of the liver. Oxidative stress causes lipid peroxidation of membranes (Braganza 1983, 1996; van Gossum et al. 1996; Norton et al. 1998). Over many years, Sarles has investigated the chemical composition of protein precipitates in pancreatic ducts. He raises the hypothesis that chronic pancreatitis is a *lithiasis.* These protein plaques obstruct the pancreatic ducts; this leads to ductal hypertension, which in turn causes the destruction of acini (Sarles 1986; Guy et al. 1983; Multigner et al 1985; Sarles et al. 1965, 1989). According to Sarles, chronic damage to acinar cells by alcohol leads to a reduction of both synthesis and secretion of low-molecular-weight proteins, called lithostathines. According to their in vitro data, lithostathines are necessary to prevent precipitation of proteins and calcium carbonate from the supersaturated pancreatic secretions (Bernard et al. 1992, 1995; Giorgi et al. 1985; Geider et al. 1996; Provansal-Cheylan et al. 1989; Yamadera et al. 1998). This hypothesis is not uniformly accepted, since others were unable to confirm a decrease of lithostathine concentration in the pancreatic juice of patients with chronic pancreatitis (Schmiegel et al. 1990) or an inhibitory function of lithostathine on calcium carbonate precipitation (Bimmler et al. 1997). According to Klöppel and Maillet, chronic pancreatitis is a sequela of repeated episodes of acute pancreatitis. Focal fat necrosis and necrosis of the pancreatic parenchyma leads to infiltration by lymphocytes, macrophages, and fibroblasts. *Fibrosis* is assumed to be the *sequence of necrosis.* (Ammann et al. 1996; Klöppel and Maillet 1991; Longnecker 1996).

Risk Factor Alcohol

According to the studies by the Marseille group, the logarithm of the relative risk of chronic pancreatitis increases linearly as a function of the quantity of alcohol and protein consumed (Durbec and Sarles 1978). There seems to be no threshold for toxicity of alcohol. Furthermore, the type of alcoholic beverage, i.e., beer or wine, is irrelevant. Patients with chronic pancreatitis and alcohol-induced liver cirrhosis do not differ with regard to their daily dose of alcohol. However, the duration of alcohol consumption is shorter in chronic pancreatitis. In most studies the time between the onset of alcohol abuse and first symptoms is 18±11 years (Almela et al. 1997). The prevalence of chronic pancreatitis is clearly correlated to the alcohol consumption of a given population (Johnson and Hosking 1991).

Further Risk Factors: Nutrition, Nicotine, Genetics

A diet rich in protein and fat or rich in protein but very low in fat seems to be a risk factor (Durbec and Sarles 1978; Levy et al. 1995; Noel-Jorand and Bras 1994). However, it has also been reported that diet has no influence on the risk of developing chronic pancreatitis (Mezey et al. 1988).

Nicotine abuse could be a further risk factor (Bourliere et al. 1991; Talamini et al. 1996). However, since most alcoholics smoke, it is difficult to separate the two factors. One will not find a group of alcoholics who do not smoke and a group of smokers who do not drink but both having chronic pancreatitis.

Certain, so far unknown, genes may contribute to an elevated risk for the development of alcohol-induced chronic pancreatitis. The Marseille group has reported that dolichomorphic types have a greater risk for the disease as compared with brachymorphic types (Pietri et al. 1991).

Malnutrition (Tropical Chronic Pancreatitis)

The pathogenesis of tropical chronic pancreatitis is also poorly understood. Diet, pancreatic function, and chronic pancreatitis were compared in southern India and France (Balakrishnan et al. 1988). Kwashiorkor and consumption of cassava do not seem to be responsible for tropical chronic pancreatitis. The authors speculate that a diet poor in fat may play an etiological role. However, in tropical regions chronic pancreatitis may also be caused by a diet rich in fat, protein, and alcohol (Uscanga et al. 1985; Laugier et al. 1993).

Chronic Pancreatitis and Cystic Fibrosis

Pancreatic lesions of cystic fibrosis closely resemble those of chronic pancreatitis. In an exciting recent report mutations of the cystic fibrosis transmembrane conductance regulator (CFTR) have also been found on one chromosome in about 13% and the 5T allele in intron 8 in about 10% of patients with either idiopathic or alcohol-induced chronic pancreatitis who nevertheless had no signs of cystic fibrosis, such as lung disease (Sharer et al. 1998). Thus, an altered electrolyte secretion of pancreatic ducts with subsequent changes in the viscosity of pancreatic secretions may play a role in the pathogenesis of chronic pancreatitis, and not only in cystic fibrosis.

Pathogenesis of Chronic Pancreatitis: an Immunological Disease?

Inflammatory cells, mainly CD4- and CD8-positive lymphocytes, are usually found in patients with chronic pancreatitis (Bedossa et al. 1989). Cytotoxic T cells are activated, as demonstrated by elevated perforin mRNA expression (Hunger et al. 1997). The exocrine pancreas does not express major histocompatibility complex class I or II. However, in chronic pancreatitis elevated expression of MHC class II has been reported (Jalleh et al. 1993). The type of inflammatory cells found in chronic pancreatitis is rather common, with a predominance of CD8-positive cells, and not typical for an autoimmunological reaction (Emmrich et al. 1998). Immune cell infiltration of nerves seems to play a major role in the pathogenesis of pain (Di Sebastiano et al. 1997).

Classical autoimmune pancreatitis is an extremely rare disease (Ito et al. 1997). In some patients with idiopathic chronic pancreatitis and Sjögren's syndrome, carbonic anhydrase II has been described as a possible antigen of autoantibodies (Kino-Ohsaki et al. 1996).

Hereditary Chronic Pancreatitis

In the rare cases of hereditary chronic pancreatitis, mutations of the gene on chromosome 7q35 coding for cationic trypsinogen have been described. Most patients with this disease, and only about 10% of their relatives who have no symptoms indicative of chronic pancreatitis, have either an arginine-histidine substitution (R117H) on exon 3 (Whitcomb et al. 1996 a, b) or an asparagine-isoleucine substitution (N21I) on exon 2 (Gorry et al. 1997; Teich et al. 1998). It is hypothesized that these point mutations may either cause autoactivation of trypsinogen or render trypsinogen more stable against degradation. Thus, activation of trypsinogen within the pancreas may be a cause of chronic pancreatitis. However, we were unable to identify any acquired mutations of trypsinogen in alcohol-induced chronic pancreatitis (Teich et al. 1999). Activation of trypsinogen may also be the leading pathomechanism in rare cases of pancreatitis due to alpha-1-antitrypsin deficiency (Blackstone 1996).

Patients with hereditary pancreatitis have a high risk of developing pancreatic cancer (Lowenfels et al. 1997). It is not known whether this risk is due to an inheritance pattern or to decades of an inflammatory process. The risk of developing pancreatic carcinoma in alcohol-induced chronic pancreatitis has been discussed controversially (Lowenfels et al. 1993). Confounding factors such as smoking and alcohol per se may play a role (Karlson et al. 1997).

Chronic Obstructive Pancreatitis

Chronic obstructive pancreatitis may be caused by scars after acute pancreatitis or trauma, tumor invasion, odditis, or anatomical variations such as pancreas divisum (Bradley 1991; Lowes et al. 1988; Odaira et al. 1987; Tarnasky et al. 1997). According to the definition, chronic obstructive pancreatitis should be reversible after removal of obstruction. In animal models, such as the opossum, obstruction of the main pancreatic duct causes acute pancreatitis but not chronic pancreatitis. In man the pathological features of chronic obstructive pancreatitis can be differentiated from alcohol-induced chronic pancreatitis (Sahel et al. 1986). However, formation of ductal stones has also been reported in chronic obstructive pancreatitis (Cavallini et al. 1996). Thus, stone formation is not only a characteristic finding in alcohol-induced pancreatitis. However, others report that chronic obstructive pancreatitis is not associated with protein plugs (Suda et al. 1990).

Fibroblast Activation

Fibroblasts and extracellular matrix synthesis are stimulated by the action of various growth factors on their respective receptors, such as epidermal growth factor (EGF), transforming growth factor β (TGFβ), fibroblast growth factor, and platelet-derived growth factor (Gress et al. 1994; van Laethem et al. 1996; Ebert et al. 1998).

It has recently been reported that urokinase (u-) plasminogen activator may play a role in the pathogenesis of chronic pancreatitis. Using Northern blot hybridization, in situ hybridization, and immunohistochemistry, the authors found elevated expression of u-plasminogen activator and transforming growth factor β in pancreatic resections from patients with chronic pancreatitis in contrast to normal pancreas, i.e., donor organs (Friess et al. 1997). They concluded that pancreatic acini are damaged by u-plasminogen activator due to its lytic capacity. Furthermore, the activation of TGFβ may lead to fibrosis.

Idiopathic Chronic Pancreatitis

Some cases of idiopathic chronic pancreatitis may be due to a low individual threshold for the damaging effect of alcohol. In others, mutations of the trypsinogen gene may have been overlooked. In children and young adults the rare disease of idiopathic fibrosing chronic pancreatitis with obstructive jaundice has been reported (Barkin et al. 1994). There is no doubt about the existence of idiopathic forms. Protein precipitates and calcifications are found as frequently in idiopathic chronic pancreatitis as in the alcohol induced forms (De Angelis et al. 1992).

Clinical Outcome in Relation to the Etiology of Chronic Pancreatitis

In a retrospective analysis the clinical courses of early- and late-onset idiopathic and alcoholic chronic pancreatitis were compared. The gender distribution was equal in both types of idiopathic chronic pancreatitis. As expected, 72% of patients with alcoholic chronic pancreatitis were men. Calcifications and exocrine and endocrine insufficiency developed more slowly in early-onset idiopathic than in late-onset idiopathic and alcoholic chronic pancreatitis. However, pain was more severe and more frequent in early onset idiopathic chronic pancreatitis. Thus, the clinical course of these three diseases seems to be different (Layer et al. 1994; Layer and DiMagno 1996).

Summary and Conclusion

The early steps in the pathogenesis of chronic pancreatitis, irrespective of its etiology, are still incompletely understood. All etiologies of chronic pancreatitis lead sooner or later to a similar pathohistological picture: protein precipitations which may calcify, fibrosis and atrophy of the acinar and endocrine tissue, and irregularities of the pancreatic ducts with dilatations, rarifications, and multiple stenoses.

References

Adler G, Schmid RM (1997) Chronic pancreatitis: still puzzling? Gastroenterology 112:1762–1765

Almela P, Aparisi L, Grau F, Sempere J, Rodrigo JM (1997) Influence of alcohol consumption on the initial development of chronic pancreatitis. Rev Esp Enferm Dig 89:741–746

Ammann RW, Heitz PU, Klöppel G (1996) Course of alcoholic chronic pancreatitis: a prospective clinicomorphological long-term study. Gastroenterology 111:224–231

Balakrishnan V, Sauniere JF, Hariharan M, Sarles H (1988) Diet, pancreatic function, and chronic pancreatitis in south India and France. Pancreas 3:30–35

Barkin JS, Stollman N, Friedman J, Willis I, Robbins E (1994) Idiopathic fibrosing pancreatitis causing obstructive jaundice in young adults: two case reports and literature review. Am J Gastroenterol 89:2063–2065

Bedossa P, Bacci J, Lemaigre G, Martin E (1989) Lymphocyte subsets and HLA-DR expression in normal pancreas and chronic pancreatitis. Pancreas 5:415–420

Bernard JP, Adrich Z, Montalto G, De Caro A, De Reggi M, Sarles H, Dagorn JC (1992) Inhibition of nucleation and crystal growth of calcium carbonate by human lithostathine. Gastroenterology 103:1277–1284

Bernard JP, Barthet M, Gharib B, Michel R, Lilova A, Sahel J, Dagorn JC, De Reggi M (1995) Quantification of human lithostathine by high performance liquid chromatography. Gut 36:630–636

Bimmler D, Graf R, Scheele GA, Frick TW (1997) Pancreatic stone protein (lithostathine), a physiologically relevant pancreatic calcium carbonate crystal inhibitor? J Biol Chem 272:3073–3082

Blackstone MO (1996) Chronic pancreatitis with alpha 1-antitrypsin deficiency: from uncontrolled trypsin activation? Dig Dis Sci 41:549–551

Bordalo O, Goncalves D, Noronha M, Cristina ML, Salgadinho A, Dreiling DA (1977) Newer concept for the pathogenesis of chronic alcoholic pancreatitis. Am J Gastroenterol 68:278–285

Bourliere M, Barthet M, Berthezene P, Durbec JP, Sarles H (1991) Is tobacco a risk factor for chronic pancreatitis and alcoholic cirrhosis? Gut 32:1392–1395

Bradley EL 3rd (1991) Chronic obstructive pancreatitis as a delayed complication of pancreatic trauma. HPB Surg 5:49–59

Braganza JM (1983) Pancreatic disease: a casualty of hepatic "detoxification"? Lancet 2:1000–1003

Braganza JM (1996) The pathogenesis of chronic pancreatitis. QJM 89:243–250

Cavallini G, Bovo P, Vaona B, DiFrancesco V, Frulloni L, Rigo L, Brunori MP, Andreaus MC, Tebaldi M, Sgarbi D, Angelini G, Talamini G, Procacci C, Pederzoli P, Filippini M (1996) Chronic obstructive pancreatitis in humans is a lithiasic disease. Pancreas 13:66–70

De Angelis C, Valente G, Spaccapietra M, Angonese C, Del Favero G, Naccarato R, Andriulli A (1992) Histological study of alcoholic, nonalcoholic, and obstructive chronic pancreatitis. Pancreas 7:193–196

Di Sebastiano P, Fink T, Weihe E, Friess H, Innocenti P, Beger HG, Büchler MW (1997) Immune cell infiltration and growth-associated protein 43 expression correlate with pain in chronic pancreatitis. Gastroenterology 112:1648–1655

Durbec JP, Sarles H (1978) Multicenter survey of the etiology of pancreatic diseases. Relationship between the relative risk of developing chronic pancreatitis and alcohol, protein and lipid consumption. Digestion 18:337–350

Ebert M, Kasper HU, Hernberg S, Friess H, Büchler MW, Roessner A, Korc M, Malfertheiner P (1998) Overexpression of platelet-derived growth factor (PDGF). B chain and type beta PDGF receptor in human chronic pancreatitis. Dig Dis Sci 43:567–574

Emmrich J, Weber I, Nausch M, Sparmann G, Koch K, Seyfarth M, Lohr M, Liebe S (1998) Immunohistochemical characterization of the pancreatic cellular infiltrate in normal pancreas, chronic pancreatitis and pancreatic carcinoma. Digestion 59:192–198

Friess H, Cantero D, Graber H, Tang WH, Guo X, Kashiwagi M, Zimmermann A, Gold L, Korc M, Büchler MW (1997) Enhanced urokinase plasminogen activation in chronic pancreatitis suggests a role in its pathogenesis. Gastroenterology 113:904–913

Geider S, Baronnet A, Cerini C, Nitsche S, Astier JP, Michel R, Boistelle R, Berland Y, Dagorn JC, Verdier JM (1996) Pancreatic lithostathine as a calcite habit modifier. J Biol Chem 271:26302–26306

Giorgi D, Bernard JP, De Caro A, Multigner L, Lapointe R, Sarles H, Dagorn JC (1985) Pancreatic stone protein. I. Evidence that it is encoded by a pancreatic messenger ribonucleic acid. Gastroenterology 89:381–386

Gorry MC, Gabbaizedeh D, Furey W, Gates LK Jr, Preston RA, Aston CE, Zhang Y, Ulrich C, Ehrlich GD, Whitcomb DC (1997) Mutations in the cationic trypsinogen gene are associated with recurrent acute and chronic pancreatitis. Gastroenterology 113:1063–1068

Gress T, Müller-Pillasch F, Elsässer HP, Bachem M, Ferrara C, Weidenbach H, Lerch M, Adler G (1994) Enhancement of transforming growth factor $\beta 1$ expression in the rat pancreas during regeneration from cerulein-induced pancreatitis. Eur J Clin Invest 24:679–685

Guy O, Robles-Diaz G, Adrich Z, Sahel J, Sarles H (1983) Protein content of precipitates present in pancreatic juice of alcoholic subjects and patients with chronic calcifying pancreatitis. Gastroenterology 84:102–107

Hunger RE, Mueller C, Z'graggen K, Friess H, Büchler MW (1997) Cytotoxic cells are activated in cellular infiltrates of alcoholic chronic pancreatitis. Gastroenterology 112:1656–1663

Ito T, Nakano I, Koyanagi S, Miyahara T, Migita Y, Ogoshi K, Sakai H, Matsunaga S, Yasuda O, Sumii T, Nawata H (1997) Autoimmune pancreatitis as a new clinical entity. Three cases of autoimmune pancreatitis with effective steroid therapy. Dig Dis Sci 42:1458–1468

Jalleh RP, Gilbertson JA, Williamson RCN, Slater SD, Foster CD (1993) Expression of major histocompatibility antigens in human chronic pancreatitis. Gut 34:1452–1457

Johnson CD, Hosking S (1991) National statistics for diet, alcohol consumption, and chronic pancreatitis in England and Wales, 1960–1988. Gut 32:1401–1405

Karlson BM, Ekbom A, Josefsson S, McLaughlin JK, Fraumeni JF jr, Nyren O (1997) The risk of pancreatic cancer following pancreatitis: an association due to confounding? Gastroenterology 113:587–592

Kino-Ohsaki J, Nishimori I, Morita M, Okazaki K, Yamamoto Y, Onishi S, Hollingsworth MA (1996) Serum autoantibodies to carbonic anhydrase I and II in patients with idiopathic chronic pancreatitis and Sjögren's syndrome. Gastroenterology 110:1579–1586

Klöppel G, Maillet B (1991) Chronic pancreatitis: evolution of the disease. Hepatogastroenterology 38:408–412

Laugier R, Bernard JP, Laroche R, Kadende P, N'Dabaneze E, Sauniere JF, Dupuy P (1993) Exocrine pancreatic secretion in normal controls and chronic calcifying pancreatitis patients from Burundi: possible dietary influences. Digestion 54:54–60

Layer P, Yamamoto H, Kalthoff L, Clain JE, Bakken LJ, DiMagno EP (1994) The different courses of early- and late-onset idiopathic and alcoholic chronic pancreatitis. Gastroenterology 107:1481–1487

Layer PH, DiMagno EP (1996) Natural histories of alcoholic and idiopathic chronic pancreatitis. Pancreas 12:318–320

Levy P, Mathurin P, Roqueplo A, Rueff B, Bernades P (1995) A multidimensional case-control study of dietary, alcohol, and tobacco habits in alcoholic men with chronic pancreatitis. Pancreas 10:231–238

Longnecker DS (1996) Role of the necrosis-fibrosis sequence in the pathogenesis of alcoholic chronic pancreatitis. Gastroenterology 111:258–259

Lowenfels AB, Maisonneuve P, Cavallini G, Ammann RW, Lankisch PG, Andersen JR, DiMagno EP, Andren-Sandberg A, Domellof L (1993) Pancreatitis and the risk of pancreatic cancer. International Pancreatitis Study Group. N Engl J Med 328:1433–1437

Lowenfels AB, Maisonneuve P, DiMagno EP, Elitsur Y, Gates LK Jr, Perrault J, Whitcomb DC (1997) Hereditary pancreatitis and the risk of pancreatic cancer. International Hereditary Pancreatitis Study Group. J Natl Cancer Inst 89:442–446

Lowes JR, Rode J, Lees WR, Russell RC, Cotton PB (1988) Obstructive pancreatitis: unusual causes of chronic pancreatitis. Br J Surg 75:1129–1133

Mezey E, Kolman CJ, Diehl AM, Mitchell MC, Herlong HF (1988) Alcohol and dietary intake in the development of chronic pancreatitis and liver disease in alcoholism. Am J Clin Nutr 48:148–151

Multigner L, Sarles H, Lombardo D, De Caro A (1985) Pancreatic stone protein. II. Implication in stone formation during the course of chronic calcifying pancreatitis. Gastroenterology 89:387–391

Noel-Jorand MC, Bras J (1994) A comparison of nutritional profiles of patients with alcohol-related pancreatitis and cirrhosis. Alcohol 29:65–74

Norton ID, Apte MV, Haber PS, McCaughan GW, Pirola RC, Wilson JS (1998) Cytochrome P4502E1 is present in rat pancreas and is induced by chronic ethanol administration. Gut 42:426–430

Odaira C, Choux R, Payan MJ, Bockman DE, Sarles H (1987) Chronic obstructive pancreatitis, nesidioblastosis, and small endocrine pancreatic tumor. Dig Dis Sci 32:770–774

Pietri H, Rizzo L, Teleechea J, Bernard JP, Berthezene P, Sarles H (1991) Liver cirrhosis and chronic calcifying pancreatitis are associated with different morphotypes. Digestion 48:173–178

Provansal-Cheylan M, Mariani A, Bernard JP, Sarles H, Dupuy P (1989) Pancreatic stone protein: quantification in pancreatic juice by enzyme-linked immunosorbent assay and comparison with other methods. Pancreas 4:680–689

Sahel J, Cros RC, Durbec JP, Sarles H, Bank S, Marks IN, Bettarello A, Duarte I, Guarita D, Machado M, et al (1986) Multicenter pathological study of chronic pancreatitis. Morphological regional variations and differences between chronic calcifying pancreatitis and obstructive pancreatitis. Pancreas 1:471–477

Sarles H (1986) Etiopathogenesis and definition of chronic pancreatitis. Dig Dis Sci 31 [Suppl 9]:91 S–107 S

Sarles H, Sarles JC, Camatte R, Muratore R, Gaini M, Guien C, Pastor J, Le Roy F (1965) Observations on 205 confirmed cases of acute pancreatitis, recurring pancreatitis, and chronic pancreatitis. Gut 6:545–559

Sarles H, Bernard JP, Johnson C (1989) Pathogenesis and epidemiology of chronic pancreatitis. Annu Rev Med 40:453–468

Schmiegel W, Burchert M, Kalthoff H, Roeder C, Butzow G, Grimm H, Kremer B, Soehendra N, Schreiber HW, Thiele HG, et al (1990) Immunochemical characterization and quantitative distribution of pancreatic stone protein in sera and pancreatic secretions in pancreatic disorders. Gastroenterology 99:1421–1430

Sharer N, Schwarz M, Malone G, Howarth A, Painter J, Super M, Braganza J (1998) Mutations of the cystic fibrosis gene in patients with chronic pancreatitis. N Engl J Med 339:645–652

Sparmann G, Merkord J, Jaschke A, Nizze H, Jonas L, Lohr M, Liebe S, Emmrich J (1997) Pancreatic fibrosis in experimental pancreatitis induced by dibutyltin dichloride. Gastroenterology 112:1664–1672

Suda K, Mogaki M, Oyama T, Matsumoto Y (1990) Histopathologic and immunohistochemical studies on alcoholic pancreatitis and chronic obstructive pancreatitis: special emphasis on ductal obstruction and genesis of pancreatitis. Am J Gastroenterol 85:271–276

Talamini G, Bassi C, Falconi M, Frulloni L, Di Francesco V, Vaona B, Bovo P, Rigo L, Castagnini A, Angelini G, Vantini I, Pederzoli P, Cavallini G (1996) Cigarette smoking: an independent risk factor in alcoholic pancreatitis. Pancreas 12:131–137

Tarnasky PR, Hoffman B, Aabakken L, Knapple WL, Coyle W, Pineau B, Cunningham JT, Cotton PB, Hawes RH (1997) Sphincter of Oddi dysfunction is associated with chronic pancreatitis. Am J Gastroenterol 92:1125–1129

Teich N, Mössner J, Keim V (1998) Mutations of the cationic trypsinogen in hereditary pancreatitis. Hum Mutat 12:39–43

Teich N, Mössner J, Keim V (1999) Screening of mutations of the cationic trypsinogen: are they of relevance in chronic alcoholic pancreatitis? Gut (in press)

Uscanga L, Robles-Diaz G, Sarles H (1985) Nutritional data and etiology of chronic pancreatitis in Mexico. Dig Dis Sci 30:110–113

Van Gossum A, Closset P, Noel E, Cremer M, Neve J (1996) Deficiency in antioxidant factors in patients with alcohol-related chronic pancreatitis. Dig Dis Sci 41:1225–1231

Van Laethem JL, Robberecht P, Resibois A, Deviere J (1996) Transforming growth factor beta promotes development of fibrosis after repeated courses of acute pancreatitis in mice. Gastroenterology 110:576–582

Whitcomb DC, Gorry MC, Preston RA, Furey W, Sossenheimer MJ, Ulrich CD, Martin SP, Gates LK Jr, Amann ST, Toskes PP, Liddle R, McGrath K, Uomo G, Post JC, Ehrlich GD (1996) Hereditary pancreatitis is caused by a mutation in the cationic trypsinogen gene. Nat Genet 14:141–145

Whitcomb DC, Preston RA, Aston CE, Sossenheimer MJ, Barua PS, Zhang Y, Wong-Chong A, White GJ, Wood PG, Gates LK Jr, Ulrich C, Martin SP, Post JC, Ehrlich GD (1996) A gene for hereditary pancreatitis maps to chromosome 7q35. Gastroenterology 110:1975–1980

Yamadera K, Wada K, Goto M, Yokoyama K, Morita Y, Kitano Y, Makino I (1998) Quantification of human lithostathine S2–5 forms using the antibody to the N-terminal peptide region. Pancreas 16:475–480

CHAPTER 10

Exocrine Pancreatic Secretion, Pain, and Malabsorption

G.H. ELTA

Introduction

Chronic pancreatitis is defined as an inflammatory disease of the pancreas characterized by persistent and often progressive lesions. Its prevalence ranges from 0.04% to 5.0% in autopsy series. Most epidemiologic data are from retrospective studies, with large differences in incidence noted between different areas. This variance in incidence has been attributed to societal alcohol consumption, regional differences in diagnostic criteria, and unknown environmental or hereditary factors. The only prospective study of chronic pancreatitis is from Copenhagen in 1978–1979 [1]. It showed an incidence of 8.2 cases per 100,000 individuals per year and a prevalence of 26.4 cases per 100,000 inhabitants. Valid figures for incidence and prevalence of chronic pancreatitis await prospective epidemiologic studies based on uniformly accepted diagnostic criteria.

Exocrine Pancreatic Secretion

The exocrine pancreas secretes digestive enzymes and bicarbonate, which affect the digestion and absorption of nutrients. Approximately 80% of the pancreas consists of acini, which are clustered into lobules separated by connective tissue. Each acinus is a sphere of 20–50 cells with their apices pointed toward a central lumen. Each acinus is drained by a ductule which connects to a series of ducts of increasing size. The acinar cells secrete digestive enzymes, and the ductular cells are responsible mainly for bicarbonate-rich electrolyte secretion (Fig. 1).

The major cations in pancreatic juice are Na^+ and K^+; these are secreted in concentrations similar to plasma and reach the duct by paracellular routes. They move down an electronegative luminal gradient. The major anions in pancreatic juice are HCO_3 and Cl^-, the concentrations of which depend on flow rates. Bicarbonate concentration rises asymptotically with increased secretory rates, with a reciprocal fall in Cl^- secretion. There is electrophysiologic evidence for an HCO_3-Cl exchange on the apical membrane; this is coupled with chloride channels that allow recirculation of the Cl^- that

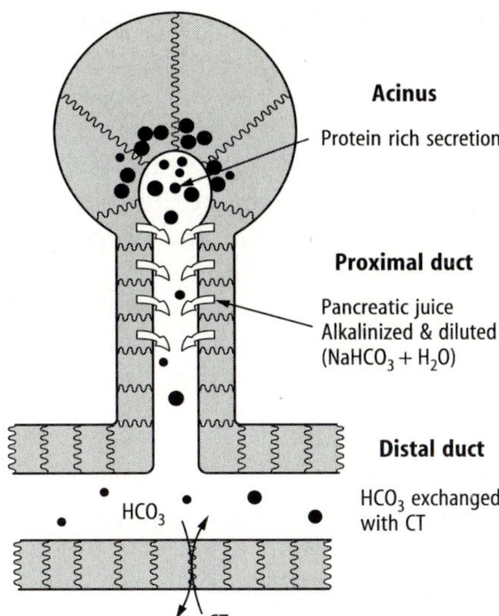

Fig. 1. Pancreatic enzymes are secreted from the acinar cells while the alkaline pancreatic juice originates from the intralobular and small interlobular ducts. Some of the secreted HCO_3^- is exchanged with Cl^- in the distal ducts

has entered the cell [2]. The secreted HCO_3^- is derived from CO_2 in the circulation, although the driving force for the secretion of HCO_3^- is not known. It has been proposed that secretin stimulates exocytosis of tubulovesicles to the basolateral membrane; these contain H^+-ATPase which initiates primary electrogenic H^+ secretion into the interstitial fluid, with secondary active HCO_3^- extrusion into the pancreatic juice [3].

Human pancreatic juice contains 0.7–10% protein, and most of these proteins are enzymes and proenzymes. The four major enzyme groups are amylolytic, lipolytic, proteolytic, and nucleolytic. The proteolytic enzymes, which include trypsinogen, chymotrypsin, procarboxypeptidase, and proaminopeptidase, account for the largest quantity of enzymes and are secreted in the proenzyme form. Enterokinase, an enzyme secreted by the duodenal mucosa, converts trypsinogen to trypsin, which then activates the other proteolytic enzymes. In pancreatic juice there is also a small quantity of a trypsin inhibitor which, in addition to secreting proenzymes, protects the pancreas against autodigestion. The other enzymes, lipase, amylase, and ribonuclease, are secreted by the acini in their active forms. A small peptide, colipase, which facilitates lipase action by binding to bile salt-lipid surfaces, thereby increasing the interaction of lipase with triglyceride, is also secreted.

Pancreatic enzymes are synthesized in the acinar cells and packaged into zymogen granules [4]. Protein synthesis occurs in the ribosomes with an amino acid terminal peptide extension called the signal peptide, which recognizes the endoplastic reticulum (ER) and allows attachment of the polysome to the membrane at the docking protein [5]. Once translation is complete the protein is released into the cisterna, where conformational changes occur. Then vesicles of the rough ER pinch off and are transported to the Golgi complex, where they undergo further modification and concentration. From the Golgi complex, secretory granules move by a mechanism involving microtubules to the apical portions of the acinar cell and remain there until a neurohumoral stimulus to secretion occurs. The entire process, from synthesis to being ready for secretion, takes about 50 min. It has been estimated that 10 million enzyme molecules are synthesized per acinar cell per minute. Pancreatic enzymes from a single cell appear to be secreted in a fixed ratio that is independent of the stimulus. However, nonparallel secretion from the pancreas can occur and is probably explained by different enzymatic contents within populations of acinar cells [6]. Differences in morphology of the acinar cells and wide variation in the enzyme ratios in granules from the same animal support this theory. Long-term adaptation of the proportion of secreted enzymes to diet has been demonstrated in animals.

Control of Pancreatic Secretion

Hormonal Mechanisms

The classic regulatory mechanism for pancreatic secretion has been the hormones secretin and cholecystokinin (CCK) and the vagovagal reflexes that activate cholinergic neurons in the pancreas. However, the picture has become increasingly complex, with other regulatory peptides and neurotransmitters.

The most potent stimulant of pancreatic fluid and bicarbonate secretion is secretin. The major control of its release is duodenal pH, the threshold value for stimulation of pancreatic bicarbonate release being pH 4.5 [7]. This appears to be controlled by a secretin-releasing factor in the upper intestinal lumen [8]. Nonacid factors which may affect secretin release include digestive products of fat and bile in the upper intestine, although these are not very important, since achlorhydric individuals do not have a postprandial increase in secretin release. The amount of postprandial secretin released is very small but sufficient to account for some of the pancreatic bicarbonate secretory release. When given simultaneously with vagal and CCK stimulation the response is much greater, suggesting that synergistic effects occur.

Cholecystokinin is the other major gut hormone that controls pancreatic secretion. It is released by hydrolytic products of digestion such as amino acids and fatty acids. The mechanism by which nutrients release CCK is not clear; there may be several. Proteins may bind or inhibit endopeptidases which otherwise inactivate CCK-releasing peptide [9]. This makes more free CCK-releasing peptide available for action. Alternatively, some of the release of CCK-releasing peptide may be mediated by cholinergic input. In addition, tryptophan and HCl may stimulate CCK cells directly. CCK release occurs within 10–30 min of ingestion of a protein- or fat-rich meal. It appears in several molecular forms; their relative contribution to the activity of CCK in plasma remains to be determined. The mechanism of CCK-induced pancreatic secretion remains somewhat controversial. It appears that it can act through both atropine-sensitive and -insensitive pathways. Under physiologic conditions in human beings, it appears that CCK affects mainly the stimulation of vagal afferents originating in the duodenal mucosa [10]. This vagovagal pathway is via a muscarinic receptor on the pancreatic acini.

Other hormones affecting pancreatic secretion include gastrin, which is not surprising, given its structural similarity to CCK. In the dog, gastrin is about one third as potent a stimulus to the pancreas as CCK. Bombesin (i.e., gastrin-releasing peptide in mammals) acts directly on pancreatic acinar cells to stimulate secretion. It remains unclear how important this is physiologically. Neurotensin, which is released by intestinal fatty acids, also stimulates pancreatic secretion. The mechanism appears to be neurally mediated, although the physiologic role of this hormone in meal-stimulated pancreatic secretion is also questionable.

Neural Mechanisms

Parasympathetic innervation of the pancreas is through the vagus nerves, the celiac ganglion, the splanchnic nerves, and perhaps through the intramural plexus of the duodenum. The role of the parasympathetics varies between species and with different experimental conditions. In man, it seems that the cholinergic effects modulate the action of gut peptides on pancreatic secretion, although they do not affect the release of CCK or secretin. Vagotomy reduces pancreatic secretory response to intestinal stimulants and food [11]. There are both volume and osmoreceptors in the human duodenum which stimulate pancreatic secretion mediated by cholinergic neurons. Intrapancreatic postganglionic cholinergic neurons are activated by central input during the cephalic phase and by vagovagal reflexes initiated by gastric- and intestinal-phase stimulation. They stimulate both enzyme secretion by acinar cells and bicarbonate secretion from duct cells. It has been estimated that the enteropancreatic reflex is responsible for approximately 50% of postprandial secretion.

Sympathetic innervation of the pancreas occurs through the splanchnic nerves and is primarily inhibitory in nature. Most of the adrenergic fibers in the pancreas are distributed to the blood vessels. The pancreatic secretion inhibitory effect is dependent on α-adrenergic stimulation of intense vasoconstriction. This vasoconstriction mediates inhibition of pancreatic fluid and bicarbonate secretion.

Several peptides in nerve cell bodies or fibers have been identified in the pancreas. VIP fibers surround the intrapancreatic ganglia and innervate duct cells and have variable effects in different species [12]. In man, VIP is a weak agonist to pancreatic secretion. The neuropeptide galanin has also been found in intrapancreatic neurons and appears to have weak modulatory effects on both endocrine and exocrine pancreas. Several other peptidergic neurotransmitters have been identified in the pancreas, although their physiologic significance remains unknown.

Inhibition of Pancreatic Secretion

Pancreatic secretion depends on a balance between inhibitory and stimulatory influences. Both hyperglycemia and intravenous infusion of amino acids inhibit pancreatic enzyme secretion. This inhibition is presumably mediated by hormones and the autonomic nervous system.

Glucagon inhibits pancreatic secretion that is stimulated by secretin and CCK or by ingestion of a test meal. Release of pancreatic glucagon is mediated by serum glucose and amino acids and has both an endocrine and a paracrine mode of action. Another pancreatic hormone, somatostatin, also inhibits pancreatic secretion and is stimulated by elevated glucose and amino acids in serum [13]. These observations may provide a theoretical basis for hyperalimentation, providing "rest" for the pancreas during severe acute pancreatitis. Factors in the distal gut also inhibit pancreatic secretion [14]. Carbohydrate in the ileum both slows gastric emptying and increases pancreatic amylase secretion relative to that of other enzymes. The proposed mechanism of this effect is the neurally mediated release of peptide YY [15]. These late postprandial events may serve as physiologic signals to reduce pancreatic secretion after digestion and absorption are completed. An intestinal glucagon present in the lower intestine is much more potent than pancreatic glucagon in inhibiting secretion of bicarbonate and enzymes. Peptide YY is present in the distal small intestine and colon and is released by fat and, to a lesser degree, protein in the gut. It is also a potent inhibitor of pancreatic secretion [16]. Another hormone which is closely related to peptide YY is pancreatic polypeptide. This is localized in the islets of Langerhans and its secretion is controlled by cholinergic pathways. It is proposed that pancreatic polypeptide modulates pancreatic secretion stimulated by the enteropancreatic reflex.

Feedback Regulation of Pancreatic Secretion

Several observations have shown that activated pancreatic proteases inhibit the release of CCK and therefore exocrine pancreatic secretion. Diversion of pancreatic juice from the duodenum increases plasma CCK. This appears to be mediated by a peptide called CCK-releasing factor (CCK-RF), which is inactivated when trypsin is present. Dietary protein in the lumen competes for luminal trypsin, which allows CCK-RF to enhance CCK release [17]. Bile has also been shown to participate in the feedback regulation of CCK release. It may act via protection of pancreatic proteases from autodigestion in the lumen and by a mechanism that is independent of luminal protease activity. The increased pancreatic enzyme secretion caused by duodenal distention or the administration of hyperosmolar substances is not controlled by CCK or CCK-RF. This is entirely under cholinergic control.

The feedback regulation of pancreatic enzyme secretion has clinical implications. Large doses of pancreatic extract given with meals may reduce pancreatic stimulation by inactivating CCK-RF (Fig. 2). This could lead to de-

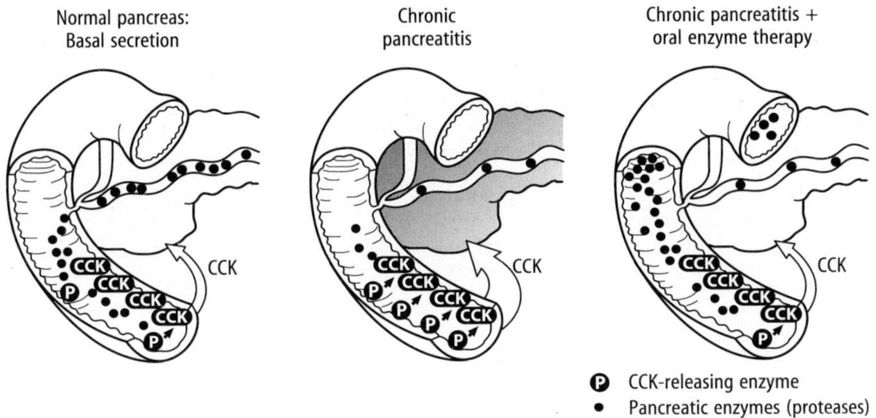

Fig. 2. The feedback inhibition of pancreatic secretion by luminal proteases forms the basis for the treatment of chronic pancreatitis pain with oral enzyme therapy. This inhibitory loop is mediated by luminal inactivation of CCK-releasing factor by the ingested pancreatic enzymes

creased pancreatic secretion and, hopefully, less pain and inflammation in patients with chronic pancreatitis [18].

Patterns of Secretion

Pancreatic secretion of enzymes and bicarbonate occurs at very low rates under basal conditions, at approximately 10% and 2% of maximal levels, respectively. There is a cyclic pattern to this fasting-state pancreatic secretion which recurs every 60–120 min. It coincides with the increased motor activity of the stomach and proximal intestine or the interdigestive migrating motor complexes (IMMC) [19]. There are also brief increases in biliary secretion associated with the IMMC. It is postulated that this cyclic secretion may be important in the digestion of residual food in the intestine in the interdigestive period. The control of cyclic pancreatic secretion is unclear, but it appears to be related to both motilin and cholinergic stimulation. It has been hypothesized that following ingestion of a meal, nutrients increase pancreatic enzyme secretion by converting cyclical interdigestive secretion to a noncyclical pattern. However, it has recently been shown in human subjects that duodenal nutrients do not abolish cycles but rather modulate them by increasing their nadir [20]. Pancreatic secretion can be separated into cephalic, gastric, and intestinal phases (Table 1).

The sight, smell, and taste of appetizing food stimulates pancreatic secretion. In human beings, the contribution of the cephalic phase to postprandial secretion appears to be 50% of the maximal responses induced by exogenous CCK and secretin stimulation [21]. Several experiments have shown that the cephalic phase is mediated by the vagus acting directly on the pancreas. The gastric phase of pancreatic secretion is caused by gastric distention. Balloon

Table 1. Three phases of postprandial pancreatic secretion

Phases	Pancreatic response (%)	Stimulants	Mediators
Cephalic	25	Sight, smell, taste, eating	Vagal innervation
Gastric	10	Distention	Vagal-cholinergic pathways
Intestinal	50–75	Amino acids	Cholecystokinin, secretion
		Fatty acids	Enteropancreatic reflexes
		Ca^{2+}, H^+	Other hormones (?)
		Distention	

distention to 250–400 ml can double the basal pancreatic output. It is unclear how much the gastric phase contributes to postprandial secretion in man, although it accounts for 20% of the maximal CCK response in dogs [22]. The mechanoreceptors are located in the body and fundus; distention of the antrum does not stimulate pancreatic secretion. This gastric phase is mediated by vagal cholinergic pathways, since it can be abolished or reduced by vagotomy and atropine. Some of the abnormal postprandial pancreatic secretion following gastric surgery is due to changes in the delivery of nutrients and acid into the duodenum. Gastric emptying rates and control of food particle size have important effects on the pattern and magnitude of the intestinal phase of pancreatic secretion.

The intestinal phase is the most important stimulus to postprandial pancreatic secretion, accounting for 70% of the maximal level. It is mediated by the hormones CCK and secretin and by vagal cholinergic reflexes. The stimulation of bicarbonate secretion is controlled primarily by secretin, which is released by luminal acid and, with a small stimulus, by fatty acids and bile. Amino acids and oligopeptides are the most potent stimulants of CCK release and are dependent on load rather than concentration, probably due to the longer segment of intestine stimulated with larger loads [23]. This response is confined to the duodenum and jejunum, with no effect of amino acid perfusion into the ileum. Fatty acids and monoglycerides stimulate pancreatic secretion, although undigested fats do not. Fatty acid stimulation of the pancreas is greater with longer chain lengths, increased saturation, larger total loads, and an increased ratio of bile salts to fatty acids. Intraduodenal calcium also stimulates pancreatic secretion via CCK release. Intestinal glucose does not affect pancreatic secretion, although it may eventually affect enzyme secretion via its effect on insulin release. The cholinergic enteropancreatic reflex is stimulated by duodenal volume distention, by increased osmolality, and by fat emulsions and amino acids.

Clinical Presentation of Chronic Pancreatitis

Pain

The most common presenting symptom of chronic pancreatitis is pain. It is epigastric and dull in nature, with frequent radiation directly through to the back. It is aggravated by food intake almost instantaneously, this short interval between eating and the onset being fairly specific for pancreatic pain. The pain may be brought on by alcohol intake, although many patients report that it occurs after 12–24 h of abstinence. Chronic pancreatitis pain may occur in "attacks" that last several days or may be almost continuous. Despite the fact that pain is the predominant symptom of chronic pancreatitis, the condition is painless or relatively painless in about 15% of patients. This painless variety of chronic pancreatitis appears to be more common in patients with an idiopathic than in those with an alcoholic etiology.

Pain in chronic pancreatitis may be intermittent; it may increase, decrease, or disappear entirely over years of follow-up. It has been widely accepted that pain tends to decrease as the severity of the chronic pancreatitis increases. The onset of exocrine insufficiency and diabetes often coincides with this pain relief, presumably due to the fact that the ongoing pancreatic inflammation in a nonfunctioning pancreas is insufficient to cause pain [24]. This "burn-out" may take 5–20 years to occur and may never happen in some patients. Some studies suggest that this spontaneous pain relief is uncommon [25]. More long-term studies of the natural history of chronic pancreatitis are needed in order to assess the utility of the various chronic pancreatitis pain treatment methods available.

Pain assessment in chronic pancreatitis, particularly chronic alcoholic pancreatitis, is often clouded by drug-dependent personalities. It may be impossible to sort out the impact of pancreatic pain in patients with addiction to alcohol and narcotics. Many of them have underlying personality disorders which make the treatment of pain very difficult.

The mechanisms of pain in chronic pancreatitis are unclear. Proposed causes include inflammation of the pancreas and peripancreatic tissues, increased pancreatic pressure, and neural inflammation. The increased pancreatic ductal pressures which have been documented in chronic pancreatitis are often associated with dilated pancreatic ducts and form the basis for surgical and endoscopic decompression as a means of pain control [26].

Weight Loss

Weight loss is extremely common in chronic pancreatitis. It is usually much more significant and common in these patients than in those with other types of food-aggravated pain such as irritable bowel syndrome or peptic ulcer disease. The major cause of weight loss in chronic pancreatitis is decreased caloric intake due to the fear of pain aggravation with eating. The frequently associated symptoms of nausea and vomiting in chronic pancreatitis probably also contribute to this weight loss. Other factors that occasionally play a role are malabsorption or uncontrolled diabetes.

Malabsorption

Malabsorption does not occur until enzyme secretion is reduced to less than 10% of normal [27]. Therefore, diarrhea and steatorrhea occur relatively late in the course of chronic pancreatitis. In addition to fat, protein and starch are also malabsorbed, although lipase secretion decreases more rapidly than the secretion of proteolytic enzymes. Hence, steatorrhea is often an earlier and more severe problem than azotorrhea. Concurrent with the reduction of pancreatic enzyme secretion there is decreased bicarbonate secretion in advanced chronic pancreatitis. Duodenal pH may fall to 4 or less, leading to inactivation of pancreatic enzymes and precipitation of bile acids.

The fecal weight is lower in pancreatic malabsorption than in other conditions with comparable levels of steatorrhea. This lower fecal weight reflects less fecal water and is likely due to the better absorption of carbohydrates than occurs with mucosal diseases like celiac sprue. This low fecal weight leads to the passage of formed, bulky stools instead of watery diarrhea. As with all malabsorption, the stools are described as particularly foul in odor. Patients may see oil droplets on the toilet bowel water. Malabsorption of fat-soluble vitamins is much less frequent than it is in celiac sprue, reflecting the unimportance of lipolysis in the absorption of these compounds.

Pancreatic Diabetes

Although glucose intolerance is common early in the course of chronic pancreatitis, clinically evident diabetes occurs late in the disease. In most patients the diagnosis of chronic pancreatitis occurs long before the presentation of diabetes. However, in patients with painless or relatively painless pancreatitis, diabetes may be the initial presenting symptom. Endocrine insufficiency eventually occurs in 60% of patients with chronic pancreatitis.

References

1. Copenhagen Pancreatic Study (1981) An interim report from a prospective epidemiological multicenter study. Scand J Gastroenterol 16:305
2. Novak J, Greger R (1988) Properties of the luminal membrane of isolated perfused rat pancreatic ducts. Effect of cyclic AMP and blockers of chloride transport. Pflugers Arch 411:546
3. Veel T, Buaner T, Engeland E, Raeder MG (1990) Colchicine inhibits the effects of secretin on pancreatic duct cell tubulovesicles and HCO_3 secretion in the pig. Acta Physiol Scand 138:487
4. Gorelick FS, Jamieson JD (1994) The pancreatic acinar cell-structure-function relationship of the pancreas. In: Johnson LR (ed) Physiology of the gastrointestinal tract, 3rd edn. Raven, New York, pp 1353

5. Meyer D, Krause E, Dobberstein B (1982) Secretory protein translocation across membranes: the role of docking protein. Nature 297:647
6. Sommer H, Schrezenmeir J, Kasper H (1985) Output dependent non-parallel enzyme secretion of the human pancreas. Hepatogastroenterology 32:246
7. Fahrenkrog J, Schaffalitzkyde Mackadell OB, Rune SJ (1978) pH threshold for release of secretin in normal subjects and in patients with duodenal ulcer and patients with chronic pancreatitis. Scand J Gastroenterol 13:177
8. Li P, Leek Y, Chang TM, Chey WY (1990) Mechanism of acid-induced release of secretin in rats. Presence of a secretin-releasing peptide. J Clin Invest 86:1474
9. Lu L, Louie D, Owyang C (1989) A cholecystokinin releasing peptide mediates feedback regulation of pancreatic secretion. Am J Physiol 256:G430
10. Soudah H, Lu Y, Owyang C (1992) Physiological action of CCK on pancreatic enzyme secretion is mediated by a cholinergic pathway. Am J Physiol 263:G102
11. Malagelada JR, Go VLW, Summerskill WHJ (1974) Altered pancreatic and biliary function after vagotomy and pyloroplasty. Gastroenterology 66:22
12. Fahrenkrug J, Schaffalitzky de Muchadell OB, Holst JJ, et al. (1979) Vasoactive intestinal polypeptide in vagally mediated pancreatic secretive of fluid and HCO_3. Am J Physiol 237:E535
13. Dollinger HC, Raptis S, Pfeiffer EF (1976) Effects of somatostatin on exocrine and endocrine function stimulated by intestinal hormones in man. Horm Metab Res 8:74
14. Tohno H, Sarr MG, Dimagno EP (1995) Intraileal carbohydrate regulates canine postprandial pancreaticobiliary secretion and upper gut motility. Gastroenterology 109:1977
15. Sarr MB, Foley MK, Winters RC, Dvenes JA, Dimagno EP (1997) Role of extrinsic innervation in carbohydrate-induced ileal modulation of pancreatic secretion and upper gut function. Pancreas 14:166
16. Pappas TN, Debas HT, Goto Y, et al (1985) Peptide YY inhibits meal stimulated pancreatic and gastric secretion. Am J Physiol 248:G118
17. Nakamura R, Miyasaka K, Kuyama Y, Kitani K (1990) Luminal bile regulates cholecystokinin release in conscious rats. Dig Dis Sci 35:55
18. Holtmann G, Kelly DG, Dimagno EP (1996) Nutrients and interdigestive pancreatic enzyme secretion in humans. Gut 38:920
19. Isaksson G, Ihse IH (1983) Pain reduction by an oral pancreatic enzyme preparation in chronic pancreatitis. Dig Dis Sci 28:97
20. Owyang C, Achem-Kavam SR, Vinik AJ (1983) Pancreatic polypeptide and intestinal migratory motor complex in humans. Effect of pancreaticobiliary secretion. Gastroenterology 84:10
21. Defillipi C, Solomon TE, Valenzuela JE (1982) Pancreatic secretory response to sham feeding in humans. Digestion 23:217
22. Vagne M, Grossman MI (1969) Gastric and pancreatic secretion in response to gastric distension in dogs. Gastroenterology 57:300
23. Meyer JH, Kelly GA, Spingola LJ, et al (1976) Canine gut receptors mediating pancreatic responses to luminal L-amino acids. Am J Physiol 231:669
24. Ammann RW (1991) Acintical appraisal of interventional therapy in chronic pancreatitis. Endoscopy 23:191
25. Lankisch PG, Seidensticker F, Lohr-Happe A, Otto J, Creutzfeldt W (1995) The course of pain is the same in alcohol and non-alcohol induced chronic pancreatitis. Pancreas 10:338
26 Bradley EL III (1982) Pancreatic duct pressure in chronic pancreatitis. Am J Surg 144:313
27. Dimagno EP, Go VLW, Summerskill WHJ (1973) Relations between pancreatic enzyme outputs and malabsorption in severe pancreatic insufficiency. N Engl J Med 288:813

CHAPTER 11

Intestinal Transit of Chyme and its Regulatory Role: Clinical Implications

P. Layer and J. Keller

Introduction

The crucial importance of pancreatic exocrine function is reflected by the detrimental malabsorption which occurs as a consequence of untreated pancreatic exocrine insufficiency, a typical complication of progressive chronic pancreatitis [1, 2]. Therapeutic options to treat pancreatic insufficiency have improved during recent years, due mainly to our growing understanding of the underlying physiologic and pathophysiologic mechanisms and improved pharmacologic and pharmaceutical strategies for enzyme replacement therapies. In most patients, however, luminal lipid digestion cannot be completely normalized. Moreover, it has to be kept in mind that chronic pancreatitis not only leads to intraluminal enzyme deficiency but also may cause complex and interacting alterations of secretory, motor, and endocrine functions in the course of the disease. This chapter deals with the intraluminal fate of enzymes and nutrients in health and in pancreatic exocrine insufficiency. In particular, the pathophysiologic role of malabsorbed nutrients for the regulation of gastrointestinal secretory and motor functions is discussed.

Development of Steatorrhea

Fate of Pancreatic Enzymes During Small Intestinal Transit

Clinically manifest nutrient malabsorption as a consequence of progressively decreasing pancreatic enzyme output is a characteristic late feature of chronic pancreatitis. For steatorrhea to occur, more than 90%–95% of the secreting parenchyma need to be destroyed [1, 3, 4]. In chronic pancreatitis of alcoholic etiology, this usually takes more than 10 years after the onset of clinical symptoms [2, 3, 5] due to the high reserve capacity of the normal pancreas, although more rapid courses are not uncommon. The capacity of the pancreas to synthesize and secrete lipase is impaired earlier and more

---

Our own cited studies were supported by the *Deutsche Forschungsgemeinschaft* grant DFG La 483/5-3.

Table 1. Clinical importance of fat maldigestion in chronic pancreatitis: pathophysiologic mechanisms

Earlier impairment of pancreatic lipase synthesis and secretion
Low effectiveness of compensating enzyme systems
Decreased bicarbonate output leading to more rapid and complete inactivation of lipase in the acidic duodenum
Greater susceptibility of lipase to proteolytic destruction
Further impairment of lipid absorption by decreased duodenal bile acid concentrations (due to precipitation within the acidic duodenum and inhibition of secretion by malabsorbed nutrients)

severely compared with other enzymes in the course of chronic pancreatitis. Thus, in the same patient, a decrease in lipase secretion to less than 5% of normal may be present, causing steatorrhea, while protease output is maintained in a range between 10% and 20% of normal, which is sufficient to prevent protein malabsorption [1, 3, 5]. In addition, several other pathophysiologic mechanisms interact which decrease the quantity and availability of luminal lipase and further impair lipid digestion [6] (Table 1). Consequently, steatorrhea (associated with malabsorption of the lipid-soluble vitamins A, D, E, and K) is usually more severe and develops several years prior to overt malabsorption of protein or starch.

However, not only the amount of enzymes released into the duodenum but also the survival of enzymatic activity within the intestinal lumen has an important impact on the extent and main site of nutrient hydrolysis, because it determines how long enzymes are available for digestion during the duodenoileal transit of chyme.

In healthy human beings, the activities of all major pancreatic enzymes present in postprandial chyme decrease during aboral small intestinal transit [7]. However, the velocity and rate of intraluminal enzyme degradation vary widely due to differing stability against inactivating mechanisms [8]. Moreover, we observed that among the same enzymes disappearance rates of enzymatic activities and immunoreactivities may be different [8].

Mostly because of its high resistance against enzymatic proteolysis [9], pancreatic amylase is relatively stable, and most of its enzymatic activity released into the duodenum survives duodenoileal transit [8, 10–12]. By contrast, about 40% of protease activity is already lost during duodenojejunal transit and only 20%–30% of the amount released into the duodenum is delivered to the terminal ileum. Interestingly, trypsin enzymatic activity is preserved better than trypsin immunoreactivity. These findings suggest that structural integrity of the trypsin molecule may not be essential for its proteolytic activity [8, 9].

Lipase is most susceptible to inactivation during small intestinal transit. In the absence of triglycerides, a large proportion of lipase activity is lost even between the duodenum and the jejunum, and only small quantities are delivered to the terminal ileum [8, 9]. In the presence of its substrate, the stability of the lipase molecule appears to be increased both in vitro and in vivo [9–13].

Proteolytic degradation is the main cause of inactivation of pancreatic enzymes within the small intestinal lumen. In vitro studies and in vivo studies in healthy human subjects suggest that chymotrypsin is of special importance for the destruction of lipase activity [10, 14]. This is in accordance with the observation that inhibition of the major pancreatic proteases, including trypsin and chymotrypsin, markedly increases the survival of lipase activity during duodenoileal transit [10]. Conversely, protease inactivation decreases the postprandial delivery of unabsorbed fat to the terminal ileum by more than 80% [12, 15]. This suggests that small amounts of ingested lipids are physiologically malabsorbed due to the rapid proteolytic inactivation of intraluminal lipase during small intestinal transit.

In summary, the earlier and more severe impairment of lipase secretion compared with other enzymes during the course of chronic pancreatitis and more rapid proteolytic degradation of lipase during small intestinal transit are important reasons why, from a clinical point of view, lipase deficiency is by far the most important digestive malfunction in pancreatic exocrine insufficiency.

Lack of Compensatory Mechanisms

Digestion of triglycerides fully depends on the presence of sufficient amounts of pancreatic lipase, because there are no effective nonpancreatic enzyme systems which might compensate for lipase deficiency in man [16]. This is in contrast to the hydrolysis of other substrates. For example, protein digestion is initiated by intragastric proteolytic activity and continued by the intestinal brush border peptidases. Therefore, protein digestion is maintained even if pancreatic proteolytic activity is blocked under experimental conditions [11]. Similarly, in the absence of pancreatic amylase activity, starch digestion is delayed, but about 80% of it is preserved quantitatively by salivary amylase and by brush border oligosaccharidases [17].

Importance of Intraduodenal Acidity

Pancreatic bicarbonate secretion, which serves to protect pancreatic enzymes from denaturation by gastric acid, is markedly diminished in exocrine pancreatic insufficiency. As a result, intraduodenal pH may fall below 4 late postprandially [18]. Since lipase is particularly susceptible to acidic destruction [18], the small residual quantities of lipase secreted into the duodenum may be inactivated [3]. Precipitation of bile acids by low intraduodenal pH and, possibly, inhibition of digestive bile secretion by malabsorbed nutrients [6] likely compromise lipid absorption further.

Fate of Nutrients During Small Intestinal Transit in Health and Pancreatic Insufficiency

In healthy human beings, digestion and absorption of nutrients takes place primarily in the upper small intestine. More than 80% of lipids are usually absorbed proximal to the mid jejunum. However, even in healthy persons ingesting a normal Western diet, considerable amounts of nutrients pass the small intestine unabsorbed. The extent of this physiologic malabsorption is influenced by the quantity and type of meal nutrients. Depending upon the type of starch ingested, varying proportions of a carbohydrate meal ranging between 1% for rice starch and 20%–30% for beans are delivered to the colon; with most other types of carbohydrates, physiologic malabsorption amounts to about 10% [19, 20]. Following ingestion of a mixed meal, ileal lipid concentrations of up to 10 mg/ml were measured [7, 21, 22].

In untreated severe pancreatic exocrine insufficiency, the amount of nutrients passing the distal small intestine unabsorbed increases dramatically. We observed a sevenfold increase in cumulative ileal nutrient delivery even in response to a low-caloric, easily digestible test meal [23]. However, not only in patients with overt malabsorption but also during the early stages of chronic pancreatitis [4] and in patients receiving enzyme supplementation [6] there is evidence that the site of maximal digestion and absorption of nutrients is shifted from the duodenum to the more distal small intestine [6].

Regulatory Role of Nutrients in the Distal Small Intestine

Effects of Malabsorbed Nutrients

Physiologically malabsorbed nutrients contribute to maintain normal gastrointestinal functions. First, they serve as an energy source for the colonic flora. Second, they participate in the regulation of upper gastrointestinal functions. Experimental ileal lipid perfusion inhibits secretory and motor functions of upper gastrointestinal organs both in the fasting state [24] and during weak or moderate endogenous stimulation [25–30]. In healthy human subjects we observed a significant negative correlation between intraileal lipid concentrations within the physiologic range and digestive pancreatic lipase and protease outputs [31]. In addition, there are several studies suggesting comparable inhibitory effects of equicaloric amounts of carbohydrates, especially glucose [24, 26, 32, 33]. By contrast, perfusion of proteins or protein hydrolysates has no [34, 35] or only weak inhibitory effects [28].

Even more importantly, the effects of ileal nutrients are not limited to unspecific inhibition of secretory responses; rather, they seem to modulate the integrated functional state of the entire gastrointestinal system. Thus, late postprandial ileal nutrient exposure correlates tightly with the termination of digestive secretory and motor responses [36]. Hence, these findings suggest that physiologic ileal nutrient exposure plays a pivotal regulatory role by

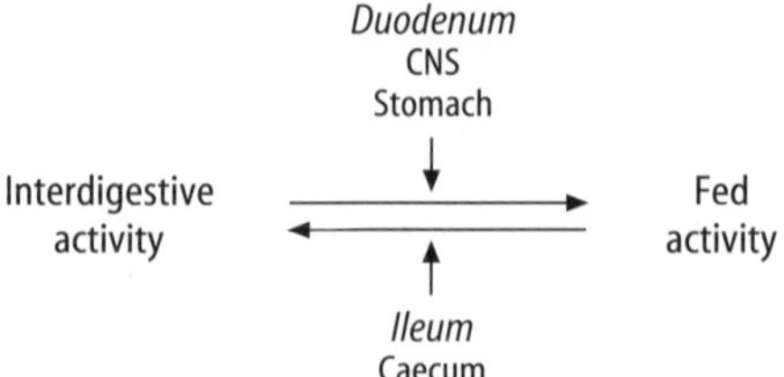

Fig. 1. Regulatory role of physiologically malabsorbed nutrients

controlling the transition from the fed to the subsequent fasting state (Fig. 1).

Intermediary Mechanisms

Inhibition of gastrointestinal secretory and motor functions by the distal small intestine may be mediated by neural or hormonal mechanisms. Based on former observations, peptide YY (PYY) and glucagon-like peptide-1 (GLP-1) are particularly attractive candidate hormones because they are released from the distal intestinal mucosa in response to a meal or intraileal nutrients [23, 31, 37–40] and have profound regulatory effects on gastrointestinal secretion and motility. We have shown that increases in GLP-1 and PYY plasma levels in response to ileal nutrient perfusion correlate indirectly, not only with gastric emptying and gastric acid secretion [38], but also with lipase and protease outputs [31]. Experimental GLP-1 infusion reproducing postprandial GLP-1 levels significantly inhibits digestive secretion of all major pancreatic enzymes; similarly, postprandial PYY plasma levels decrease pancreatic enzyme outputs in response to weak exogenous stimulation by CCK [41]. Inhibition of digestive pancreatic exocrine secretion by GLP-1 has been attributed solely to decreased gastric emptying rates [40]. Nevertheless, recent observations have shown that it also occurs during complete aspiration of gastric contents [42]. Therefore, GLP-1 seems to be directly involved in the regulation of pancreatic exocrine secretion. Since no GLP-1 receptors have been found on pancreatic acinar cells so far, mediation of its inhibitory effect on pancreatic exocrine secretion is still unclear. Overall, inhibitory mechanisms induced by ileal nutrient exposure appear to act, at least in part, on the level of the pancreas, and not only indirectly by inhibition of stimulating mechanisms, because they are also active in the presence of exogenous stimulation with CCK [43].

Pathophysiologic Regulatory Role of Malabsorbed Nutrients in Pancreatic Insufficiency

In states of malabsorption, postprandial plasma levels of inhibitory distal intestinal hormones are markedly increased compared with healthy subjects [23]. Disturbed regulation of gastrointestinal secretory and motor functions

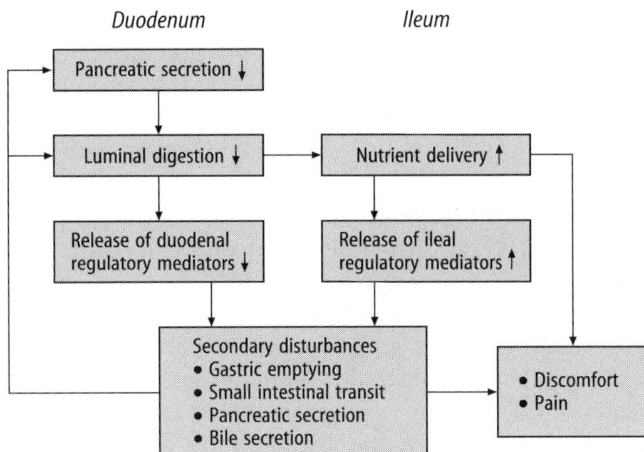

Fig. 2. Contribution of nutrient malabsorption to regulatory disturbances in chronic pancreatitis

by increased distal intestinal nutrient exposure is an important consequence of maldigestion (Fig. 2). Even in the absence of overt malabsorption during the early stages of chronic pancreatitis [4] there is evidence that the site of maximal digestion and absorption is shifted from the duodenum to the distal small intestine [6]. As a result, increased amounts of nutrients may be delivered to the distal ileum, causing disturbed regulation of motor and secretory functions of upper gastrointestinal organs [24, 26, 28, 30, 36]. We have shown that in healthy persons ileal nutrient exposure decreases digestive pancreatic enzyme response as well as biliary secretion [31]. Therefore, in patients with chronic pancreatitis, malabsorbed nutrients may further impair nutrient digestion – in particular lipid digestion – by decreasing residual pancreatic exocrine secretion and biliary secretion.

In addition, we have recently demonstrated another feature of pancreatic insufficiency which likely contributes to intraluminal maldigestion: Small intestinal transit is significantly accelerated in patients with pancreatic insufficiency compared with healthy subjects, resulting in a 50% reduction of intestinal transit time [23]. As a consequence, the available time for digestion and absorption is markedly decreased. Enzyme replacement corrects disturbance of not only digestion but also gastrointestinal transit [23]. These findings suggest that malabsorption likely is both a consequence and a cause of abnormal motor function [23].

Clinical Implications

The available experimental data and clinical evidence suggest that "subclinical" pancreatic exocrine insufficiency (i.e., residual secretory capacity significantly decreased but sufficient to prevent manifest steathorrhea) causes a delay and aboral shift of maximal digestion and absorption of a meal. As a consequence, distal segments of the small intestine, in particular the ileum, are exposed to excessive (or supraphysiologic) quantities of unabsorbed nutrients. This in turn has marked pathophysiologic regulatory effects on both secretory and motor responses to the meal. These pathophysiologic mechanisms likely contribute to some of the symptoms of patients who have no manifest malabsorption, and they explain the (hitherto unexplained) symptom-relieving effects of pancreatic enzyme supplementation (Fig. 2) in a subgroup of patients [23, 44].

In the future course of the disease, deterioration of lipid absorption is a result of several interacting pathomechanisms (Table 1). As outlined above, the ability of the pancreas to synthesize and secrete lipase is impaired earlier and more severely than secretion of other enzymes. Second, in contrast to pancreatic amylase and proteases, there are no effective substitution systems for pancreatic lipase. Moreover, lipase is more susceptible to proteolytic destruction and to inactivation within the duodenum, which has an acidic milieu due to decreased bicarbonate output. Finally, lipid absorption is impaired by bile acid precipitation within the acidic duodenum and additionally by inhibition of bile acid secretion due to malabsorbed ileal nutrients.

Taken together, pancreatic insufficiency due to chronic pancreatitis not only causes intraluminal enzyme deficiency but also induces complex and interacting alterations of secretory, motor, and endocrine functions. Therefore, future therapeutic concepts for patients with chronic pancreatitis should consider both quantitative replacement of enzymes within the intestinal lumen and correction of disturbed integration of digestive functions.

References

1. DiMagno EP, Clain JE, Layer P (1993) Chronic pancreatitis. In: Go VLW, et al (eds) The pancreas: biology, pathobiology, and diseases, 2nd edn. Raven, New York, pp 665–706
2. Layer P, DiMagno EP (1996) Natural histories of alcoholic and idiopathic chronic pancreatitis. Pancreas 12:318–319
3. DiMagno EP, Layer P (1993) Human exocrine pancreatic enzyme secretion. In: Go VLW, et al (eds): The pancreas: biology, pathobiology, and diseases, 2nd edn. Raven, New York, pp 275–300
4. DiMagno EP, Go VLW, Summerskill WHJ (1973) Relations between pancreatic enzyme outputs and malabsorption in severe pancreatic insufficiency. N Engl J Med 288:813–815
5. DiMagno EP, Malagelada JR, Go VLW (1975) Relationship between alcoholism and pancreatic insufficiency. Ann NY Acad Sci 252:200–207
6. Layer P, von der Ohe M, Gröger G, Dicke D, Goebell H (1992) Luminal availability and digestive efficacy of substituted enzymes in pancreatic insufficiency. Pancreas 7:745
7. Borgström B, Dahlqvist A, Lundh G, Sjövall J (1957) Studies of intestinal digestion and absorption in the human. J Clin Invest 36:1521–1536
8. Layer P, Go VLW, DiMagno EP (1986) Fate of pancreatic enzymes during aboral small intestinal transit in humans. Am J Physiol 251:G475–G480
9. Granger M, Abadie B, Marchis-Mouren G (1975) Limited action of trypsin on porcine pancreatic amylase: characterization of the fragments. FEBS Lett 56:189–193
10. Layer P, Jansen JBMJ, Cherian L, Lamers CBHW, Goebell H (1990) Feedback regulation of human pancreatic secretion: effects of protease inhibition on duodenal delivery and small intestinal transit of pancreatic enzymes. Gastroenterology 98:1311–1319
11. Layer P, Baumann J, Hellmann C, v.d. Ohe M, Gröger G, Goebell H (1990) Effect of luminal protease inhibition on prandial nutrient digestion during small intestinal chyme transit. Pancreas 5:718
12. Holtmann G, Kelly DG, Sternby B, DiMagno EP (1997) Survival of human pancreatic enzymes during small bowel transit: effect of nutrients, bile acids, and enzymes. Am J Physiol 273:G553–G558

13. Kelly DG, Sternby B, DiMagno EP (1991) How to protect human pancreatic enzyme activities in frozen duodenal juice. Gastroenterology 100:189–195
14. Thiruvengadam R, DiMagno EP (1988) Inactivation of human lipase by proteases. Am J Physiol 255:G476–481
15. Layer P, Hellmann C, Baumann J, v.d. Ohe M, Gröger G, Goebell H (1990) Modulation of physiologic fat malabsorption in humans. Digestion 46:153
16. Sternby B, Holtmann G, Kelly DG, DiMagno EP (1992) Effect of gastric or duodenal nutrient infusion on gastric and pancreatic lipase secretion. Gastroenterology 102:A292
17. Layer P, Zinsmeister AR, DiMagno EP (1986) Effects of decreasing intraluminal amylase activity on starch digestion and postprandial gastrointestinal function in humans. Gastroenterology 91:41–48
18. DiMagno EP, Malagelada JR, Go VLW, Moertel CG (1977) Fate of orally ingested enzymes in pancreatic insufficiency: comparison of two dosage schedules. N Engl J Med 296:1318–1322
19. Levitt MD, Hirsh P, Fetzer CA, Sheahan M, Levine AS (1987) H2 excretion after ingestion of complex carbohydrates. Gastroenterology 92:383–389
20. Stephen AM, Haddad AC, Phillips SF (1983) Passage of carbohydrate into the colon. Gastroenterology 85:589–595
21. Fields M, Duthie HL (1965) Effect of vagotomy on intraluminal digestion of fat in man. Gut 6:301–310
22. Hofman AF, Borgström B (1964) The intraluminal phase of fat digestion in man: the lipid content of the micellar and oil phases of intestinal content obtained during fat digestion and absorption. J Clin Invest 43:247–257
23. Layer P, von der Ohe MR, Holst JJ, Jansen JBMJ, Grandt D, Holtmann G, Goebell H (1997) Altered postprandial motility in chronic pancreatitis: role of malabsorption. Gastroenterology 112:1624–1634
24. Layer P, Schlesinger T, Gröger G, Goebell H (1993) Modulation of periodic interdigestive gastrointestinal motor and pancreatic function by the ileum. Pancreas 8:426–432
25. Holgate AM, Read NW (1985) Effect of ileal infusion of intralipid on gastrointestinal transit, ileal flow rate, and carbohydrate absorption in humans after ingestion of a liquid meal. Gastroenterology 88:1005–1011
26. Layer P, Peschel S, Schlesinger T, Goebell H (1990) Human pancreatic secretion and intestinal motility: effects of ileal nutrient perfusion. Am J Physiol 258:G196–G201
27. Layer P, Gröger G, Ohe M, Goebell H (1991) Ileal carbohydrates alter intestinal fed motor pattern in response to weak but not strong endogenous stimulation. (Abstr) Gastroenterology 100:A462
28. Read NW, McFarlane A, Kinsman RI, Bates TE, Blackhall NW, Farrar GB, Hall JC, Moss G, Morris AP, Neill BO, Welch I, Lee Y, Bloom SR (1984) Effect of infusion of nutrient solutions into the ileum on gastrointestinal transit and plasma levels of neurotensin and enteroglucagon. Gastroenterology 86:274–280
29. Soper NJ, Chapman NJ, Kelly KA, Brown ML, Phillips SF, Go VLW (1990) The 'ileal brake' after ileal pouch-anal anastomosis. Gastroenterology 98:111–116
30. Spiller RC, Trotman IF, Higgins BE, Ghatei MA, Grimble GK, Lee YC, Bloom SR, Misiewicz JJ, Silk DBA (1984) The ileal brake – inhibition of jejunal motility after ileal fat perfusion in man. Gut 25:365–374
31. Keller J, Conrads H, Goebell H, Layer P (1998) Differential responses of human pancreatic and biliary secretion to graded ileal lipid perfusion. Digestion 59:206
32. Jain NK, Boivin M, Zinsmeister AR, Brown ML, Di Magno EP (1989) Effect of ileal perfusion of carbohydrates and amylase inhibitor on gastrointestinal hormones and emptying. Gastroenterology 96:177–187
33. Layer P, VanKrieken A, Daecke W, Grandt D, Goebell H (1993) Non-parallel responses of human pancreatic enzyme outputs to ileal nutrient exposure. Digestion 54:289
34. Layer P, Gröger G, Grandt D, Cherian L (1993) Das terminale Ileum als Koregulator der zyklischen interdigestiven Pankreassekretion beim Menschen. Med Klin 88:15–17
35. Welch IM, Cunningham KM, Read NW (1988) Regulation of gastric emptying by ileal nutrients in humans. Gastroenterology 94:401–404
36. Keller J, Rünzi M, Goebell H, Layer P (1997) Duodenal and ileal nutrient deliveries regulate human intestinal motor and pancreatic responses to a meal. Am J Physiol 272:G632–G63
37. Adrian T, Ferri GL, Bacarese-Hamilton AJ, Fuessl HS, Polak JM, Bloom SR (1985) Human distribution and release of a putative new gut hormone, peptide YY. Gastroenterology 89:1070–1077

38. Layer P, Holst JJ, Grandt D, Goebell H (1995) Ileal release of glucagon-like-1 peptide (GLP-1): association with inhibition of gastric acid secretion in humans. Dig Dis Sci 40:1074–108
39. Savage AP, Adrian TE, Carolan G, Chatterjee VK, Bloom SR (1987) Effects of peptide YY (PYY) on mouth to caecum intestinal transit time and on the rate of gastric emptying in healthy volunteers. Gut 28:166–170
40. Wettergren A, Schjoldager B, Mortensen PE, Myhre J, Christiansen J, Holst JJ (1993) Truncated GLP-1 (proglucagon 78-107-amide) inhibits gastric and pancreatic functions in man. Dig Dis Sci 38:665–673
41. Grandt D, Gschossmann JM, Schimiczek M, Beglinger C, Goebell H, Layer P (1995) Peptide YY inhibits low-dose but not high-dose CCK-stimulated pancreatic enzyme secretion in humans. Gastroenterology 108:A972
42. Layer P, Franke A, Keller J, Holst JJ, Grandt D, Goebell H (1996) Glucagonlike peptide-1 (GLP-1) inhibits pancreatic enzyme secretion in humans. Gastroenterology 110:A409
43. Gröger G, Unger A, Holst JJ, Goebell H, Layer P (1997) Ileal carbohydrates inhibit cholinergically stimulated exocrine pancreatic secretion in humans. Int J Pancreatol 22:23–29
44. Slaff J, Jacobson D, Tillmann CR, Curington C, Toskes PP (1984) Protease-specific suppression of pancreatic exocrine secretion. Gastroenterology 87:44–52

CHAPTER 12

Treatment of Exocrine Pancreatic Insufficiency in Chronic Pancreatitis

M. J. Bruno

Introduction

The treatment of exocrine pancreatic insufficiency has come a long way. Presently, many patients can be treated satisfactorily with high-strength (≥20,000 Ph.Eur.U. [units of enzyme activity according to the European Pharmacopeia] of lipase per capsule) enteric-coated mini-dose-unit preparations. In some cases, however, treatment remains difficult and a true challenge to the clinician. Insight into the gastrointestinal (patho)physiology of exocrine pancreatic insufficiency and properties of the pharmaceutical preparations is prerequisite to the achievement of optimal treatment results.

This chapter will give an overview of how pancreatic enzyme replacement therapy, based on a better understanding of the (patho)physiology of the exocrine pancreas, has evolved during the past decades. We will discuss the state of the art with respect to both drug therapy and dietary counseling. Taking into consideration the limitations of present therapeutic possibilities, we will point out areas of research that may improve treatment efficacy in terms of both pharmacology and patient comfort.

Exocrine Pancreatic Insufficiency

There are only very few data on the natural history of exocrine pancreatic insufficiency in patients with chronic pancreatitis. Thirty to 40% of patients will develop exocrine pancreatic insufficiency at some point during their illness, usually after 8–15 years, and may need pancreatic enzyme replacement therapy to correct maldigestion [1]. This supplementation therapy is usually for life and involves considerable costs, amounting to a total of Fl. 2190 (ca. $1050) per year for a Dutch patient taking six capsules of an enteric-coated mini-dose-unit preparation daily.

The consequences of maldigestion and steatorrhea should not be underestimated. There are unpleasant and discomforting symptoms such as cramps, foul-smelling voluminous stools, and diarrhea, but also major medical consequences. Because fat has the highest caloric density (38 kJ/g) compared with proteins (17 kJ/g) and carbohydrates (17 kJ/g), it is an important source for the daily uptake of energy. Steatorrhea causes weight loss through caloric losses and, in extreme cases, may lead to emaciation. Steatorrhea may also induce deficiencies of magnesium, calcium, essential fatty acids, and fat-soluble vitamins [2]. Its treatment may even have consequences in terms of morbidity and mortality. In patients with chronic pancreatitis reduced plasma levels of factors protective against atherogenesis such as high-density lipoprotein C, Apo A-I, and lipoprotein A were observed [3]. The higher incidence of atheromatous large-vessel disease and cardiovascular events in patients with exocrine pancreatic insufficiency are associated with a significantly shorter life span [4, 5].

Pathophysiology

Since the early 1970s, knowledge about the (patho)physiology of exocrine pancreatic insufficiency and its treatment has expanded rapidly, due mainly to the work of DiMagno's group at the Mayo Clinics.

Exocrine pancreatic insufficiency includes decreased activity of amylase, trypsin, and lipase and involves maldigestion of carbohydrate, protein, and fat. As endogenous pancreatic enzymes move from the duodenum to the ileum during intestinal transit in healthy volunteers, 74% of amylase activity, 22% of trypsin activity, and only 1% of lipase activity survive [6]. When patients were treated with non-enteric-coated pancreatin, large amounts of these enzymes were already inactivated before the site of action was reached, and only 22% of trypsin and 8% of lipase were delivered at the level of the ligament of Treitz [7]. This high loss of lipase activity is attributed mainly to fast and irreversible inactivation of lipase below pH 4.0 [8]. Moreover, lipase is also inactivated by proteases [9]. Trypsin is relatively acid stable, and its inactivation is mainly a function of peptic destruction [8]. The clinical picture of exocrine pancreatic insufficiency, therefore, is dominated by the consequences of deficient lipase activity. Azotorrhea is usually easily abolished during enzyme replacement therapy [7, 10].

In 1973, DiMagno et al. showed that patients with chronic pancreatitis do not have steatorrhea until maximal stimulated lipase outputs are below 10% of normal [11]. Consequently, supplementation of lipase in patients with exocrine pancreatic insufficiency to a level of 10% of normal should theoretically abolish steatorrhea. Indeed, treatment with oral pancreatin abolished fat malabsorption when postprandial duodenal lipase levels 7%–8% of normal were reached [7, 10]. Another important issue to consider is the intraluminal pH of the upper gastrointestinal tract. In patients with severe exocrine pancreatic insufficiency due to chronic pancreatitis (secretin-cerulein test: lipase output below 6100 IU/30 min) there was an early postprandial drop in intraluminal gastric pH with significantly lower peak values and longer periods when pH was below 2.0 [12]. It has also been shown that the intraduodenal pH is reduced and that periods during which it is below 4.0 are longer compared with healthy volunteers [13–16]. These conditions are more favorable for acidic inactivation of lipase. Moreover, low intestinal pH causes bile salts to precipitate, which leads to a reduction in postprandial duodenal lipid solubilization and further impairs lipolysis and absorption of lypolytic products [17].

Treatment

Treatment of exocrine pancreatic insufficiency includes drug therapy and dietary counseling. Its goals are to prevent loss of body weight and maintain an adequate nutritional status and to abolish subjective symptoms associated with steatorrhea. Body weight is the most important clinical parameter for monitoring treatment efficacy.

Drugs

Despite all the research undertaken to maximize the treatment efficacy of enzyme preparations over the past decades, the key issue in the treatment of exocrine pancreatic insufficiency is still how to get sufficient amounts of enzymes, in particular lipase, at the right time and the right place.

Undisputed indications for pancreatic enzyme replacement therapy are progressive weight loss and/or complaints associated with steatorrhea. Whether patients with steatorrhea but without symptoms and/or weight loss should be treated is unclear. It is generally accepted that when steatorrhea exceeds 15–20 g/day enzyme replacement therapy is indicated. The amount of lipase activity that abolishes steatorrhea in achlorhydric patients is approximately 30,000 IU [18]. In patients with chronic pancreatitis who may have normal or even increased gastric acid outputs and decreased bicarbonate production this amount is insufficient because of acidic inactivation of lipase. Ways to account for this acidic loss are either to increase the dose of lipase activity or to protect lipase from acidic inactivation. It is important to note that there is no clear-cut linear relationship between the amount of ingested lipase and corresponding fecal fat excretion. Furthermore, increasing the dosage of lipase will not lead to abolishment of steatorrhea in all patients. Protection of lipase against acidic inactivation can be achieved by adjunct treatment with either an H_2-receptor antagonist or a proton pump inhibitor, or by using enteric-coated mini-dose-unit preparations. The latter preparations consist of multiple mini-dose units with a diameter of 1–2 mm, contained in a gelatin capsule. In the stomach the gelatin capsule quickly dissolves and the enteric-coated mini-dose units are released. The enteric coat protects the pancreatic enzymes from acidic destruction. Liberation of enzymes occurs only when a preparation-specific pH threshold (commonly 5.0–5.5) is reached. This is intended to happen in the proximal small intestine. In most patients adequate enzyme supplementation is achieved with one to three capsules of an enteric-coated mini-dose-unit preparation with high lipase content per meal.

Stronger suppression of gastric acid secretion improves the efficacy of conventional non-enteric-coated enzyme preparations, but even with 60 mg omeprazole daily steatorrhea is rarely abolished [19]. Treatment with enteric-coated mini-dose-unit preparations is either equally effective or superior to conventional non-enteric-coated enzyme preparations [20–25]. Where treatment efficacy was equal, fewer units of lipase were needed with enteric-coated mini-dose-unit preparations. With the introduction of enteric-coated mini-dose-unit preparations with high lipase content, even fewer capsules need to be ingested for comparable treatment efficacy, which contributes to patients' acceptance and compliance [26]. The addition of a proton pump inhibitor during treatment with enteric-coated multi-dose-unit preparations can significantly improve treatment efficacy [27]. By increasing the intraduodenal pH, these adjunct preparations prevent the enteric coat from dissolving too distally. Patients with cystic fibrosis in particular, who have even more markedly reduced intraduodenal pH values than patients with chronic pancreatitis [17, 28], often benefit from this kind of adjunct therapy.

Sphere Size, Gastric Emptying, and Treatment Efficacy

With respect to the treatment efficacy of enteric-coated mini-dose-unit preparations, there has been discussion about the optimal sphere size in relation to their gastric emptying rate compared with a meal. In vitro and in vivo studies showed that, compared with a meal, preparations with a diameter of 1.8–2.0 mm emptied more slowly from the stomach than preparations with a diameter of 1.0–1.2 mm. However, these experiments were performed in healthy volunteers, used artificial microspheres, or used indirect measurements to assess gastric emptying [29–31]. We performed an in vivo experiment in which we simultaneously assessed the gastric transit profile of a 2-mm enteric-coated pancreatin minitablet preparation in comparison to a pancake meal and the resulting pancreatic enzyme activities by means of indirect pancreatic function tests [32]. This experiment showed that a high-strength 2-mm enteric-coated mini-dose-unit preparation ingested after the first bite of a meal does not pass through the stomach more slowly than a pancake meal; in fact, it emptied significantly faster. Timing of ingestion of the preparation (e.g., at the beginning of the meal or halfway through) may have an effect on the gastric transit profile and the mixture of the mini-dose-units with the meal, but it was not possible to evaluate this from these data. Digestion of ester lipids and proteins showed an improvement to subnormal and normal levels, respectively. Comparative clinical trials have always failed to show a difference in the efficacy of treatment among various commercially available enteric coated mini-dose-unit preparations with different sphere sizes [21, 33–39].

Dosage Recommendations

Although treatment in exocrine pancreatic insufficiency should be cause related and patient tailored, some general guidelines can be given [40]. The required dose for a main meal (breakfast, lunch, or dinner) ranges from about 20,000 to 75,000 Ph.Eur.U. lipase and for in-between snacks from about 5,000 to 25,000 Ph.Eur.U. lipase of an enteric-coated mini-dose-unit preparation. Consequently, one to three capsules of a high-strength preparation during main meals will usually suffice. Individual patients, however, may require lower or higher doses. If more capsules are taken per meal, their ingestion should be divided over the meal. In selected patients, compared with a fixed dosage recommended by the manufacturer, self-administration of pancreatic enzymes achieved the highest relieve of symptoms [41]. The mean number of capsules that were taken by patients increased significantly from five to 11.5. This illustrates that many patients are prescribed a dosage of pancreatic enzymes that is too low.

Adverse Events

Pancreatic enzyme preparations are relatively safe and only a few adverse effects have been reported, such as hypersensitivity, nausea, bloating, and diarrhea. A case report was published in 1994 in which children with cystic fibrosis using high doses of the enteric-coated mini-dose-unit preparations had developed bowel obstruction due to colonic stricture formation [42]. This adverse event has occurred only in young children (<12 years) with cystic fibrosis and not in patients with chronic pancreatitis. In a recent case-control study it was shown that the total daily dose of pancreatic enzymes is the major risk factor, rather than exposure to a high-strength preparation [43]. Among predisposing clinical characteristics were prior histories of colitis and distal intestinal obstruction syndrome. An increased risk for fibrosing colonopathy was found when a daily dosage of more than 24,000 units of lipase/kg was used. It was shown that the enteric coat composed of Eudragit L was not the causative agent, as had been suggested in earlier reports.

Diets

As opposed to earlier treatment recommendations, fat intake should not be restricted. Restrictions of fat intake may seriously compromise caloric intake and lead to loss of body weight. In fact, fat intake should be encouraged within limits of individual tolerance during carefully balanced enzyme replacement therapy. If the latter fails to control steatorrhea, restrictions in fat intake may be imposed but should be monitored by a dietitian. Whenever appropriate, a loss in caloric intake should be compensated by a carbohydrate-enriched diet (65–70% of total daily energy intake) When feasible, both meal density and frequency should be increased (≥6).

If both enzyme replacement therapy and fat restriction fail to control steatorrhea, it has been suggested that patients may benefit from substitution of long-chain triglycerides (LCTs) by medium-chain triglycerides (MCTs), i.e., fatty acids with 6–12 carbons. A recent study, however, showed that although MCTs are absorbed better than LCTs they do require pancreatic extracts for optimal absorption [44]. No significant difference in fat absorption was observed between LCTs or MCTs during pancreatic enzyme therapy. These results make the clinical use of MCTs questionable.

Deficiencies of fat-soluble vitamins, especially vitamin A and E, are frequent despite pancreatic enzyme treatment because steatorrhea is hardly ever completely abolished [2]. Folate absorption was shown to be inhibited by pancreatic extracts, probably because of the formation of insoluble complexes [45]. In clinical practice, however, folic acid deficiency is uncommon [46]. Genuine cobalamin deficiency is extremely rare [46, 47]. Patients on pancreatic enzyme replacement therapy should avoid a fiber-enriched diet. Dietary fibers are capable of altering enzyme activity, presumably by binding of enzymes to the fiber or by the presence of enzyme inhibitors [48]. This counteracts pancreatic enzyme supplementation therapy and may result in an increase in fecal weight and fecal fat excretion [49].

Failure of Treatment

If treatment fails there are several causes that should be considered. A common reason for treatment failure is prescription of a dose of pancreatic enzymes that is too low. Moreover, ignorance of patients with respect to the proper use of enzyme medication should not be underestimated. Patient compliance can be an issue, because some patients feel embarrassed about taking multiple capsules during each meal. For patient education, the help of an experienced dietitian is indispensable. Acidic inactivation of pancreatic enzymes is probably the most important reason for failure of therapy. We have already discussed how to deal with it. Last but not least, other (concomitant) diseases that may lead to maldigestion and steatorrhea should be considered, such as celiac disease and bacterial overgrowth [50, 51].

Future Expectations and Areas for Research

Modification/Adaptation of Presently Available Enzyme Preparations

The optimum pH level for liberation of enzyme activity from the enteric coat of the mini-dose-unit preparations is difficult to set. Theoretically, this should happen at a pH level that is present in the duodenum postprandially in health. In chronic pancreatitis, however, the intragastric pH is lower and periods during which the intraduodenal pH is below 4.0 are longer compared with those in healthy volunteers [12–16]. If the threshold at which the enteric coat dissolves is set too low, pancreatic enzymes may be released prematurely because of a transient rise of the (intragastric) pH, especially as a result of acidic buffering by food, and be irreversibly inactivated when the intraluminal pH subsequently drops below 4.0. If the threshold at which the enteric coat dissolves is set too high, pancreatic enzymes are released beyond the proximal jejunum, and absorption of nutrients is impaired [52]. An in vitro study showed that there are marked differences between commercially available enzyme preparations concerning the properties of the enteric coat [53]. All preparations prevented release of enzyme activity below pH 4.0 but the dissolution profiles (pH level at which enzyme release starts and the rate of dissolution) varied significantly. Instead of using one preparation for all causes of exocrine pancreatic insufficiency, fine-tuning of the properties of the enteric coat for chronic pancreatitis and cystic fibrosis may improve treatment efficacy. A mixture of enteric-coated mini-dose-units with various pH dissolution profiles may ensure optimal availability of enzymes to all components of a meal.

Other Sources of Lipase

For decades the source of commercial pancreatic enzyme preparations has been pancreatin, an alcoholic extract obtained mainly from porcine pancreatic glands. Its composition resembles that of the human pancreas. Since porcine pancreatic lipase is vulnerable to acidic inactivation and proteolytic denaturation, the search for other sources of lipase has received more and more attention in the past few years. The ideal lipase should not be inactivated by acid or proteases, should be independent of co-lipase, and should maintain activity at low to physiological levels of bile salts. Fungal lipase is more resistant to acidic and proteolytic degradation than porcine lipase but is inactivated by bile salts and offers no significant reduction of steatorrhea [22, 54, 55]. The use of bacterial lipase seems to more promising. The superior properties of bacterial lipase (secreted by *Burkholderia plantasii*, previously called *Pseudomonas Glumae*, during fermentation) over porcine lipase were shown in a series of gastric and duodenal incubation studies [56]. Assays of enzyme activity of porcine and bacterial lipase in both gastric and duodenal juice were performed under various conditions: with and without nutrients, different lipase concentrations, different pH levels, and in the case of duodenal juice different bile acid concentrations. Compared with that of porcine lipase, survival of bacterial lipase was significantly higher at intragastric conditions present postprandially. Also, intraduodenal bacterial lipase activity was much greater in postprandial conditions known to be present in patients with exocrine pancreatic insufficiency, and bacterial lipase was not inactivated by bile salts. The promising results of this in vitro study encouraged the same group to conduct a study in pancreatic duct-ligated dogs to investigate the in vivo effects of different doses and formulations of bacterial lipase and diets on steatorrhea [57]. Diets varied in their relative composition of fat, protein, and carbohydrate. Powdered bacterial lipase increased fat absorption in a dose-dependent fashion. Interestingly, the amount of fat absorbed in response to powdered bacterial lipase correlated highly with increasing percentage of fat calories in meals. These are, as the authors state, iconoclastic results, because for a long time physicians and patients tended to keep fat intake as low as possible to avoid symptoms associated with steatorrhea. A logical step would be to conduct a trial to assess the efficacy of bacterial lipase in human subjects. However, treatment of maldigestion should not be limited to correction of fat maldigestion. Impaired digestion of proteins and starch should be treated with proteolytic enzymes and amylase. Further studies are needed to determine the optimal treatment regimen with respect to composition of such a new enzyme preparation and the optimal dietary recommendations.

Gene Therapy

The most exciting prospects for the treatment of exocrine pancreatic insufficiency are those supplied by gene therapy. These are not just theoretical possibilities anymore. In an exciting article in *Gastroenterology* in 1994, Meada et al. investigated the feasibility of adenovirus vector-mediated transfer of human pancreatic complementary DNA (AdCMV.lip) by in vitro infection to a human gallbladder epithelial cell line and by ex vivo infection to freshly excised sheep gallbladder [58]. Their choice of the single-layer gallbladder epithelium as the primary target for the human complementary DNA was based on several considerations. First, adenovirus will infect most epithelia, and the slow renewal rate of the gallbladder epithelium may minimize the need for repeat treatment. Second, its release from the gallbladder into the duodenum is triggered by the same mechanisms as the release of pancreatic juice and also occurs at the same site, the papilla of Vater in the second part of the duodenum. This may ensure conditions that best approximate the normal physiology of upper gastrointestinal digestive events and their timing. The results of this study were exciting. Supernatants from a human gallbladder epithelial cell line infected with AdCMV.lip showed lipase activity up to 14 days after infection, whereas sham-infected epithelial cells did not. Fluid from intact sheep gallbladders infected with AdCMV.lip showed a significant 15-fold increase in lipase activity as compared with sham-infected gallbladders. Although promising, these are preliminary experiments only. For one thing, the amount of enzyme activity recovered was very low and far below levels needed for treatment of exocrine pancreatic insufficiency. Clinical implementation of gene therapy for exocrine pancreatic insufficiency still has a long way to go, and there are many obstacles to be overcome [59]. The first practical point is how to get human pancreatic lipase cDNA to its target in vivo. Direct installation into the gallbladder is cumbersome, especially when there is need for repeat treatments. Obviously, the need for repeat treatment should be as infrequent as possible, and expression of the human pancreatic lipase cDNA must be high enough to reach adequate levels of enzyme activity in the small bowel, in order to abolish signs and symptoms of pancreatic maldigestion. Put more practically , many patients do not have a gallbladder because they have undergone cholecystectomy, and others have an abnormal gallbladder (function), such as some patients with cystic fibrosis who have microgallbladders. Therefore, other target areas must also be investigated. Enterocytes may prove to be an alternative.

In conclusion, the treatment of exocrine pancreatic insufficiency has come a long way. Due to a better understanding of the (patho)physiology of the exocrine pancreas, together with the development of high-strength enteric-coated mini-dose-unit preparations, we are at a point in time where many patients can be treated satisfactorily. However, there is still room for improvement. New and exciting developments already are taking place which ultimately will revolutionize the management of exocrine pancreatic insufficiency.

References

1. DiMagno EP, Layer P, Clain JE (1993) Chronic pancreatitis. In: Go VLW, DiMagno EP, Gardner JD, Lebenthal E, Reber HA, Scheele GA (eds) The pancreas: biology, pathobiology, and disease, 2nd edn. Raven, New York, pp 665–706
2. Dutta SK, Bustin MP, Russell RM, Costa BS (1982) Deficiency of fat-soluble vitamins in treated patients with pancreatic insufficiency. Ann Intern Med 97:549–552
3. Montalto G, Soresi M, Carroccio A, et al (1994) Lipoproteins and chronic pancreatitis. Pancreas 9:137–138
4. Gullo L, Stella A, Labriola E, Costa PL, Descovich G, Labo G (1982) Cardiovascular lesions in chronic pancreatitis: a prospective study. Dig Dis Sci 27:716–722
5. Gullo L, Tassoni U, Mazzoni G, Stefanini F (1996) Increased prevalence of aortic calcification in chronic pancreatitis. Am J Gastroenterol 91:759–761
6. Layer P, Go VL, DiMagno EP (1986) Fate of pancreatic enzymes during small intestinal aboral transit in humans. Am J Physiol 251:G475–G480
7. DiMagno EP, Malagelada JR, Go VL, Moertel CG (1977) Fate of orally ingested enzymes in pancreatic insufficiency. Comparison of two dosage schedules. N Engl J Med 296:1318–1322
8. Heizer WD, Cleaveland CR, Iber FL (1965) Gastric inactivation of pancreatic supplements. Bull John Hopkins Hosp 116:261–270
9. Thiruvengadam R, DiMagno EP (1988) Inactivation of human lipase by proteases. Am J Physiol 255:G476–G481
10. Regan PT, Malagelada JR, DiMagno EP, Glanzman SL, Go VL (1977) Comparative effects of antacids, cimetidine and enteric coating on the therapeutic response to oral enzymes in severe pancreatic insufficiency. N Engl J Med 297:854–858
11. DiMagno EP, Go VL Summerskill WH (1973) Relations between pancreatic enzyme outputs and malabsorption in severe pancreatic insufficiency. N Engl J Med 288:813–815
12. Bovo P, Cataudella G, Di Francesco V, et al (1995) Intraluminal gastric pH in chronic pancreatitis. Gut 36:294–298
13. Regan PT, Malagelada JR, DiMagno EP, Go VL (1979) Postprandial gastric function in pancreatic insufficiency. Gut 20:249–254
14. Dutta SK, Russell RM, Iber FL (1979) Impaired acid neutralization in the duodenum in pancreatic insufficiency. Dig Dis Sci 24:775–780
15. Dutta SK, Russell RM, Iber FL (1979) Influence of exocrine pancreatic insufficiency on the intraluminal pH of the proximal small intestine. Dig Dis Sci 24:529–534
16. Andersen JR, Bendtsen F, Ovesen L, Pedersen NT, Rune SJ, Tage-Jensen U (1990) Pancreatic insufficiency. Duodenal and jejunal pH, bile acid activity, and micellar lipid solubilization. Int J Pancreatol 6:263–270
17. Zentler-Munro PL, Fitzpatrick WJ, Batten JC, Northfield TC (1984) Effect of intrajejunal acidity on aqueous phase bile acid and lipid concentrations in pancreatic steatorrhoea due to cystic fibrosis. Gut 25:500–507

18. DiMagno EP (1982) Controversies in the treatment of exocrine pancreatic insufficiency. Dig Dis Sci 27:481–484
19. Bruno MJ, Rauws EA, Hoek FJ, Tytgat GN (1994) Comparative effects of adjuvant cimetidine and omeprazole during pancreatic enzyme replacement therapy. Dig Dis Sci 39:988–992
20. Graham DY (1979) An enteric-coated pancreatic enzyme preparation that works. Dig Dis Sci 24:906–909
21. Dutta SK, Tilley DK (1983) The pH-sensitive enteric-coated pancreatic enzyme preparations: an evaluation of therapeutic efficacy in adult patients with pancreatic insufficiency. J Clin Gastroenterol 5:51–54
22. Schneider MU, Knoll-Ruzicka ML, Domschke S, Heptner G, Domschke W (1985) Pancreatic enzyme replacement therapy: comparative effects of conventional and enteric-coated microspheric pancreatin and acid-stable fungal enzyme preparations on steatorrhoea in chronic pancreatitis. Hepatogastroenterology 32:97–102
23. Lankisch PG, Lembcke B, Goke B, Creutzfeldt W (1986) Therapy of pancreatogenic steatorrhoea: does acid protection of pancreatic enzymes offer any advantage? Z Gastroenterol 24:753–757
24. Dutta SK, Rubin J, Harvey J (1983) Comparative evaluation of the therapeutic efficacy of a pH-sensitive enteric-coated pancreatic enzyme preparation with conventional pancreatic enzyme therapy in the treatment of exocrine pancreatic insufficiency. Gastroenterology 84:476–482
25. Jorgensen BB, Pedersen NT, Worning H (1991) Monitoring the effect of substitution therapy in patients with exocrine pancreatic insufficiency. Scand J Gastroenterol 26:321–326
26. Delhaye M, Meuris S, Gohimont AC, Buedts K, Cremer M (1996) Comparative evaluation of a high lipase pancreatic enzyme preparation and a standard pancreatic supplement for treating exocrine pancreatic insufficiency in chronic pancreatitis. Eur J Gastroenterol Hepatol 8:699–703
27. Lamers CB, Jansen JB (1986) Omeprazole as adjunct to enzyme replacement treatment in severe pancreatic insufficiency. Br Med J 293:994–994
28. Youngberg CA, Bernardi RR, Howatt WF (1987) Comparison of gastrointestinal pH in cystic fibrosis and healthy subjects. Dig Dis Sci 32:472–480
29. Meyer JH, Elashoff J, Porter-Fink V, Dressman J, Amidon GL (1988) Human postprandial gastric emptying of 1- to 3-millimeter spheres. Gastroenterology 94:1315–1325
30. Mundlos S, Kuhnelt P, Adler G (1990) Monitoring enzyme replacement treatment in exocrine pancreatic insufficiency using the cholesteryl octanoate breath test. Gut 31:1324–1328
31. Kuhnelt P, Mundlos S, Adler G (1991) Effect of pellet size of a pancreas enzyme preparation on duodenal lipolytic activity. Z Gastroenterol 29:417–421
32. Bruno MJ, Borm JJ, Hoek FJ, et al (1998) Gastric transit and pharmacodynamics of a two-millimeter enteric-coated pancreatin microsphere preparation in patients with chronic pancreatitis. Dig Dis Sci 43:203–213
33. Gottschalk B, Wiesemann HG, Stephan U (1988) Comparison of 2 pancreatic enzyme preparations in the treatment of digestive insufficiency in mucoviscidosis (cystic fibrosis). Monatsschr Kinderheilkd 136:626–629
34. Stern M, Plettner C, Gruttner R (1988) Pancreatic enzyme replacement in mucoviscidosis (CF): clinical evaluation of a gastric acid-resistant pancreatin preparation in encapsulated microtablet form. Klin Padiatr 200:36–39
35. Lankisch PG, Lembcke B, Kirchhoff S, Hilgers R, Creutzfeldt W (1988) Therapy of pancreatogenic steatorrhea. Comparison of 2 acid-protected enzyme preparations. Dtsch Med Wochenschr 113:15–17
36. Beverley DW, Kelleher J, MacDonald A, Littlewood JM, Robinson T, Walters MP (1987) Comparison of four pancreatic extracts in cystic fibrosis. Arch Dis Child 62:564–568
37. Braggion C, Borgo G, Faggionato P, Mastella G (1987) Influence of antacid and formulation on effectiveness of pancreatic enzyme supplementation in cystic fibrosis. Arch Dis Child 62:349–356
38. Williams J, MacDonald A, Weller PH, Fields J, Pandov H (1990) Two enteric-coated microspheres in cystic fibrosis. Arch Dis Child 65:594–597
39. Thomson M, Clague A, Cleghorn GJ, Shepherd RW (1993) Comparative in vitro and in vivo studies of enteric-coated pancrelipase preparations for pancreatic insufficiency. J Pediatr Gastroenterol Nutr 17:407–413
40. Bruno MJ, Haverkort EB, Tytgat GN, van Leeuwen DJ (1995) Maldigestion associated with exocrine pancreatic insufficiency: implications of gastrointestinal physiology and

properties of enzyme preparations for a cause-related and patient-tailored treatment. Am J Gastroenterol 90:1383–1393
41. Ramo OJ, Puolakkainen PA, Seppala K, Schroder TM (1989) Self-administration of enzyme substitution in the treatment of exocrine pancreatic insufficiency. Scand J Gastroenterol 24:688–692
42. Smyth RL, van Velzen D, Smyth AR, Lloyd DA, Heaf DP (1994) Strictures of ascending colon in cystic fibrosis and high-strength pancreatic enzymes. Lancet 343:85–86
43. FitzSimmons SC, Burkhart GA, Borowitz D, et al (1997) High-dose pancreatic-enzyme supplements and fibrosing colonopathy in children with cystic fibrosis. N Engl J Med 336:1283–1289
44. Caliari S, Benini L, Sembenini C, Gregori B, Carnielli V, Vantini I (1996) Medium-chain triglyceride absorption in patients with pancreatic insufficiency. Scand J Gastroenterol 31:90–94
45. Russell RM, Dutta SK, Oaks EV, Rosenberg IH, Giovetti AC (1980) Impairment of folic acid absorption by oral pancreatic extracts. Dig Dis Sci 25:369–373
46. Glasbrenner B, Malfertheiner P, Büchler M, Kuhn K, Ditschuneit H (1991) Vitamin B_{12} and folic acid deficiency in chronic pancreatitis: a relevant disorder? Klin Wochenschr 69:168–172
47. Henderson JT, Simpson JD, Warwick RR, Shearman DJ (1972) Does malabsorption of vitamin B_{12} occur in chronic pancreatitis? Lancet 2:241–243
48. Leng-Peschlow E (1989) Interference of dietary fibres with gastrointestinal enzymes in vitro. Digestion 44:200–210
49. Dutta SK, Hlasko J (1985) Dietary fiber in pancreatic disease: effect of high fiber diet on fat malabsorption in pancreatic insufficiency and in vitro study of the interaction of dietary fiber with pancreatic enzymes. Am J Clin Nutr 41:517–525
50. Regan PT, DiMagno EP (1980) Exocrine pancreatic insufficiency in celiac sprue: a cause of treatment failure. Gastroenterology 78:484–487
51. Lembcke B, Kraus B, Lankisch PG (1985) Small intestinal function in chronic relapsing pancreatitis. Hepatogastroenterology 32:149–151
52. Guarner L, Rodriguez R, Guarner F, Malagelada JR (1993) Fate of oral enzymes in pancreatic insufficiency. Gut 34:708–712
53. Gan KH, Geus WP, Bakker W, Lamers CB, Heijerman HG (1996) In vitro dissolution profiles of enteric-coated microsphere/microtablet pancreatin preparations at different pH values. Aliment Pharmacol Ther 10:771–775
54. Zentler-Munro PL, Assoufi BA, Balasubramanian K, et al (1992) Therapeutic potential and clinical efficacy of acid-resistant fungal lipase in the treatment of pancreatic steatorrhoea due to cystic fibrosis. Pancreas 7:311–319
55. Moreau J, Bouisson M, Saint MGM, Pignal F, Bommelaer G, Ribet A (1988) Comparison of fungal lipase and pancreatic lipase in exocrine pancreatic insufficiency in man. Study of their in vitro properties and intraduodenal bioavailability. Gastroenterol Clin Biol 12:787–792
56. Raimondo M, DiMagno EP (1994) Lipolytic activity of bacterial lipase survives better than that of porcine lipase in human gastric and duodenal content. Gastroenterology 107:231–235
57. Suzuki A, Mizumoto A, Sarr MG, DiMagno EP (1997) Bacterial lipase and high-fat diets in canine exocrine pancreatic insufficiency: a new therapy of steatorrhea? Gastroenterology 112:2048–2055
58. Maeda H, Danel C, Crystal RG (1994) Adenovirus-mediated transfer of human lipase complementary DNA to the gallbladder. Gastroenterology 106:1638–1644
59. Ramakrishna J, Grand RJ (1994) Gene therapy for exocrine pancreatic insufficiency. Gastroenterology 106:1711–1713

CHAPTER 13

Mechanisms of Fibrosis and Potential Antifibrotic Agents

A. Menke, R. Vogelmann, M. Bachem, and G. Adler

Introduction

Fibrosis is a pathological process resulting from injury and can occur in any organ. The biological cause of fibrosis is the accumulation of excessive amounts of extracellular matrix, leading to tissue dysfunction and organ failure. There is a growing body of evidence for the concept that fibrosis represents a dysregulation of the normal repair process following tissue injury [1, 2]. This idea is based on the overwhelming evidence that fibrosis and tissue repair involve similar biological reactions regulated by the same group of molecules. The best-characterized example for these molecules are the members of the transforming growth factor beta family (TGFβ) [3].

TGFβ_1 represents the prototype of this family of highly similar growth factors with the unique ability to stimulate the expression and deposition of extracellular matrix. This seems to be propagated by four separate but simultaneous effects. TGFβ enhances expression of all important ECM proteins including collagen, fibronectin, and proteoglycans. At the same time, this growth factor inhibits the degradation of ECM by blocking the secretion of proteases and the stimulation of protase inhibitor production. Furthermore, TGFβ is able to modulate the concentration of integrins, the most important cellular matrix receptors, and alters cell-matrix adhesion and by this process also the matrix deposition. Finally, TGFβ induces its own production and the expression of its own receptors, causing a high amplification of its biological actions. All these effects leading to fibrosis have been demonstrated in several types of cultured cells. In the review presented here we summarize the data regarding the influence of different growth factors, but mainly TGFβ, on the fibrogenic process during pancreatitis, and we discuss potential antifibrotic strategies.

Pancreatitis

Pancreatitis is characterized by inflammation, acinar and ductal cell injury, and fibrosis. In the affected areas proliferation of fibroblasts and production of collagen can be observed, resulting in a transient or persistent fibrosis.

The connective tissue which replaces parts of the pancreas is the result of increased biosynthesis and deposition but reduced destruction of extracellular matrix proteins, namely collagens type I and III, fibronectin, and to a lesser extent, collagen type IV and laminin. The importance of collagen turnover during pancreatitis was demonstrated by measuring the procollagen type III peptide (PIIINP), which is released during extracellular polymerization of collagen type III fibers. Serum levels of this peptide may be a useful marker for monitoring the inflammatory process within the pancreas [4].

The identification of pancreatic stellate cells (PSC), named for their structural and functional similarities to hepatic stellate cells, represents an important step in understanding the fibrotic reaction in pancreatic regeneration. These myofibroblast-like cells, in connection with normal fibroblasts, seem to be responsible for the production of collagen types I and III, laminin, and fibronectin in the regeneration from acute pancreatitis and in the development of chronic fibrosis of the pancreas [5, 6].

In addition to the production of ECM proteins, the collagen content is regulated by degradative events. Matrix metalloproteases (MMPs) as well as their natural inhibitors (TIMPs) are involved in this coordinated turnover. The family of MMPs now contains 17 known members, all characterized by a zinc ion in their catalytic center [7]. During regeneration after experimentally induced acute pancreatitis in rats MMP2 (the 72-kDa collagenase type IV) and MMP3 (stromelysin) were overexpressed; this was accompanied by a parallel rise in transcript levels of TIMP2, the MMP2 inhibitor. In correlation with the expression data, MMP2 and MMP3 activities detected by zymography were elevated in the regenerative process. Thus, MMP2 and MMP3 seem to be involved in the removal of extracellular matrix during regeneration from acute pancreatitis [8].

In contrast to acute pancreatitis, which is characterized by succeeding degradation of the extracellular matrix and complete functional and structural regeneration after a few weeks [9, 10], chronic pancreatitis is a progressive inflammatory disease in which irreversible morphological damage and loss of organ-function are accompanied by continuous fibrosis [11, 12]. At present, the mechanisms leading to the fibrotic events remain unclear. One postulate is that relapsing attacks of acute pancreatitis may result in a chronic form, suggesting a relationship between acute and chronic pancreatitis [11, 13]. In chronic pancreatitis, only MMP2 and its inhibitor TIMP2 were reported to be overexpressed, while neither MMP1 nor MMP3 expression was changed [14]. The reduced expression of degradative enzymes may contribute to the differences between acute and chronic pancreatitis.

TGFβ in Acute and Chronic Pancreatitis

The basic cellular mechanisms triggering the development of transient or progressive fibrosis are not very well understood. Mediators of fibrotic events during regeneration in many tissues such as liver, kidney, and skin are the transforming growth factors beta (TGFβ) [15–17]. An overproduction of

TGFβ_1 is thought to play a key role in idiopathic lung fibrosis, liver cirrhosis, glomerulosclerosis, and cardiac fibrosis. In most diseases of the pancreas, such as acute or chronic pancreatitis and pancreatic cancer, enhanced concentrations of TGFβ_1 were also found.

TGFβ_{1-3} – the three isoforms in mammals – are highly conserved and interchangeable in most biological assays [18]. TGFβ stimulates the transcription and synthesis of extracellular matrix proteins. Additionally, it is involved in the regulation of cell proliferation [19]. The ability of TGFβ to induce gene expression, leading to increased extracellular matrix deposition during the regeneration of different organs, has been characterized by many groups.

The low constitutive expression of TGFβ_{1-3} in normal pancreas and its overexpression in acute and chronic pancreatitis, as well as in different experimental models for these diseases, has been demonstrated in conjunction with increased deposition of collagen and other ECM components [20, 21]. Expression of TGFβ_1 is more extensively distributed throughout the ductular epithelium and also in mononuclear cells in chronic pancreatitis, as compared with normal tissue. In obstructive chronic pancreatitis, all ductular cells adjacent to the lesions were stained, while in unaffected regions distant from the sites of obstruction, only single cells were stained [22, 23]. In all studies so far, TGFβ_1 has not been expressed in interstitial fibroblasts.

Only very few data are available regarding TGFβ overexpression in human acute pancreatitis [21, 24]. In tissue samples taken after cerulein-induced acute pancreatitis in rats a very early increase (12–24 h) in TGFβ transcription and secretion was shown. In situ hybridization revealed acinar and ductal cells as sources for TGFβ production in pancreatitis [20, 25, 26].

TGFβ in the Development of Pancreatic Fibrosis

The enhanced concentration of TGFβ in pancreatic diseases, including acute and chronic pancreatitis and pancreatic cancer, is paralleled by elevated production and deposition of extracellular matrix. The detailed mechanisms by which TGFβ_1 is involved in the regulation of ECM turnover are barely understood. Whether TGFβ exerts its effects by direct or indirect mechanisms is the subject of controversy. Recently, the connective tissue growth factor (CTGF) was described as a factor acting downstream of TGFβ and responsible for the enhanced production of ECM, even in the pancreas [27, 28]. Although an increase in gene transcription of type-I collagen and some other matrix proteins has been observed, post-transcriptional and post-translational regulatory events have not been ruled out. It is also suggested that the stimulated proliferation of fibroblasts by TGFβ is responsible for the enhanced ECM production, rather than having a direct influence on collagen expression [29]. Furthermore, there are data supporting the idea that TGFβ_1 reduces the expression of extracellular matrix degrading proteases (MMPs) [30]. Administration of TGFβ together with repeated induction of pancreatitis by cerulein promotes the development of extensive fibrosis. The transgenic production of TGFβ_1 in pancreatic islet cells of mice results in continuous pancreatic inflammation and progressive accumulation of ECM. These transgenic pancreata are affected by multifocal fibrosis, characterized by an enormous deposition of collagen, fibronectin, and elastin fibers replacing the acinar tissue [31, 32]. Following the same line of evidence, it is reported that the hepatic expression of mature TGFβ_1 not only results in hepatic fibrosis but also elevates TGFβ_1 levels in serum and produces a mild pancreatic fibrosis [33, 34]. Many aspects of the phenotype developed in the TGFβ_1-transgenic mouse are reminiscent of chronic pancreatitis. Interestingly, animals transgenic for TGFα, which is not associated with fibrotic reactions, also develop a prominent pancreatic fibrosis [35, 36].

The recently described pancreatic stellate cells (PSC) may represent the target cells of the elevated TGFβ_1 concentrations in the transgenic mouse model as well as in pancreatitis. As described for the hepatic stellate cells, TGFβ stimulates PSC to produce large amounts of collagen and fibronectin. Interestingly, not only TGFβ but also basic FGF and – less effectively – PDGF and TGFα stimulated fibronectin mRNA and protein concentrations in isolated PSC [37].

Before a causal link can be postulated between PSC and pancreatic fibrosis, further analyses are required to find out how TGFβ_1 and other peptide growth factors influence the matrix production in the pancreas.

Antifibrotic Treatment

Progressive fibrosis represents a major clinical problem in various diseases. Different strategies have been developed or are under current investigation to influence the development of fibrosis. Besides pharmacological intervention in the process of collagen synthesis and fibrillogenesis, the manipulation of collagen gene expression seems to be a worthwhile approach (Table 1).

Table 1. Potential antifibrotic agents

Mediators	Modulators
Interferon α, β, and γ	Growth factor-binding proteins
Endothelin receptor antagonists	Modulators of collagen biosynthesis and polymerization
Prostaglandin E	Inducers of stress relaxation in fibrogenic cells
Anti-TGFβ, anti-CTGF, anti-FGF2	

TGFβ as a Therapeutic Target

There is a strong body of evidence for the hypothesis that TGFβ is a key mediator of fibrosis in both experimental and human pancreatitis. This provides a basis for choosing TGFβ as a therapeutic target for the development of an antifibrotic agent. The complex regulation of TGFβ production and activation offers a number of targets for TGFβ suppression.

The therapeutic effect of inhibiting TGFβ by numerous injections of neutralizing antibody during the early phase of acute pancreatitis has been demonstrated [20]. Three injections of anti-TGFβ antiserum, before, during, and after the cerulein infusion, resulted in reduced autocrine TGFβ production in the regenerating pancreas and, furthermore, in a significantly diminished ECM content in the disease model. Collagen type I and type III as well as fibronectin contents were reduced by about 30%, as demonstrated on mRNA, protein, and the immunofluorescence level [20].

Similar results have been reported by Border and co-workers, who described a reduction of TGFβ_1 mRNA and expression of extracellular matrix components in experimental glomerulonephritis after treatment with a neutralizing TGFβ_1 antibody and decorin [38, 39]. The proteoglycan decorin, a natural inhibitor of TGFβ_1, may be more suitable than antibodies for clinical use. Border and colleagues tested a model of decorin gene therapy to treat the experimentally induced glomerulonephritis. The background for this study was muscle-based gene therapy [40], where a decorin expression vector was injected into skeletal muscles. These cells do not integrate the cDNA into their genome, but produce the protein product and secrete it into the blood for several months. Using this approach, the authors were able to show a markedly reduced manifestation of the glomerulonephritis as compared with nontreated rats [41].

Inhibition of Collagen Synthesis and Deposition

While only a few studies have been aimed at the prevention of pancreatic fibrosis, several studies have been performed in models of liver cirrhosis and lung fibrosis. In rat models of liver fibrosis prostaglandin E, as well as interferon γ, α, and β, suppressed collagen synthesis and proliferation of fibroblasts.

The phytopharmacon silymarin is effective in reducing fibrosis, at least in liver cirrhosis, probably by inhibiting the inflammation and following proliferation of stellate cells [42, 43]. An interesting antifibrotic effect was observed using endothelin receptor antagonists in liver fibrosis. There is evidence that activation of the endothelin system is necessary for the activation of hepatic stellate cells. Schuppan and collaborators reported a moderate antifibrotic effect of oral endothelin receptor antagonists in a rat model of liver fibrosis [44].

Another plausible strategy for preventing fibrosis would be causal treatment by inhibition of collagen biosynthesis (Fig. 1). This process contains

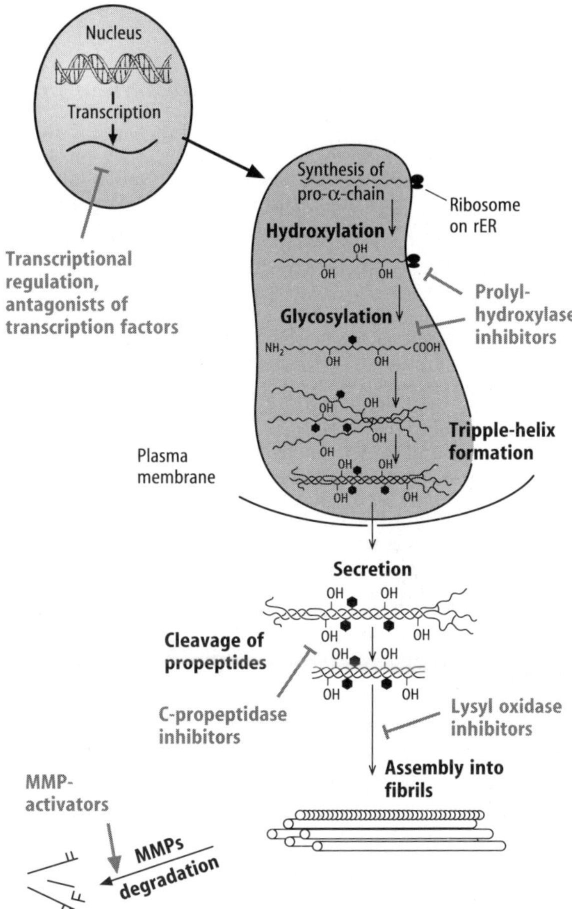

Fig. 1. Collagen biosynthesis and possible targets for antifibrotic strategies

several intracellular and extracellular post-transcriptional modifications of the proteins which represent possible therapeutic targets. First attempts were made to inhibit proline hydroxylation, a critical reaction in collagen synthesis, by inhibition of the responsible enzyme prolyl-4-hydroxylase. However, the administration of HOE 077, a specific inhibitor of this enzyme, failed to reduce the fibrotic reaction during regeneration from cerulein-induced pancreatitis in the rat model [45].

In conclusion, significant progress has been made in understanding the cellular and molecular events occurring during the induction and progression of fibrosis. However, detailed investigations are necessary to elucidate the basic regulatory events.

References

1. Border WA, Ruoslahti E (1992) Transforming growth factor-beta in disease: the dark side of tissue repair. J Clin Invest 90:1–7
2. Rodemann HP, Binder A, Burger A, Guven N, Loffler H, Bamberg M (1996) The underlying cellular mechanism of fibrosis. Kidney Int Suppl 54:S32–36
3. Roberts AB, Heine UI, Flanders KC, Sporn MB (1990) Transforming growth factor-beta. Major role in regulation of extracellular matrix. Ann N Y Acad Sci 580:225–232
4. Adler G, Kropf J, Grobe E, Gressner AM (1990) Follow-up of the serum levels of extracellular matrix components in acute and chronic pancreatitis. Eur J Clin Invest 20:494–501
5. Bachem MG, Schneider E, Gross H, Weidenbach H, Schmid RM, Menke A, Siech M, Beger H, Grünert A, Adler G (1998) Identification, culture, and characterization of pancreatic stellate cells in rats and humans. Gastroenterology 115:421–432
6. Kato Y, Inoue H, Fujiyama Y, Bamba T (1996) Morphological identification of and collagen synthesis by periacinar fibroblastoid cells cultured from isolated rat pancreatic acini. J Gastroenterol 31:565–571
7. Woessner JF (1994) The family of matrix metalloproteinases. Ann N Y Acad Sci 732:11–21
8. Müller-Pillasch F, Gress TM, Yamaguchi H, Adler G, Menke A (1997) The influence of transforming growth factor β1 on the expression of genes coding for extracellular matrix metalloproteinases and tissue inhibitors of metalloproteinases during regeneration from caerulein-induced pancreatitis. Pancreas 15:168–175
9. Elsässer HP, Adler G, Kern HF (1989) Fibroblast structure and function during regeneration from hormone-induced acute pancreatitis in the rat. Pancreas 4:169–178
10. Elsässer HP, Adler G, Kern HF (1986) Time course and cellular source of pancreatic regeneration following acute pancreatitis in the rat. Pancreas 1:421–429
11. DiMagno EP, Layer P, Clain JE (1993) Chronic pancreatitis. In: Go VLW, DiMagno EP, Gardner JD, Lebenthal E, Scheele GA (eds) The pancreas: biology, pathobiology, and disease. Raven, New York, pp 665–706
12. Forsmark CE, Toskes PP (1995) Chronic pancreatitis. Curr Opin Gastroenterol 11:407–413
13. Klöppel G, Maillet B (1992) The morphological basis for the evolution of acute pancreatitis into chronic pancreatitis. Virchows Archiv A Pathol Anat 420:1–4
14. Gress TM, Müller-Pillasch F, Lerch MM, Friess H, Büchler M, Beger HG, Adler G (1994) Balance of expression of genes coding for extracellular matrix proteins and extracellular matrix degrading proteases in chronic pancreatitis. Z Gastroenterol 32:221–225
15. Bachem MG, Meyer D, Melchior R, Sell KM, Gressner AM (1992) Activation of rat liver perisinusoidal lipocytes by transforming growth factors derived from myofibroblast-like cells. A potential mechanism of self-perpetuation in liver fibrogenesis. J Clin Invest 89:19–27
16. Border WA (1994) Transforming growth factor-beta and the pathogenesis of glomerular diseases. Curr Opin Nephrol Hypertens 3:54–58
17. Shah M, Foreman DM, Ferguson MW (1994) Neutralising antibody to TGF-beta 1,2 reduces cutaneous scarring in adult rodents. J Cell Sci 107:1137–1157
18. Sporn MB, Roberts AB (1992) Transforming growth factor-β: recent progress and new challenges. J Cell Biol 119:1017–1021
19. Roberts AB, Flanders KC, Heine UI, Jakowlew S, Kondaiah P, Kim SJ, Sporn MB (1990) Transforming growth factor-beta: multifunctional regulator of differentiation and development. Philos Trans R Soc Lond B Biol Sci 327:145–154
20. Menke A, Yamaguchi H, Gress TM, Adler G (1997) Extracellular matrix is reduced by inhibition of transforming growth factor β1 in pancreatitis in the rat. Gastroenterology 113:295–303
21. Friess H, Lu Z, Riesle E, Uhl W, Brundler AM, Horvath L, Gold LI, Korc M, Büchler MW (1998) Enhanced expression of TGF-betas and their receptors in human acute pancreatitis. Ann Surg 227:95–104
22. Slater SD, Williamson RC, Foster CS (1995) Expression of transforming growth factor-beta 1 in chronic pancreatitis. Digestion 56:237–241
23. van Laethem JL, Deviere J, Resibois A, Rickaert F, Vertongen P, Ohtani H, Cremer M, Miyazono K, Robberecht P (1995) Localization of transforming growth factor β1 and its latent binding protein in human chronic pancreatitis. Gastroenterology 108:1873–1881
24. Berberat P, Friess H, Uhl W, Schilling M, Zimmermann A, Büchler MW (1997) Is TGF-beta a repair and regeneration promotor after acute pancreatitis? Langenbecks Arch Chir Suppl Kongressbd 114:387–393

25. Gress TM, Müller-Pillasch F, Elsässer HP, Bachem M, Ferrara C, Weidenbach H, Lerch M, Adler G (1994) Enhancement of transforming growth factor beta 1 expression in the rat pancreas during regeneration from caerulein-induced pancreatitis. Eur J Clin Invest 24:679–685
26. Riesle E, Friess H, Zhao L, Wagner M, Uhl W, Baczako K, Gold LI, Korc M, Büchler MW (1997) Increased expression of transforming growth factor beta s after acute oedematous pancreatitis in rats suggests a role in pancreatic repair. Gut 40:73–79
27. Grotendorst GR (1997) Connective tissue growth factor: a mediator of TGF-beta action on fibroblasts. Cytokine Growth Factor Rev 8:171–179
28. Wenger C, Ellenrieder V, Alber B, Lacher U, Menke A, Hameister H, Wilda M, Iwamura T, Beger HG, Adler G, Gress TM (1999) Expression and differential regulation of connective tissue growth factor in pancreatic cancer cells. Oncogene 18:1073–1080
29. Robey PG, Young MF, Flanders KC, Roche NS, Kondaiah P, Reddi AH, Termine JD, Sporn MB, Roberts AB (1987) Osteoblasts synthesize and respond to transforming growth factor-type beta (TGF-beta) in vitro. J Cell Biol 105:457–463
30. Kerr LD, Miller DB, Matrisian LM (1990) TGF-β1 inhibition of transin/stromelysin gene expression is mediated through a fos binding sequence. Cell 61:267–278
31. Sanvito F, Nichols A, Herrera PL, Huarte J, Wohlwend A, Vassalli JD, Orci L (1995) TGF-beta 1 overexpression in murine pancreas induces chronic pancreatitis and, together with TNF-alpha, triggers insulin-dependent diabetes. Biochem Biophys Res Commun 217:1279–1286
32. Lee MS, Gu D, Feng L, Curriden S, Arnush M, Krahl T, Gurushanthaiah D, Wilson C, Loskutoff DL, Fox H, et al (1995) Accumulation of extracellular matrix and developmental dysregulation in the pancreas by transgenic production of transforming growth factor-beta 1. Am J Pathol 147:42–52
33. Sanderson N, Factor V, Nagy P, Kopp J, Kondaiah P, Wakefield L, Roberts AB, Sporn MB, Thorgeirsson SS (1995) Hepatic expression of mature transforming growth factor beta 1 in transgenic mice results in multiple tissue lesions. Proc Natl Acad Sci U S A 92:2572–2576
34. Kopp JB, Factor VM, Mozes M, Nagy P, Sanderson N, Bottinger EP, Klotman PE, Thorgeirsson SS (1996) Transgenic mice with increased plasma levels of TGF-beta 1 develop progressive renal disease. Lab Invest 74:991–1003
35. Sandgren EP, Luetteke NC, Palmiter RD, Brinster RL, Lee DC (1990) Overexpression of TGFα in transgenic mice: induction of epithelial hyperplasia, pancreatic metaplasia, and carcinoma of the breast. Cell 61:1121–1135
36. Jhappan C, Stahle C, Harkins RN, Fausto N, Smith GH, Merlino GT (1990) TGFα overexpression in transgenic mice induces liver neoplasia and abnormal development of the mammary gland and pancreas. Cell 61:1137–1146
37. Hahn SA, Bartsch D, Schroers A, Galehdari H, Becker M, Ramaswamy A, Schwarte-Waldhoff I, Maschek H, Schmiegel W (1998) Mutations of the DPC4/Smad4 gene in biliary tract carcinoma. Cancer Res 58:1124–1126
38. Border WA, Noble NA, Yamamoto T, Harper JR, Yamaguchi Yu, Pierschbacher MD, Ruoslahti E (1992) Natural inhibitor of transforming growth factor-beta protects against scarring in experimental kidney disease. Nature 360:361–364
39. Border WA, Okuda S, Languino LR, Sporn MB, Ruoslahti E (1990) Suppression of experimental glomerulonephritis by antiserum against transforming growth factor beta 1. Nature 346:371–374
40. Blau HM, Springer ML (1995) Muscle-mediated gene therapy. N Engl J Med 333:1554–1556
41. Isaka Y, Brees DK, Ikegaya K, Kaneda Y, Imai E, Noble NA, Border WA (1996) Gene therapy by skeletal muscle expression of decorin prevents fibrotic disease in rat kidney. Nat Med 2:418–423
42. Fuchs EC, Weyhenmeyer R, Weiner OH (1997) Effects of silibinin and of a synthetic analogue on isolated rat hepatic stellate cells and myofibroblasts. Arzneimittelforschung 47:1383–1387
43. Boigk G, Stroedter L, Herbst H, Waldschmidt J, Riecken EO, Schuppan D (1997) Silymarin retards collagen accumulation in early and advanced biliary fibrosis secondary to complete bile duct obliteration in rats. Hepatology 26:643–649
44. Cho JJ, Boigk G, Hocher B, Rühl M, Somasundaram R, Riecken EO, Schuppan D (1998) Deletäre Auswirkungen einer Blockierung des ET-1/WTA-Rezeptorsystems bei der sekundären biliären Zirrhose der Ratte. Z Gastroenterol 36:769
45. Weidenbach H, Lerch MM, Turi S, Bachem M, Adler G (1997) Failure of a prolyl 4-hydroxylase inhibitor to alter extracellular matrix deposition during experimental pancreatitis. Digestion 58:50–57

CHAPTER 14

Mechanisms of Pain and its Medical Management, Including Neurolytic Treatments

L. Gullo

Introduction

Pain is the most frequent and most important symptom in patients with chronic pancreatitis [1, 2]. Usually, it is intense and recurrent, and it is the main reason for hospitalization of these patients. Medical treatment of pain is usually simple, but in some cases it is complicated or without effect, and surgery is necessary. A high percentage of these patients, generally 30%–40%, are operated on for pain [1, 2]. While the clinical characteristics of this symptom are well known, the mechanisms responsible for its appearance and persistence are not completely understood. In this paper I will review the main mechanisms which are believed to be responsible for pain in chronic pancreatitis and I will discuss its medical management.

The presumed mechanisms of pain in chronic pancreatitis are increased ductal and interstitial pressure, enlarging pseudocysts, damage to pancreatic nerves, and pancreatic ischemia.

Increased Ductal and Interstitial Pressure

Several studies have shown that in patients with painful chronic pancreatitis, the pancreatic intraductal pressure is greatly elevated as compared with that of normal subjects [3–7]. In 19 patients with chronic pancreatitis and dilated pancreatic ducts who underwent surgery for pain, Bradley [4] found that the average pressure recorded in the duct of Wirsung was 35.4±3.4 cm H_2O (range 23–57 cm H_2O). In control patients the pressure was significantly lower: 14.5±1.8 cm H_2O. This investigator noted that the patients with more severe pain had higher pressure in the pancreatic duct. Furthermore, each patient with ductal dilatation and significant preoperative pain experienced dramatic relief following internal drainage of the pancreatic ductal system. Bradley concluded that, in view of the dramatic relief of pain by operative internal decompression of the pancreatic ductal system, pancreatic ductal hypertension is clearly at least one important mechanism for the production of pain in these patients with chronic pancreatitis.

Ebbehoj et al. [5–7] performed a series of studies regarding pancreatic tissue fluid pressure and pain in chronic pancreatitis. In one study of nine patients with painful chronic pancreatitis [5], the median pressure was increased in patients (27 mmHg; range 19–34 mmHg) as compared with controls (7 mmHg; range 2–13 mmHg). The drainage operations led to a 45% pressure decrease. In a 1 year follow-up study, the pressure was increased in patients with recurrent pain, and there was a significant relation between pressure and pain. The duration of the pain-free period was significantly related to the magnitude of the intraoperative pressure decrease. In another study [7], these investigators measured pancreatic tissue fluid pressure in 25 patients who had chronic pancreatitis and pain and in 14 without pain. The pressure was significantly higher in patients with pain than in those without pain. Moreover, patients with pancreatic pseudocysts had both higher pressure and a higher pain score than those without.

In our department, most of the patients with chronic pancreatitis and persistent pain who underwent Wirsung jejunostomy experienced pain relief after surgery. This effect was definitive in about 80% of them.

It is therefore clear that increased ductal and interstitial pressure is an important factor in the pathogenesis of pain in patients with chronic pancreatitis. The fact that pain tends to disappear spontaneously in the advanced phases of chronic pancreatitis [1, 2], when there is severe exocrine insufficiency, further supports the role of ductal hypertension in the pathogenesis of pain. The mechanism by which increased pressure in ducts causes pain is not clear.

Enlarging Pseudocysts

Enlarging pseudocysts are usually the cause of intense and persistent pain. We have shown that in the majority of cases, i.e., 60%, treatment with octreotide results in a reduction in size and in the eventual disappearance of the pseudocysts together with a rapid, definitive disappearance of pain [8, 9]. Increased pressure in the pseudocyst is the factor responsible for pain in these patients.

Damage to Pancreatic Nerves

Damage to the pancreatic nerves is frequent in chronic pancreatitis. An accurate description of nerve lesions in this disease was made by Bockman et al. [10]. They found that the mean diameter of the nerves was significantly greater, and the mean area of tissue served per nerve less than in controls. Foci of inflammatory cells were associated with nerves and ganglia, and there was invasion of nerve tissue by inflammatory cells. The perineural sheath was altered so that it no longer provided a barrier between the surrounding connective tissue and the internal neural components. This loss of barrier function between neural elements and the surrounding inflammatory cells was interpreted as structural evidence for a mechanism of pain generation and continuation in chronic pancreatitis [10].

In a subsequent study carried out by Büchler et al. [11], the number and diameter of intra- and interlobular nerve bundles were found to be increased in patients with chronic pancreatitis. These nerves contained a very large number of fibers staining intensely for substance P and calcitonin gene-related peptide, which are considered to be neurotransmitters of pain.

More recently, Di Sebastiano et al. [12] found that immune cell infiltration and growth-associated protein 43 expression are correlated with pain in chronic pancreatitis. These investigators studied pancreatic tissue samples from 29 patients with chronic pancreatitis operated on for pain. They found that perineural immune cell infiltration was correlated with the intensity of pain, and that growth-associated protein 43 was significantly increased in pancreatic nerve fibers and intrinsic neurons. They concluded that infiltration of pancreatic nerves by immune cells and neuronal plasticity are pathogenetic factors for the generation of pain. Based on these studies [10–12], it seems that damage to pancreatic nerves is an important factor for pain in chronic pancreatitis.

Pancreatic Ischemia

Decreased pancreatic blood flow, ischemia, and local changes in parenchymal pH are believed to contribute to pain in chronic pancreatitis [13, 14]. However, most studies in this regard have been performed using the cat, so it is difficult to extend the results to man. The fact that pain appears early in chronic pancreatitis, when the pancreatic lesions are very scarce, and tends to disappear in the advanced stages of the disease when vascular lesions and ischemia are more pronounced than in the initial phases, tends to exclude the role of this factor in the pathogenesis of pain. It was very recently shown that the administration of isosorbide mononitrate, a potent vasodilator, to chronic pancreatitis patients with pain has no analgesic effect [15].

In conclusion, of the various factors so far believed to be the cause of pain in chronic pancreatitis, increased ductal and interstitial pressure is the most likely. Damage to pancreatic nerves is also probable, but further studies are necessary to confirm this assumption.

Medical Management of Pain

Pain in chronic pancreatitis poses problems of prevention and treatment. Prevention is difficult, and there are no measures capable of reaching this objective with certainty. However, the most important measure that can be taken in alcoholic pancreatitis is the suppression of alcohol use. Generally, this tends to reduce the frequency of painful attacks and contributes to a better prognosis of the disease [1, 2]. In the nonalcoholic forms of chronic pancreatitis, the cause of pancreatitis should be identified and treated.

The treatment of pain may be a simple procedure, but in some cases it may be difficult, requiring surgery. The common analgesics are usually effective in the treatment of pain. We use the nonsteroidal anti-inflammatory drugs (ketoprofen, diclofenac) two to three times daily with good success in most cases. If these drugs are not effective, we use meperidine or pentazocine, which usually block pain. If pain is due to an enlarging pseudocyst we use octreotide, which is helpful in 60% of cases, both in relieving pain and in treating the pseudocyst [8, 9].

The use of pancreatic extracts for pain and its prevention is controversial. So far, five studies have been published; in two of these some benefit was reported [16, 17], whereas in the remaining three [18–20] no beneficial effect was found. The reason for this difference is not clear; however, it should be noted that in the first two studies an enzyme preparation in tablet form was used, whereas in the other three studies microspheres were used. Whether the type of enzyme preparation may have a role in determining its analgesic efficacy is difficult to say.

For patients whose pain persists, a celiac plexus block is a good measure. Unfortunately, there have been only a few studies on this technique, but they show that this measure is usually effective in relieving pain, at least for some months. Bell et al. [21] treated 16 patients with chronic pancreatitis and disabling abdominal pain using this procedure. They showed that severe pain recurred within 6 months of nerve block in three patients, but recurrence of pain at a later stage was not observed. Madsen and Hansen [22] performed a controlled randomized trial of celiac plexus block versus pancreaticogastrostomy for pain in 17 patients with chronic pancreatitis. They found that the celiac plexus block caused a disappearance of the pain, but this effect was short-lived. Finally, Pap et al. [23] made a comparison among analgesic, alcohol, and steroid blocks and concluded that alcohol blocks are not effective but steroid blocks often obtain several months (3–6 months) of pain-free life for the patient. These investigators concluded that repeated treatment may be effective. I believe that celiac plexus block is a good measure for patients with persistent pain and should be adopted more frequently.

There are no other effective neurolytic treatments for pain in these patients. Ballegaard et al. [24] studied the effect of acupuncture and transcutaneous electric nerve stimulation for the treatment of pain in 23 patients with chronic pancreatitis and found that neither technique brought about relief of pain that could substitute for or supplement medical treatment.

Medications that might modify neural transmission, including amitriptyline and doxepin, have been ineffective [25]. Other techniques for modifying neural transmission such as bilateral splanchnic nerve denervation, interpleural analgesia, and celiac plexus block using endoscopic ultrasonography are currently being evaluated [25].

Thus, at present, only the celiac plexus block is effective in the treatment of persistent pain. Unfortunately, the effect is of relatively brief duration. For patients in whom pain is severe and persisting or in whom there are complications, surgery should be performed. In any case, surgical treatment should be considered as a last resort, only after all medical measures have failed to relieve pain.

References

1. Gullo L, Costa PL, Labò G (1977) Chronic pancreatitis in Italy. Aetiological, clinical and histological observations based on 235 cases. Rendic Gastroenterol 9:97–104
2. Ammann RW, Akovbiantz A, Largiader F, Schueler G (1984) Course and outcome of chronic pancreatitis. Gastroenterology 86:820–828
3. Madsen R, Winkler K (1982) The intraductal pancreatic pressure in chronic obstructive pancreatitis. Scand J Gastroenterol 17:553–556
4. Bradley EL III (1982) Pancreatic duct pressure in chronic pancreatitis. Am J Surg 144:313–316
5. Ebbehoj N, Borly L, Bulow J, Rasmussen SG, Madsen P (1990) Evaluation of pancreatic tissue fluid pressure and pain in chronic pancreatitis. A longitudinal study. Scand J Gastroenterol 25:462–466
6. Ebbehoj N, Borly L, Madsen P, Matzen P (1990) Pancreatic tissue fluid pressure during drainage operations for chronic pancreatitis. Scand J Gastroenterol 25:1041–1045
7. Ebbehoj N, Borly L, Bulow J, Gronvall Rasmussen S, Madsen P, Matzen P, Owre A (1990) Pancreatic tissue fluid pressure in chronic pancreatitis. Relation to pain, morphology and function. Scand J Gastroenterol 25:1046–1051
8. Gullo L, Barbara L (1991) Treatment of pancreatic pseudocysts with octreotide. Lancet 338:540–541
9. Gullo L, Pezzilli R, De Giorgio R (1996) Effect of octreotide on pain in patients with chronic pancreatitis. Dig Surg 13:465–468
10. Bockman DE, Buchler M, Malfertheiner P, Beger HG (1988) Analysis of nerves in chronic pancreatitis. Gastroenterology 94:1459–1469
11. Buchler M, Weihe E, Friess H, Malfertheiner P, Bockman E, Muller S, Nohr D, Beger HG (1992) Changes in peptidergic innervation in chronic pancreatitis. Pancreas 7:183–192
12. Di Sebastiano P, Fink T, Weihe E, Friess H, Innocenti P, Beger HG, Buchler MW (1997) Immune cell infiltration and growth-associated protein 43 expression correlate with pain in chronic pancreatitis. Gastroenterology 112:1648–1655
13. Reber HA, Karanja ND, Alvarez C, Widdison AL, Leung FW, Ashley SW, Lutrin FJ (1992) Pancreatic blood flow in cats with chronic pancreatitis. Gastroenterology 103:652–659
14. Patel AG, Toyama MT, Alvarez C, Nguyen TN, Reber PU, Ashley SW, Reber HA (1995) Pancreatic interstitial pH in human and feline chronic pancreatitis. Gastroenterology 109:1639–1645
15. Vaquero E, Molero X, Guarner L, Malagelada JR (1998) Efecto de los donantes de oxido nitrico sobre el dolor abdominal cronico y la funcion pancreatica en pacientes con pancreatitis cronica. Rev Esp Enferm Dig 90:744
16. Isaksson G, Ihse I (1983) Pain reduction by an oral pancreatic enzyme preparation in chronic pancreatitis. Dig Dis Sci 28:97–102
17. Slaff J, Jacobson D, Tillman CR, Curington C, Toskes P (1984) Protease-specific suppression of pancreatic exocrine secretion. Gastroenterology 87:44–52
18. Halgreen H, Pederson NT, Worning H (1986) Symptomatic effect of pancreatic enzyme therapy in patients with chronic pancreatitis. Scand J Gastroenterol 21:104–108
19. Mossner J, Secknus R, Meyer J, Niederau C, Adler G (1992) Treatment of pain with pancreatic extracts in chronic pancreatitis: results of a prospective placebo-controlled multicenter trial. Digestion 53:54–66
20. Malesci A, Gaia E, Fioretta A, Bocchia G, Ciravegna P, Cantor E, Vantini I (1995) No effect of long-term treatment with pancreatic extracts on recurrent abdominal pain in patients with chronic pancreatitis. Scand J Gastroenterol 30:392–398
21. Bell SN, Cole R, Roberts-Thomson IC (1980) Coeliac plexus block for control of pain in chronic pancreatitis. Br Med J 281:1604
22. Madsen P, Hansen E (1985) Coeliac plexus block versus pancreaticogastrostomy for pain in chronic pancreatitis. A controlled randomized trial. Scand J Gastroenterol 20:1217–1220

23. Pap A, Nauss LA, DiMagno EP (1990) Is percutaneous celiac plexus block (PCPB) associated with pain relief in chronic pancreatitis? A comparison among analgesic, alcohol and steroid PCPB. Pancreas 5:725–729
24. Ballegaard S, Christophersen SJ, Gamwell Dawids S, Hesse J, Vestergaard Olsen N (1985) Acupuncture and transcutaneous electric nerve stimulation in the treatment of pain associated with chronic pancreatitis. A randomized study. Scand J Gastroenterol 20:1249–1254
25. Banks PA (1998) Acute and chronic pancreatitis. In: Feldman M, Scharschmidt BF, Sleisenger MH (eds) Gastrointestinal and liver disease, vol 1, 6th edn. Saunders, Philadelphia, pp 809–862

CHAPTER 15

Endoscopic Treatment of Pain and Complications of Chronic Pancreatitis

R. Jakobs, D. Apel, and J.F. Riemann

Introduction

Chronic pancreatitis (CP) is a common disease in industrialized countries, occurring with an incidence of approximately five to ten cases in 100,000. The main cause of this disease is alcohol abuse (app. 75%); other causes are rare (e.g., drug-induced CP). About 20%–25% of the cases are idiopathic. The resulting exocrine and less frequent endocrine pancreatic insufficiency can be controlled by medicament substitution [1]. Nevertheless, many patients suffer from recurrent pain attacks which lead to impairment of their life quality. Those severe abdominal pains comprise an important indication for surgical or endoscopic interventional therapy [2]. Furthermore, during disease progression there may be some morphological changes, such as pseudocysts and intraductal stone formation. These changes can also be cured with nonoperative measures.

The endoscopic treatment of CP has become increasingly important during the past 10 years. Techniques that were originally designed for the biliary system have recently been applied as well to the pancreatic system [2]. The indications for and up-to-date results of endoscopic interventional measures are presented in this report.

Pancreatic Duct Stricture: Pancreatic Duct Sphincterotomy, Pancreatic Duct Prosthesis

There are various theories about what causes pain in CP. One of the most accepted, but quite controversial [3], is that of increased intraductal and intraparenchymal pressure. Consequently, surgical drainage measures were developed; in the past 15 years these have been widely replaced by endoscopic techniques [4].

Candidates for endoscopic drainage are patients with so-called obstructive pancreatitis: ductal strictures or intraductal stone formation prohibit pancreatic excretion through the duct of Wirsung; this leads to fluid retention, with subsequent retrograde ductal dilatation [5]. Primary endoscopic treatment is pancreatic duct sphincterotomy (pEST). pEST can be the only thera-

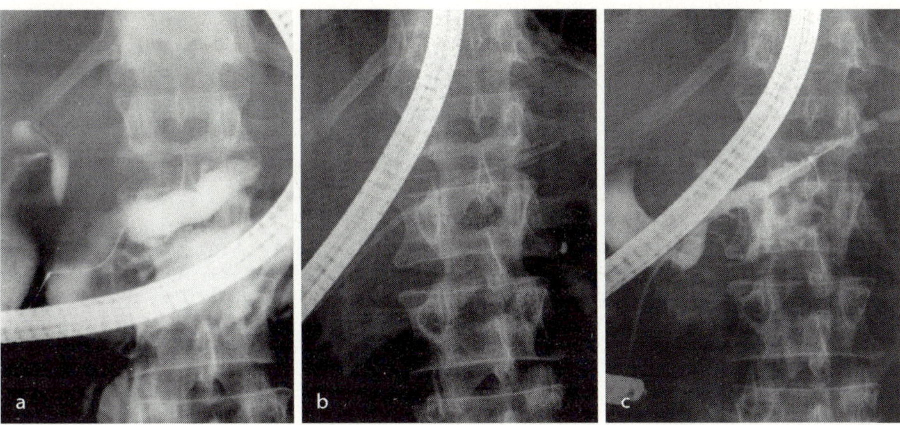

Fig. 1 a–c. a Chronic pancreatitis with duct obstruction and prestenotic dilatation. **b** After insertion of pancreatic duct endoprosthesis. **c** Reduction of the duct diameter following removal of the endoprosthesis

py applied, but in most cases it serves as a preparatory measure for further endoscopic intervention [6]. Compared with biliary duct sphincterotomy, pEST seems to be associated with a higher incidence of complications, with an up to 5% risk of bleeding in some cases. Nevertheless, in specialized gastrointestinal centers pEST is a safe procedure [6].

Fuji et al. [7] reported the results of pEST in patients with strictures in the pancreatic sphincter area or in close proximity to it; 21 of 22 patients benefited from this measure. A review of the literature shows that in 54%–88% of cases patients improved clinically after undergoing pEST for stricture or stone formation [8]. A retrospective analysis of our contingent of patients reveals that 23 of 34 (67%) with a dominant ductal stricture in the papillary area and prestenotic dilatation have shown a remarkable reduction of pain symptoms within a follow-up period of 36 months after pEST; 17 patients reported a median weight gain of approximately 4 kg [9].

In case of dominating stenosis of the duct of Wirsung in the head of the pancreas or the proximal body, a pancreatic duct prosthesis may be implanted, in analogy with biliary duct stenosis (Fig. 1). In 90% of cases this method is technically successful. In case of occlusion or migration of the stent, prosthesis replacement is indicated. In certain cases this is done at regular intervals of 2–3 months (standardized protocol of prosthesis exchange) [10]. A good prognostic parameter of the method's efficacy is the sonographically measured reduction of pancreatic duct diameter [2].

Clinical improvement is observed following successful stent implantation in 74%–94% of cases (Table 1). In a follow-up period of 7.4±6.3 months, 62% of patients are free of pain and 59% even show a weight gain of about 7±5 kg (2–22 kg) [11]. In 82% of endoscopically treated cases further stationary treatment is not required [11]. Other authors [12] report similar pain-free intervals after endoscopic therapy in as many as 66% of patients after 11 months. In a retrospective analysis we have examined 23 patients treated

Table 1. Results of pancreatic duct endoprosthesis insertion

Reference	*n*	Mean follow-up (months)	Improvement of symptoms: no./total (%)	Stent patency (months)	Complications
Binmoeller et al. [31]	93	36	69/73 (74)	6	4×p; 2×abscess
Smits et al. [14]	49	34	40/49 (82)	5	2×b, 2×p, 9×mi
Cremer et al. [18]	75	37	71/74 (94)	12	3×ch, 1×he, 2×mi, 8×in
Riemann et al. [13]	23	32	18/23 (78)	4[a]	1×ch, 1×p, 1×in

p, pancreatitis; b, bleeding; ch, cholangitis; in, pancreatic duct infection; mi, prosthesis migration; he, hemobilia.
[a] Partly standardized protocol.

with pancreatic duct prostheses. We aimed for a stent exchange every 3 months. The mean follow-up was 31.7 months (5–66 months). The result was that 65% of the patients had pain-free intervals, which was similar to the other cited results [13]. Smits et al. described a remarkable benefit upon stent removal after 28.5 months in 55% of the patients [14].

Early complications are primarily mild acute pancreatitis, which occurs in approximately 8% of cases, as well as bleeding during the procedure [6, 15]. In the long range, complications are caused mainly by the plastic stent. Stent occlusion occurs in 8%–28% of patients after a mean interval of 4–6 months. Stent migration (in-/outward) is reported in 7%–18% of cases and can be accompanied by duodenal erosion [15]. These complications can be cured in almost all cases by stent replacement.

The prosthesis can induce ductal and parenchymal changes which resemble the morphological picture of CP [16, 17]. The cause seems to be local compression and the resulting stasis in the pancreatic tree. The clinical relevancy of the ductal changes is not clear.

At present it appears that patients with pancreatic duct obstruction within the vicinity of the head should be treated primarily with an endoscopic prosthesis, so that in many cases at least a short-term benefit can be achieved. Nevertheless, a strict assessment of the indication and clinical follow-up are necessary in view of the possible complications. In a few patients surgical intervention will remain necessary for extended treatment (pancreatic head resection with duodenal retention). A future alternative might be the implantation of self-expanding metal stents. A recent report described positive results in 22 cases [18]. In any case, this method requires long-term assessment.

Pancreatic Duct Stones: Stone Extraction, Extra-/intracorporeal Lithotripsy

Stenosis of the duct of Wirsung in CP is often accompanied by intraductal calculi, which cause temporary or permanent obturation of the duct lumen. Stone extraction by balloon or dormia basket is indicated in this case. Suit-

Table 2. ESWL: technical and clinical success rates in the treatment of pancreatic duct stones

Reference	*n*	Fragmentation/stone clearance *n* (%)	Improvement of symptoms *n* (%)	Mortality
Delhaye et al. [21]	123	122 (99)/72 (58)	85 (69)	0
Sauerbruch et al. [22]	24	17 (71)/10 (42)	12 (70)	0
Adamek et al. [19]	65	41 (63)/21 (33)	24 (58)	0
Schneider et al. [23]	50	43 (86)/30 (60)	36 (83)	0
van de Hul et al. [24]	17	13 (76)/7 (41)	11 (85)	0

able candidates for this procedure are patients with solitary [3, 19, 20] stones with a diameter of less than 10 mm in the proximal ductal system [5]. If primary stone extraction fails, extracorporeal shock-wave lithotripsy is an option for stone fragmentation. Depending on the shock-wave generation and the possibility of targeting the stone, success rates of the procedure vary between 60% and 99%. Clinical improvement after stone fragmentation and eventual extraction is reported to be between 59% and 94%. [19, 21–24]. Lithotripsy equipment with radiological focusing facilities is more effective than that with sonographic facilities (Table 2). On the other hand, intracorporeal fragmentation methods are being developed and practiced at the moment only at a few treatment centers. Currently applied methods are electrohydraulic [25] and laser lithotripsy [26]. In an experimental study we have achieved complete or partial lithotripsy in ten cases using a rhodamine 6G-laser with an integrated stone-tissue discrimination system [27]. The main problem of the intracorporeal method is to reach the stone despite the coexisting stricture. Improvement of the clinical symptoms after stone disintegration and stone extraction is observed in about 55%–85% of patients [5, 21, 22].

Pseudocysts of the Pancreas: Percutaneous Puncture or Drainage, Endoscopic Enterocystostomy, Transpapillary Drainage

During the course of CP, pseudocysts are found in 15%–35% of patients upon imaging. Therapeutic intervention is necessary if pseudocysts present with a diameter greater than 5 cm, if the pseudocyst rapidly increases in size, or if it persists for longer than 6 weeks. In these cases regression is unlikely and the risk of complications (e.g., rupture, infection, bleeding) increases [20, 28]. Further indications for treatment are jaundice due to local compression, intestinal obstruction, or pain.

Percutaneous cyst puncture is easy, but percutaneous drainage often leads to only short-term resolution. It is more difficult, and success depends on many weeks of the patient's cooperation. In 50% of cases drainage is accompanied by bacterial infection of the cyst or the puncture canal, pancreatic ascites, or other complications [20].

Large pseudocysts that lead to an impression of the duodenal bulb or the stomach wall can be endoscopically drained [29]. Endoscopic ultrasound

Table 3. Results of pancreatic pseudocyst drainage

Reference	*n*	Technical success *n* (%)	Follow-up (months)	Relapse *n*	Long-term follow-up *n* (%)	Early and late complications
ECG						
Cremer et al. [29]	22	21 (95.4)	31 (3–84)	2	19 (86.4)	1×b,
Sahel [30]	40	38 (95)	37	1	–	1×death
ECD						
Cremer et al. [29]	11	11 (100)	31 (3–84)	2	9 (81.8)	2×b, 2×in
Sahel [30]	3	1	37	1	–	
Transpapillary drainage						
Catalano et al. [32]	22	21 or 17[a] (95.4)	37 (12–26)	1	16 (72.7)	1×p,
Binmoeller et al. [31]	33	33 or 31[a] (100)	11 (1.5–24)	5	26 (78.9)	2×ab, 13×oc

ECG, endoscopic cystogastrostomy; ECD, endoscopic cystoduodenostomy; b, bleeding; in, infection; p, pancreatitis; ab, abscess; oc, stent occlusion.
[a] Complete cyst resolution.

scanning has added to the safety of the procedure, as it allows assessment of the local vascular situation and the wall morphology.

Endoscopic cystogastrostomy (ECG) has a technical success rate of 89%–100% [29, 30]. Main complications are bleeding and cyst infection. The mortality lies below 1% in specialized centers. Large studies show a relapse rate of approximately 10% during a follow-up of 3 years (Table 3).

Pancreatic pseudocysts reaching the duodenum can be drained via gastroscope or duodenoscope (endoscopic cystoduodenostomy [ECD]). The primary technical success rate of ECD is 88%–96%, somewhat lower than that of ECG. On the other hand, complications, especially bleeding, were less frequent. In the long range the relapse rate of 9%–15% was similarly high for both procedures [29–31].

When pancreatic pseudocysts connect to the pancreatic duct, drainage can be achieved by transpapillary access with a nasopancreatic probe or with a pancreatic duct prosthesis. Catalano et al. [32] reported on transpapillary drainage in 21 cases. The procedure led to cyst resolution in 81%, and only one patient presented with cyst relapse within a time frame of 3 years. These data correspond to those from other studies [5, 8, 20, 31, 33].

Endoscopic drainage of pancreatic pseudocysts, either transmural or transpapillary, proves to be very successful and superior to surgical procedures, considering the complication and mortality rates [28]. Relapse rates for both surgical and endoscopic techniques are similarly high at approximately 10%–15%.

Common Bile Duct Stricture: Biliary Endoprosthesis, Metal Stent

Up to 45% of patients with CP present with narrowing of the bile duct upon ERCP. The narrowing is due to either cicatricial stricture or compression by the pseudocyst [34]. Treatment is indicated in case of cholestatic jaundice, because of possible development of secondary biliary cirrhosis and acute cholangitis. Implantation of a plastic biliary endoprosthesis is usually successful and leads to at least temporary relief of cholestasis [33].

The main problem is the long-term success of the technique in this patient group, with disappointing results. Between 1988 and 1993, 20 patients with obstructive jaundice due to CP were treated with a plastic endoprosthesis. Prosthesis replacement was performed 13 times because of occlusion and/or cholangitis. Satisfactory improvement upon prosthesis removal was observed in only five cases [34]. Another study group [35] reported on their experience with this technique in 25 cases. Two patients died due to septic complications, ten patients presented with stent migration, and eight patients presented with endoprosthesis occlusion after a mean of 6.5 months. Only three patients remained asymptomatic without stent (Table 4).

Because of the high complication rate and the frequent endoprosthesis replacements, implantation of biliary plastic stents can serve only as a short-term measure or as definitive therapy for inoperable patients. Standard treatment of stenosis of the DHC due to CP remains surgical biliodigestive anastomosis.

It is possible that implantation of self-expanding (30-French) metal stents will promote endoscopic treatment in the future. Devière et al. [36] report a medium-range success of 90%, occlusion being especially rare in the follow-up period. Short metal stents for strictures in the proximity of the papilla allow easy surgical intervention.

Table 4. Common bile duct strictures due to chronic pancreatitis and endoprostheses

Reference	Prosthetic material	*n*	Technical success *n* (%)	Follow-up (months)	Mortality	Migration, occlusion	Long-term success *n* (%)
Devière et al. [35]	Plastic	25	25 (100)	14 (7–42)	2 (sepsis)	M: 10, O: 8	3 (12)
Riemann et al. [34]	Plastic	20	20 (100)	36 (6–70)	–	M: 0, O: 13	5 (25)
Barthet et al. [3]	Plastic	19	19 (100)	18 (13–48)	–	?	8 (42)
Devière et al. [36]	Metal	20	20 (100)	20	–	M: 0, O: 2	18 (90)

Pancreas Divisum: Sphincterotomy, Pancreatic Duct Endoprosthesis

In pancreas divisum the disproportionate minor papilla and the glandular secretion of the larger dorsal part can lead to flow obstruction with painful stasis. In the early 1990s, the coincidence of pancreas divisum and CP was controversially discussed [37]. Recent studies seem to prove that patients can benefit from surgical or endoscopic drainage of the dorsal part.

In one study, 11 cases of CP and pancreas divisum were treated endoscopically [38]. Initially, all patients profited from pEST, but only three (27%) with relapsing episodes showed long-term improvement of their condition. In four of eight patients with relapsing symptoms a restenosed minor papilla was observed. Another study, analyzing 31 cases of pancreas divisum [15], reported an improvement of symptoms after pEST in 26 patients (84%). Again, patients with relapsing pain episodes were more likely to benefit.

Review articles [8, 33, 39] report technically successful prosthesis implantation in the duct of Santorini in more than 90% of cases and clinical success rates of 83%–90%. In these studies, mere pEST of the minor papilla in pancreas divisum palliated the symptoms in 62%–100% of cases [33]. There is general agreement that patients presenting with chronic pain are less likely to profit from interventional treatment of pancreas divisum than those with relapsing episodes of pain [15, 38, 39].

Conclusions

In the past decade, a large variety of nonsurgical interventional measures for the treatment of chronic pancreatitis have been developed. The endoscopic methods have become the measure of primary choice for certain conditions (e.g., pancreatic pseudocysts, endoscopic enterocystostomy), making surgical intervention superfluous. Some methods prove to be ineffective as long-term treatment (e.g., stenosis of the common bile duct, biliary plastic endoprosthesis) but offer short-term resolution or are of diagnostic value.

Some conditions (e.g., obstructive pancreatitis, pancreatic duct prosthesis, pancreas divisum) have been studied only retrospectively or with small case numbers. The promising results should be further analyzed in prospective studies and larger groups.

As all of the methods may be accompanied by possibly serious complications [40], they should be employed only at specialized gastrointestinal centers. Stringent indications for these measures should be established, and close clinical follow-up is necessary [37]. In order to enable optimal individual patient therapy, communication and consensus with surgical colleagues should be pursued.

References

1. Mössner J (1991) Therapie der chronischen Pankreatitis. Z Gastroenterol 29:541–547
2. Cremer M (1993) Endoscopy, treatment of the future in chronic pancreatitis? Gastroenterol Clin Biol 17:787–791
3. Barthet M, Bernard JP, Duval JL, Affriat C, Sahel J (1994) Biliary stenting in benign biliary stenosis complicating chronic calcifying pancreatitis. Endoscopy 26:569–572
4. Karanjia ND, Widdison AL, Leung F. Alvarez C, Lutrin FJ, Reber HA (1994) Compartment syndrome in experimental chronic obstructive pancreatitis: effect of decompressing the main pancreatic duct. Br J Surg 81:259–264
5. Sherman S, Lehman GA, Hawes RH, Ponich T, Miller LS, Cohen LB, Kortan P, Haber GB (1991) Pancreatic ductal stones: frequency of successful endoscopic removal and improvement in symptoms. Gastrointest Endosc 37:511–517
6. Rabenstein T, Ruppert T, Hahn EG, Ell C (1996) Endoskopische Papillotomie bei chronischer Pankreatitis. Endoskopie Heute 9:12–18
7. Fuji T, Amaro R, Ohmura T, Akiyama T, Aibe T (1989) Endoscopic pancreatic sphincterotomy technique and evaluation. Endoscopy 21:27–30
8. Bedford RA, Howerton DH, Geenen JE (1994) The current role of ERCP in the management of benign pancreatic disease. Endoscopy 26:113–119
9. Jakobs R, Leonhardt A, Benz C, Bregenzer N, Maier M, Riemann JF (1996) Endoscopic sphincterotomy as a therapy for chronic pancreatitis – is it worth to try? Int J Pancreatol 19:247(A)
10. Ponchon T, Bory RM, Hedelius F, Roubein LD, Paliard P, Napoleon B, Chavaillon A (1995) Endoscopic stenting for pain relief in chronic pancreatitis: results of a standardized protocol. Gastrointest Endosc 42:452–456
11. Löhr M, Schneider HT, Farnbacher M, Hahn EG, Fleig WE, Liebe S, Ell C (1997) Endoskopische interventionelle Therapie der chronischen Pankreatitis. Z Gastroenterol 35: 437–448
12. Huibregtse K, Schneider B, Vrij AA, Tytgat GN (1988) Endoscopic pancreatic drainage in chronic pancreatitis. Gastrointest Endosc 34:9–15
13. Riemann JF, Bregenzer N, Maier M, Benz C, Martin WR (1996) Interventionelle Techniken am Pankreasgangsystem. Chir Gastroenterol 12:38–42
14. Smits ME, Badiga SM, Rauws EA, Tytgat GN Huibregtse K (1995) Long-term results of pancreatic stents in chronic pancreatitis. Gastrointest Endosc 42:461–467
15. Siegel JH, Ben-Zvi JS, Pullano W, Cooperman A (1990) Effectiveness of endoscopic drainage for pancreas divisum: endoscopic and surgical results in 31 patients. Endoscopy 22:129–133
16. Smith MT, Sherman S, Ikenberry SO, Hawes RH, Lehman GA (1996) Alterations in pancreatic ductal morphology following polyethylene pancreatic stent therapy. Gastrointest Endosc 44:268–275
17. Sherman S, Hawes RH, Savides TJ, Gress FG, Ikenberry SO, Smith MT, Zaidi S, Lehman GA (1996) Stent-induced pancreatic ductal and parenchymal changes: correlation of endoscopic ultrasound with ERCP. Gastrointest Endosc 44:276–282
18. Cremer M, Devière J, Delhaye M, Balze M, Vandermeeren ATI (1992) Stenting in severe chronic pancreatitis: results of medium-term follow-up in seventy-six patients. Bildgebung 59 [Suppl 1]:20–24
19. Adamek HE, Jakobs R, Krömer MU, Buttmann A, Riemann JF (1996) Ultraschallgesteuerte extrakorporale Stoßwellenlithotripsie (ESWL) von Pankreasgangsteinen. Dtsch Med Wochenschr 121 [Suppl 1]:73
20. Adams DB, Anderson MCT (1992) Percutaneous catheter drainage compared with internal drainage in the management of pancreatic pseudocyst. Ann Surg 215:571–576
21. Delhaye M, Vandermeeren A, Baize M, Cremer M (1992) Extracorporeal shock-wave lithotripsy of pancreatic calculi. Gastroenterology 102:610–620
22. Sauerbruch T, Holl J, Sackmann M, Paumgartner G (1992) Extracorporeal lithotripsy of pancreatic stones in patients with chronic pancreatitis and pain: a prospective follow-up study. Gut 33:969–972
23. Schneider HT, May A, Benninger J, Rabenstein T, Hahn EC, Katalinic A, Ell C (1994) Piezoelectric shock wave lithotripsy of pancreatic duct stones. Am J Gastroenterol 89: 2042–2048
24. van de Hul R, Plaisier P, Jeekel J, Terpstra O, den Toom R, Bruining H (1994) Extracorporeal shock-wave lithotripsy of pancreatic duct stones: immediate and long-term results. Endoscopy 26:573–578

25. Tanaka M, Yokohata K, Kimura H, Naritomi G, Ichimaya H, Minasi JS (1992) Intraoperative endoscopic electrohydraulic lithotripsy of pancreatic stones. Int J Pancreatol 12:227–231
26. Renner IG (1991) Laser fragmentation of pancreatic stones. Endoscopy 23:166–170
27. Jakobs R, Maier M, Benz C, Riemann JF (1996) Laser lithotripsy of pancreatic duct stones using a standard or a prototype version of a stone-tissue discrimination system. Int J Pancreatol 16:248(A)
28. Rapp K, Zundler J, Walker S (1995) Nichtoperative Verfahren zur Behandlung von Pankreaspseudozysten. Dtsch Med Wochenschr 120:1129–1132
29. Cremer M, Devière J, Engelholm L (1989) Endoscopic management of cysts and pseudocysts in chronic pancreatitis: a long-term follow-up after 7 years of experience. Gastrointest Endosc 35:1–9
30. Sahel J (1991) Endoscopic drainage of pancreatic cysts. Endoscopy 23: 181–184
31. Binmoeller KE, Jue P, Seifert H, Nam WC, Izbicki J, Soehendra N (1995) Endoscopic pancreatic stent drainage in chronic pancreatitis and a dominant stricture: long-term results. Endoscopy 27:638–644
32. Catalano ME, Geenen JE, Schmalz MJ, Johnson GK, Dean RS, Hogan WJ (1995) Treatment of pancreatic pseudocysts with ductal communication by transpapillary pancreatic duct prosthesis. Gastrointest Endosc 42:214–218
33. Parikh NJ, Geenen JE (1992) Current role of ERCP in the management of benign pancreatic disease. Endoscopy 24:120–124
34. Riemann JF, Maier M, Schilling D, Kohler B (1994) Benign bile duct stenosis – conservative management as long as possible? Schweiz Rundsch Med Prax 83:883–885
35. Devière J, Devaere S, Baize M, Cremer M (1990) Endoscopic biliary drainage in chronic pancreatitis. Gastrointest Endosc 36:96–100
36. Devière J, Cremer M, Baize M, Love J, Sugai B, Vandermeeren A (1994) Management of common bile duct stricture caused by chronic pancreatitis with metal mesh self-expandable stents. Gut 35:122–126
37. Burdick JS, Hogan WJ (1991) Chronic pancreatitis: selection of patients for endoscopic therapy. Endoscopy 23:155–159
38. Lehman GA, Sherman S, Nisi R, Hawes RH (1993) Pancreas divisum: results of minor papilla sphincterotomy. Gastrointest Endosc 39:1–8
39. Huibregtse K, Smits ME (1994) Endoscopic management of diseases of the pancreas. Am J Gastroenterol 89:66–77
40. Kozarek RA (1994) Chronic pancreatitis in 1994: is there a role for endoscopic treatment? Endoscopy 26:625–628

CHAPTER 16

Surgical Treatment of Chronic Pancreatitis

H.G. Beger, M. Siech, and W. Schlosser

Introduction

The frequency of chronic pancreatitis (CP) in European countries varies between 6.7 for men and 3.2 for women per 100,000 inhabitants. Patients with CP have a much shorter life expectancy than others. Long-term follow-up revealed that patients with CP have a 5-year survival of 65% and a 10-year survival of 43%; in 19% of cases mortality was related to the patients' disease [1–3]; however, in the other 81% the causes of death were factors other than CP, such as malignancies, alcoholic hepatopathy, and severe infections. Lankisch found a 13% mortality related to chronic pancreatitis within a 14-year period [4, 5]. Epidemiological studies of chronic pancreatitis demonstrated a coincidence with pancreatic cancer; in patients who suffered from CP for more than 10 years the risk of pancreatic cancer was 3%. In our own prospective observation series of patients with CP and an inflammatory mass, 3.8% also developed pancreatic cancer. The frequency of surgical treatment due to medically intractable pain and severe local complications was 65% in the series of Ammann et al. [2] and 58–67% in that of Levy et al. [3] (Table 1). Patients with alcoholic CP frequently develop an inflammatory mass

Table 1. Natural course and prognosis of chronic pancreatitis

Factor	%	Reference
Survival after onset of CP (cumulative survival)		
5 years	65	[1]
10 years	43	[1]
20 years	50	[2]
	50	[3]
Mortality related to CP	13	[4]
	19.3	[3]
	19	[2]
Causes of death not related to CP		
Malignancies	4–19	[5]
Cardiovascular disease	19	[2]
Alcohol hepatopathy	8	[2]
Severe infections	14	[2]
Surgical treatment for pain and local complications	66.7	[6]
	58	[3]

in the head of the pancreas and, due to the inflammatory tumor, frequently severe local complications as well [7]. The subgroup of patients with CP and an inflammatory mass in the head of the pancreas are predominantly men who are below 35 years of age at the onset of their disease; they usually suffer severe abdominal pain, eventually resistant to analgesic medical treatment, and in 50% common bile duct stenosis, in 60% pancreatic main duct stenosis, in 7% severe duodenal stenosis, and in 15% compression of the portal vein with some degree of portal hypertension [8]. One quarter of the patients who are candidates for surgical treatment suffer insulin-dependent diabetes mellitus. Another 20% demonstrate impaired glucose metabolism without the need for insulin supplementation.

Indication for Surgery

In most patients weekly, daily, or even daily severe, medically intractable upper abdominal pain necessitates surgical treatment. Local complications leading to interventional management and finally to surgical treatment are common bile duct stenosis with long-lasting cholestasis, or even periodical jaundice, and development of an inflammatory tumor in the head of the pancreas, not easy to discriminate from a cancer. If the inflammatory tumor in the head causes severe duodenal stenosis, surgical decompression is unavoidable. Most of the patients demonstrated, on the basis of ERCP or MRCP investigations, a high-grade pancreatic main duct stenosis in the head, and more than one third showed multiple pancreatic main duct stenosis additionally in the duct of body and tail. Calcifications of pancreatic tissue are not an indication for surgical treatment; however, pancreatic main duct stones have to be treated surgically if interventional endoscopic or lithotripsy treatment is unsuccessful. More than 30% of the patients have pseudocystic lesions in the pancreatic tissue, most frequently in the head. This requires surgical treatment if the duodenum, the CBD, or segments of the intestine are compressed. Infection of the pseudocyst or massive bleeding into a pseudocystic cavity are conditions necessitating urgent surgical intervention if interventional drainage or radiological measures do not control these severe acute complications. The frequency of portal and splenic vein and superior mesenteric vein involvement in CP is underestimated; 15%–25% of all patients with CP have some degree of compression or encasement of the portal and superior mesenteric vein or a thrombosis of the splenic or portal vein. Decompression of the portal vein system is an indication for surgery (Table 2).

Principles of Surgical Treatment

Two different principles of surgical treatment are currently in use: duct drainage procedures and limited resections (Table 3).

Table 2. Indications for surgical treatment of patients with CP

Medically intractable abdominal pain
Local complications
CBD stenosis causing cholestasis
Severe stenosis of the duodenum (<1 cm)
Persisting inflammatory mass in the pancreatic head
Pseudocystic lesion >6 cm in diameter
CP plus pancreatic abscess
Portal vein compression
Gastric outlet syndrome
Stenosis of the transverse colon
Main duct stenosis in the head with pancreatic duct dilatation in body and tail
Pancreas divisum causing chronic pancreatitis
Suspicion of a malignant pancreatic lesion

Table 3. Surgical options in CP

Options	Resections	Drainage procedures
Historical	Whipple resection	Puestow drainage
	Subtotal left resection (Child-OP)	–
Classic	Pylorus-preserving partial pancreaticoduodenectomy	Partington-Rochelle duct drainage
Standard today	Duodenum-preserving pancreatic head resection	Frey's procedure
	Spleen-preserving pancreatic left resection	–
	Pseudocysto-gastrojejunostomy (duodenum-preserving total pancreatectomy)	–

Drainage Procedures

The first drainage operation was described by Puestow and Gillesby in 1958. This procedure combines the drainage of the tail-sided main pancreatic duct with a pancreatic tail resection. Consequently, the procedure has all the postoperative drawbacks of a pancreatic left resection. Moreover, for a drainage operation it is technically not necessary to perform a left resection. Therefore, the Puestow pancreatic drainage was replaced by the lateral pancreaticojejunostomy, first published in 1960 by Partington and Rochelle [9].

The drainage of the main pancreatic duct by lateral pancreaticojejunostomy in combination with limited resection of inflamed tissue of the head of the pancreas was described by Frey et al. in 1987 [15]. This procedure is a modification of the Partington-Rochelle drainage of the pancreatic main duct. The late outcome of the Frey procedure still needs to be evaluated.

The main pancreatic duct is incised longitudinally over the full length of the pancreatic main duct and anastomosed with a Roux-en-Y jejunal loop. The disadvantage of this procedure is that the inflammatory mass in the head of the pancreas is not treated. This inflammatory mass causes most of the mechanical problems in chronic pancreatitis, e.g., pain, biliary stenosis,

Table 4. Pain relief after pancreaticojejunostomy; >5 years follow-up

No. of patients	Complete pain relief (%)	Pain, but improved (%)	Failure (%)
205 [a]	44	31	25
85 [b]	24	31	45

[a] From White and Hart 1979 [10], Prinz and Greenlee 1981 [11], Morrow et al. 1984 [12], and Bradley 1987 [13].
[b] From Adams et al. 1994 [14].

duodenal stenosis, and vascular stenosis with portal hypertension. Because the majority of such patients suffer from mechanical problems due to an inflammatory mass in the head of the pancreas, the use of a drainage operation alone is limited. Consequently, the long-term results of this procedure are rather discouraging: 22%–44% of the patients report some but not complete improvement, and in 25%–45% of cases the results are even poorer (Table 4). Markowitz et al. [16] evaluated the reasons for failure in 15 consecutive patients at 5 months after Partington-Rochelle surgery. They reoperated on 14/15 patients (13 head resections, one left resection) and followed them up for a median of 39 months. During this follow-up ten patients became pain free and two died of pancreatic cancer which had been overlooked during the Partington-Rochelle operation. The reasons for failure of the Partington-Rochelle procedure, according to the authors, were: pancreatic cancer, inadequate duct decompression, biliary stenosis, inflammation of the head of the pancreas.

In summary, single drainage operations are effective only in patients without an inflammatory mass in the head of the pancreas but with dilatation of the pancreatic main duct of at least 6–8 mm. However, drainage operations sometimes may be helpful as an additional procedure, combined with duodenum-preserving pancreatic head resection.

Drainage of Pancreatic Pseudocysts in Chronic Pancreatitis

The first option in the treatment of pancreatic pseudocysts due to CP is US- or CT-guided interventional drainage. This procedure is inexpensive, has a low complication rate, and is done with the patient under local anesthesia. The recurrence rate after a one-time needle aspiration is high; this rate can be reduced to less than 10% by using an indwelling catheter. In cases of small pseudocysts of 4–6 cm it is possible to wait for their spontaneous disappearance. A cystic tumor must always be excluded by additional diagnostic procedures. Our own experience with pancreatic pseudocysts and their symptoms and location is that most of those larger than 6 cm cause severe pain. Other symptoms are weight loss, compression of the duodenum and common bile duct, and obstruction of the superior mesenteric vein or portal vein. As shown by Warshaw et al., the frequency of spontaneous resolution of pseudocysts larger than 4–6 cm is only 7% [17]. Even under conservative management of chronic pancreatic pseudocysts, the rate of complications can be up to 41% [18, 19]. The mortality of pancreatic pseudocysts during non-surgical management is between 12% and 14% [18, 20]. Therefore, it is suggested that pseudocysts larger than 4–6 cm be drained surgically. This is usually done by cystojejunostomy with an excluded loop and Roux-en-Y reconstruction. In 1991, all pseudocyst treatments in the literature (1142 patients) were summarized, and it was demonstrated that the mortality after surgical treatment is as high as 9%. Many patients with pseudocysts and CP require additional resection of the head of the pancreas later on. In cases of smaller cysts, the duodenum-preserving pancreatic head resection can be performed simultaneously. Pseudocysts larger than 4 cm should first be drained surgically, and the resection of the head of the pancreas may be performed as a second procedure after an interval of 6–12 months.

Duodenum-preserving Pancreatic Head Resection

The duodenum-preserving resection of the head of the pancreas was developed by Beger in 1980 and established in clinical surgical practice for patients with CP and an inflammatory mass in the head of the pancreas [7]. Resection follows three major steps: exposure of the head of the pancreas, subtotal resection of the head, and reconstruction using the upper jejunal loop for interposition (Figs. 1,2). The major advantage of duodenum-preserving head resection in comparison to the pylorus-preserving head resection and Whipple's resection of the pancreatic head is the preservation of the stomach and the duodenum and the extrahepatic common bile duct, as well as the gallbladder. It also preserves the pancreatic parenchyma to a large extent.

Early results after duodenum-preserving head resection have been very promising. The postoperative hospitalization lasts a median of approximately 14 days, and hospital mortality lies below 1%. In terms of preservation of the endocrine function of the pancreas early postoperatively, only 2% of patients developed new diabetes mellitus, whereas 9% demonstrated improvement of their postoperative glucose metabolism on the basis of an oral glucose tolerance test [21]. During the follow-up period of 6 months to 23 years it has been demonstrated that late morbidity and mortality after duodenum-preserving head resection are surprisingly low. After a median follow-up of 6 years, 75%–82% of all patients were absolutely pain free, and an additional 7%–11% did not need analgesic medication in spite of occasional upper abdominal complaints. Regarding pain recurrence, 8%–11% suffered pain requiring analgesic treatment at the re-evaluation. As to working status, more than 60% of all patients were professionally employed. Body weight increase occurred in more than 80% in the first postoperative month. Late after surgical treatment only one third of the patients were still on a full dose of enzyme supplementation. Late mortality after duodenum-preserving head resection was 7.7%. Only 10% had to be rehospitalized because of further attacks of pancreatitis. This low postoperative hospitalization rate in CP deserves special mention, because on the basis of our knowledge of the natural

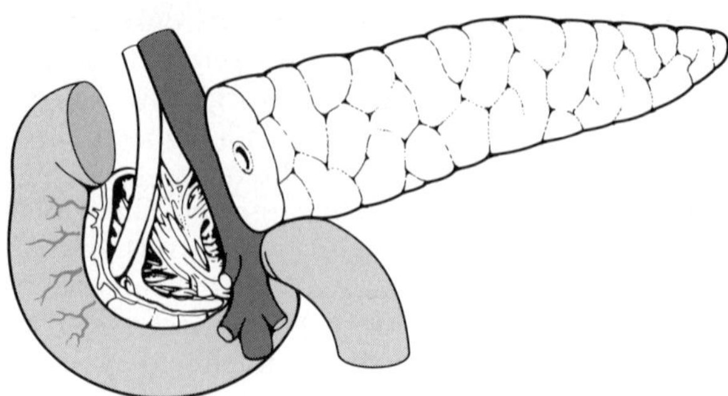

Fig. 1. Duodenum-preserving pancreatic head resection; subtotal excision of the inflammatory tumor of the pancreatic head

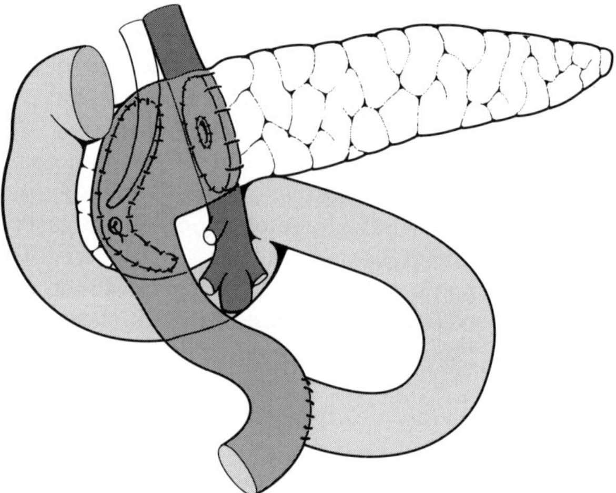

Fig. 2. Reconstruction after duodenum-preserving pancreatic head resection using an excluded upper jejunal loop

course of CP, at least 50% of patients normally experience further severe attacks of acute pancreatitis. The low late morbidity in spite of progression of the CP provides evidence that surgical excision of the inflammatory process in the head of the pancreas promotes the transformation of a clinically manifest CP into a clinically silent, nonprogressing disease (Table 5).

The rationale behind the use of the duodenum-preserving pancreatic head resection in patients with CP and an inflammatory mass in the pancreatic head is based on our present knowledge about the pathomorphological events and the natural course of CP. The inflammatory process, the pacemaker of the disease, develops in the head of the pancreas; pain is generated by the inflammatory process, which leads to a specific, pancreatitis-associated neuritis and the liberation of pain hormones in the head of the pan-

Table 5. Results of long-term follow-up after duodenum-preserving pancreatic head resection (*IDDM* insulin-dependent diabetes mellitus)

	Year of study [reference]		
	1984 [2]	1988 [8]	1994 [23]
No. of patients	57	128	298
Follow-up, range (years)	0–11	0–16	1–22
Median follow-up (years)	2.0	3.6	6.0
Follow-up rate (%)	100	96	87
Pain-free[a] (%)	92.8	89	88
Continuing abdominal pain (%)	7.2	11	12
Hospitalization due to attacks of acute pancreatitis (%)	12.3	11	10
Endocrine function improved (%)	15.8	5.5	
Incidence of IDDM (%)	5.4	13.7	
Late mortality (%)	3.6	4.7	8.9

[a] None or rare (once per month) upper abdominal complaints.

creas and to an increase of duct and tissue pressure. Preservation of the stomach, the duodenum, and the extrahepatic biliary organs represents the major advantage of duodenum-preserving head resection in CP.

Pancreatic Left Resection

Pancreatic left resection maintains the duodenal passage and therefore the normal function of the upper gastrointestinal tract. Also, left resection of the pancreas is much easier to perform than all resections of the right pancreas, and postoperative morbidity and mortality are much lower. Therefore, in the 1970s and 1980s many surgeons performed pancreatic left resections in patients with CP. The postoperative results were rather discouraging, however. Pancreatic left resection failed to improve pain in 48%–66% of patients with diffuse pancreatitis [24]. In 8%–33% of cases even patients with segmental left CP failed to become pain free and experienced recurrence (Table 6). These data from 1981 were recently confirmed by a study of Rattner et al. [25]. Because of the poor outcome of patients following pancreatic left resection this procedure is indicated only for segmental pancreatitis in the left pancreas with otherwise "normal" parenchyma. This is a very rare condi-

Table 6. Early and late results after left resection [24]

	n	Failure to improve/recurrence (%)
Segmental left CP (54 patients)		
Partial	24	33.3
Subtotal	34	8
Diffuse CP (67 patients)		
Partial	24	66.7
Subtotal	43	48.8

Table 7. Early and late results (in percent) after different types of pancreatic head resection

	Whipple [a]	Pylorus-preserving partial PD [b]
Mortality (30 days)	3.2	1.2
Late mortality	20.7	n.d.
Pain relief	64	74
Professional rehabilitation	n.d.	67
New diabetes, late	24.5	15.6

[a] Whipple: Howard and Zhang 1990 [30], Frick et al. 1987 [31], Gall et al. 1990 [32], Stone et al. 1988 [33], Morel et al. 1990 [34].
[b] PPPD: Traverso and Kozarek 1993 [27], Braasch 1990 [35], Büchler et al. 1995 [36], Morel et al. 1990 [34].

tion, which usually occurs only after pancreatic trauma. For such patients the spleen-preserving left resection should be the procedure of choice.

Pylorus-preserving Partial Duodenopancreatectomy

The pylorus-preserving technique of partial duodenopancreatectomy was developed by Watson in 1944 and introduced into clinical routine by Traverso et al. [26]. The operation avoids the typical complaint of gastric dumping, frequently observed after a Whipple resection. The mortality of 1.7% was lower than that in patients with a Whipple operation (Table 7). Also, pain relief is better in these patients than in those undergoing the Whipple operation (74% vs. 64%). The rate of surgical diabetes (15.6%) is smaller compared with the Whipple operation (24.5%).

Typical postoperative complications after pylorus-preserving Whipple are delayed gastric emptying within the first 4 weeks after surgery in 12%–32% and anastomotic ulcerations in 2%–11% of patients [27–29]. Thus, the pylorus-preserving partial pancreaticoduodenectomy offers advantages over the Whipple procedure. However, the early and late postoperative results are not as good as with duodenum-preserving pancreatic head resection. The pylorus-preserving head resection is indicated for patients with CP in whom malignancy is additionally suspected.

References

1. Thorsgaard-Pedersen N, Nyboe-Andersen B, Pedersen G, Worning H (1982) Chronic pancreatitis in Copenhagen. A retrospective study of 64 consecutive patients. Scand J Gastroenterol 17:925–931
2. Ammann RW, Akovbiantz A, Largiader F, et al (1984) Course and outcome of chronic pancreatitis. Gastroenterology 56:820–828
3. Levy P, Milan C, Pognon JP, Baetz A, Bernardes P (1989) Mortality factors associated with chronic pancreatitis. Unidimensional and multidimensional analysis of a medical-surgical series of 240 patients. Gastroenterology 96:1165–1172
4. Lankisch PG, Andrén-Sandberg Å (1993) Standards for the diagnosis of chronic pancreatitis and for the evaluation of treatment. Int J Pancreatol 14:205–212

5. Lankisch PG (1997) Natural course of chronic pancreatitis. In: Izbicki J, Binmoeller KF, Soehendra N (eds) Chronic pancreatitis. de Gruyter, Berlin, pp 1–14
6. Bernard HR (1987) Discussion of MM Connolly. Ann Surg 206:366–371
7. Beger HG, Witte C, Kraas E, Bittner R (1980) Erfahrung mit einer das Duodenum erhaltenden Pankreaskopfresektion bei chronischer Pankreatitis. Chirurg 51:303–307
8. Beger HG, Büchler M, Bittner R, Oettinger W, Roscher R (1989) Duodenum-preserving resection of the head of the pancreas in severe chronic pancreatitis. Early and late results. Ann Surg 209:273–278
9. Partington PF, Rochelle REL (1960) Modified Puestow procedure for retrograde drainage of the pancreatic duct. Ann Surg 152:1037–1043
10. White TT, Hart MJ (1979) Pancreaticojejunostomy versus resection in the treatment of chronic pancreatitis. Am J Surg 138:129–135
11. Prinz RA, Greenlee HB (1981) Pancreatic duct drainage in 100 patients with chronic pancreatitis. Ann Surg 194:313–320
12. Morrow CE, Cohen JI, Sutherland DER, Najarian JS (1984) Chronic pancreatitis: long-term surgical results of pancreatic duct drainage, pancreatic resection, and near-total pancreatectomy and islet autotransplantation. Surgery 96:608–615
13. Bradley EL (1987) Long-term results of pancreaticojejunostomy in patients with chronic pancreatitis. Am J Surg 153:207–213
14. Adams DB, Ford MC, Anderson MC (1994) Outcome after lateral pancreaticojejunostomy for chronic pancreatitis. Ann Surg 219:289–293
15. Frey CF, Smith GJ (1987) Description and rationale of a new operation for chronic pancreatitis. Pancreas 2:701–707
16. Markowitz JS, Rattner DW, Warshaw AL (1994) Failure of symptomatic relief after pancreaticojejunal decompression for chronic pancreatitis. Strategies for salvage. Arch Surg 129:374–379
17. Warshaw AL (1989) Pancreatic cysts and pseudocysts: new rules for a new game. Br J Surg 76:533–534
18. Bradley EL, Clements JL, Gonzalez AC (1979) The natural history of pancreatic pseudocysts: a unified concept of management. Am J Surg 137:135–141
19. O'Malley V, Cannon JP, Postier RG (1985) Pancreatic pseudocysts: cause, therapy and results. Am J Surg 150:680–682
20. Wade JW (1985) Twenty-five year experience with pancreatic pseudocysts. Are we making progress? Am J Surg 149:705–708
21. Beger HG, Büchler M (1990) Duodenum-preserving resection of the head of the pancreas in chronic pancreatitis with inflammatory mass in the head. World J Surg 14:83–87
22. Beger HG, Krautzberger W, Bittner R, Büchler M, Limmer J (1985) Duodenum-preserving resection of the head of the pancreas in patients with severe pancreatitis. Surgery 97:467–473
23. Büchler MW, Friess H, Bittner R, Roscher R, Krautzberger W, Müller MW, Malfertheiner P, Beger HG (1997) Duodenum-preserving pancreatic head resection: long-term results. J Gastrointest Surg 1: 3–19
24. Gebhardt C, Zirngibl H, Gossler M (1981) Pankreaslinksresektion zur Behandlung der chronischen Pankreatitis. Langenbecks Arch Chir 354:209–220
25. Rattner DW, Fernandez del Castillo C, Warshaw AL (1996) Pitfalls of distal pancreatectomy for relief of pain in chronic pancreatitis. Am J Surg 171:142–145
26. Traverso LW, Longmire WP (1978) Preservation of the pylorus during pancreaticoduodenectomy. Surg Gynecol Obstet 146:959–962
27. Traverso LW, Kozarek RA (1993) The Whipple procedure for severe complications of chronic pancreatitis. Arch Surg 128:1047–1053
28. Warshaw AL, Torchiana DL (1985) Delayed gastric emptying after pylorus-preserving pancreaticoduodenectomy. Surg Gynecol Obstet 160:1–4
29. Pellegrini CA, Heck CF, Raper S, Way LW (1989) An analysis of the reduced morbidity and mortality rates after pancreaticoduodenectomy. Arch Surg 124:778–781
30. Howard J, Zhang Z (1990) Pancreaticoduodenectomy (Whipple resection) in the treatment of chronic pancreatitis. World J Surg 14:77–82
31. Frick S, Jung K, Rückert K (1987) Chirurgie der chronischen Pankreatitis. Dtsch Med Wochenschr 112:629–635
32. Gall FP, Zirngibl H, Gebhardt C, Schneider MU (1990) Duodenal pancreatectomy with occlusion of the pancreatic duct. Hepatogastroenterology 37:290–294
33. Stone WM, Sarr MG, Nagorney DM, McIllrath DC (1988) Chronic pancreatitis. Results of Whipple's resection and total pancreatectomy. Arch Surg 123:815–819

34. Morel P, Mathey P, Corboud H, Huber O, Egeli RA (1990) Pylorus-preserving duodeno-pancreatectomy: long-term complications and comparison with the Whipple procedure. World J Surg 14:642–647
35. Braasch JW (1990) Pyloric-preserving pancreatectomy for chronic pancreatitis. In: Trede M, Saeger HD (eds): Aktuelle Pankreaschirurgie. Springer, Berlin Heidelberg New York, pp 165–169
36. Büchler MW, Friess H, Müller MM, Beger HG (1995) Randomized trial of duodenum-preserving pancreatic head resection versus pylorus-preserving Whipple in chronic pancreatitis. Am J Surg 169:65–70

Part III
Cystic Fibrosis

CHAPTER 17

Genetics and Molecular Pathology of Cystic Fibrosis

B. TÜMMLER

Cystic Fibrosis: The Most Common Severe Genetic Disease in Caucasian Populations

Cystic fibrosis (CF) is a generalized disorder of the secretory epithelia of all exocrine glands (Quinton 1990; Welsh et al. 1995). This genetic disease of autosomal recessive inheritance is caused by mutations in the cystic fibrosis transmembrane conductance regulator (*CFTR*) gene. CF is diagnosed by elevated electrolyte concentrations in sweat, reduced ion permeability of upper respiratory epithelium, and impaired luminal ion secretion in gastrointestinal epithelium upon stimulation with secretagogues. The basic defect of perturbed salt and water transport leads to secondary alterations of the pancreas and the gastrointestinal, hepatobiliary and respiratory tracts. Exocrine pancreatic insufficiency and the pulmonary manifestations determine the course and prognosis of most CF cases. Chronic infections with viral and bacterial pathogens sustain a vicious cycle of airway infection, inflammation, tissue remodeling, and destruction which ultimately leads to respiratory failure. Symptomatic treatment of disease manifestations at specialized CF centers has continuously improved during the past three decades, so that median survival is now more than 30 years.

CFTR

The *CFTR* Gene

The 230-kbp *CFTR* gene is located on chromosome 7q3.1 (Rommens et al. 1989). Its 27 exons encode the 1480-amino acid CFTR glycoprotein with a molecular weight of 170,000 (Riordan et al. 1989). There is only one single

Work in the author's laboratory was supported by the Deutsche Forschungsgemeinschaft, the BIOMED II program of the EU, the CF Selbsthilfe e.V., the Christiane-Herzog-Stiftung, the Deutsche Fördergesellschaft für die Mukoviszidoseforschung e.V., and the Mukoviszidose e.V.

copy of the *CFTR* gene in the human genome, although a 30-kbp stretch of sequence around exon 9 has been amplified during primate evolution and dispersed on at least ten different chromosomal regions (Rozmahel et al. 1997).

Transcription: Promoter and Alternative Splicing

The basal promoter encompasses a short sequence of 276 bp upstream from exon 1 of *CFTR*. The 27 exons are transcribed into a polyadenylated mRNA of approximately 6500 bp. The population of the CFTR mRNA transcripts consists of full-length and multiple alternatively spliced isoforms; of these, the exon 9^- and exon 12^- mRNA isoforms may be present in relative amounts of up to 90% of total CFTR mRNA. A polymorphism in the length of the oligo-T_n tract of the acceptor splice site of intron 8 is associated with the amount of exon 9 skipping. Individuals carrying T_7 or T_9 alleles are asymptomatic, whereas two T_5 alleles may cause mild pulmonary CF disease and infertility in males by congenital bilateral absence of the vas deferens (CBAVD) (Zielenski and Tsui 1995).

CFTR is not an abundantly expressed gene. Cells of the pancreatic duct and enterocytes or goblet cells of the gastrointestinal tract may contain up to 100 CFTR mRNA molecules per cell, but the gallbladder or renal epithelial cells have only 5–30 copies on average and respiratory epithelial cells just one or two (Bremer et al. 1992).

Post-translational Maturation and Trafficking of CFTR

After synthesis at the endoplasmic reticulum (ER), nascent CFTR is core-glycosylated (form B) and folded by chaperones such as calnexin into an ATP-sensitive conformation that is translocated to the Golgi apparatus and processed to glycosylated isoforms of the complex type (form C) (Brown et al. 1997; Qu et al. 1997; Seibert et al. 1997). However, most CFTR does not gain the correctly folded secondary and tertiary structures. These misfolded intermediates are recognized by the ER quality control, ubiquitinylated, and degraded. Mature CFTR, which is resident in the trans-Golgi network, endosomal compartments, or the apical plasma membrane, has a half-time of about 24 h. The cellular localization and lifetime of CFTR are affected by cell type and differentiation state. For example, CFTR is expressed at the apex of pseudostratified respiratory epithelium, but remodeling or dedifferentiation leads to internalization and, finally, to loss of CFTR protein, although CFTR mRNA transcript remains at wild-type levels (Dupuit et al. 1995). These properties impose an extra challenge on any attempts in CF somatic gene therapy to achieve the expression of CFTR protein at its genuine site. In the respiratory tract, for example, pseudostratified epithelium is refractory to transduction with vectors and liposomes, whereas dedifferentiated airway epithelium is more susceptible to uptake of vector DNA.

Structure: CFTR Is an ABC Transporter

CFTR belongs to the protein superfamily of ATP-binding cassette (ABC) transporters which consist of six membrane-spanning segments (TM) and cytoplasmic nucleotide-binding domains (NBD) (Schneider and Hunke 1998; Schwiebert et al. 1998; Seibert et al. 1997). CFTR has the topology TM(1–6)-NBD1-R-TM(7–12)-NBD2, whereby R represents a large regulatory domain with multiple phosphorylation sites for protein kinases A and C and tyrosine kinases. Besides the Walker motifs A and B generally found in nucleotide-binding proteins, the NBDs contain a dodecapeptide preceding Walker B that is diagnostic for all ABC transporters.

The two membrane domains form an ion channel. Amino acids of TM6 and TM12 have contact with the hydrophilic ion pore, and amino acids at the cytosolic terminus of TM6 control the ion selectivity of the pore (Akabas et al. 1997). The functionally nonequivalent NBDs can bind and probably hydrolyze ATP (Bear et al. 1997; Foskett 1998).

The closest relative of CFTR in man is the "multidrug resistance-associated protein" MRP, which translocates glutathione conjugates and arachidonic acid metabolites across membranes.

Functions of CFTR

CFTR is a 6- to 8-pS, low-conductance, ATP-activated anion channel with linear current/voltage characteristics (Devidas and Guggino 1997; Foskett 1998; Schwiebert et al. 1998; Welsh et al 1995). Ions are transported across the electrochemical gradient; i.e., chloride ions are secreted into the lumen of exocrine glands. Permeability decreases in the order $Br^{-}>Cl^{-}>I^{-}$. Channel activity is regulated by interaction with other proteins, phosphorylation, and dephosphorylation, whereby cAMP elicits the strongest response.

A paracrine mechanism of CFTR activation operates in the gut. When the peptide guanylin is secreted into the intestinal lumen, it stimulates a guanylate cyclase in the apical membrane of the enterocyte and the production of cGMP, which leads to the activation of CFTR by phosphorylation by the cGMP-dependent protein kinase cGK II.

The function of CFTR as a chloride channel in the apical membrane of epithelial cells is extensively documented. However, less is known about the molecular determinants of CFTR residence in the apical membrane, basal regulation of its activity, and its physical interplay with other transporters. The aspects of CFTR function should require specific interactions between CFTR and other proteins in the apical compartment of epithelial cells. Recently, the ERM-binding phosphoprotein EBP50 and the Na^{+}/H^{+} exchanger regulator factor NHERF have been shown to bind to the COOH-terminal DTRL sequence of CFTR (Hall et al. 1998; Short et al. 1998). Since this binding motif is found in many proteins, such as the β_2-adrenergic receptor or the purinergic P2Y1 receptor, adaptor proteins like EBP50 or NHERF could spatially link divergent signaling pathways. CFTR chloride channels also interact with syntaxin 1A. This membrane protein, which also modulates neurosecretion and calcium channel gating in the brain, regulates CFTR-mediated currents in epithelia. These interactions are blocked by a syntaxin-binding protein of the Munc18 protein family (Naren et al. 1997). Hence, CFTR function in epithelial cells seems to be tuned by an interplay between syntaxin and Munc18 isoforms and adaptor proteins that link CFTR with other elements of signal transduction cascades.

CFTR is not only a chloride channel but also transports glutathione (Linsdell and Hanrahan 1998) and amphiphilic organic compounds, like the related ABC transporters MRP and MDR1. The question of whether ATP is translocated by CFTR is a current and still controversial issue. CFTR-associated ATP channels exhibit slow gating kinetics that depend on the presence of protein kinase A and cytoplasmic ATP, similar to CFTR chloride channels. The phosphorylation- and nucleotide-hydrolysis-dependent gating of CFTR is directly involved in gating of an associated ATP channel. However, the permeation pathways for chloride and ATP are distinct, and the ATP conduction pathway is not obligatorily associated with the expression of CFTR (Sugita et al. 1998).

In addition to its transport function, CFTR regulates the activities of sodium, potassium, and the outwardly rectifying chloride channels, is involved in the trafficking between trans-Golgi network and apical membrane, and influences protein secretion, exo- and endocytosis of vesicles, and the pH in endosomal compartments (Mall et al. 1998; Schwiebert et al. 1998; Tümmler and Puchelle 1997). The physiological relevance of these findings is under investigation. Other ongoing issues are the roles of CFTR in cell growth, apoptosis and the first line of bacterial defense. CFTR has been ascribed to the function of an apical receptor for *Pseudomonas aeruginosa* in airway epithelial cells and for *Salmonella typhi* in intestinal epithelium (Pier et al. 1998).

Genetics of Cystic Fibrosis

CF is observed mainly in Caucasian populations, where the frequency of asymptomatic carriers varies between 1:20 and 1:30. Carriers are about ten times less frequent among black Africans and very rare among Asians (Welsh et al. 1995).

Up to the summer of 1998, more than 800 disease-causing lesions had been identified in the *CFTR* gene. The majority of CF mutations are substitutions of single nucleotides, followed by small deletions or insertions. Large deletions of more than 1000 bp are rare, and intragenic rearrangements have not yet been reported. The *CFTR* mutation database of the Cystic Fibrosis Genetic Analysis Consortium, run by Dr. Lap-Chee Tsui (Kerem et al 1989), one of the discoverers of the CF gene, is available on-line in the internet under the address HYPERLINK http://www.genet.sickkids.on.ca./cftr.

The most frequent *CFTR* mutation is a 3-bp in-frame deletion of codon 508, ΔF508, which is present on 67% of all CF chromosomes in Europe. ΔF508 is more frequent in the Northern, Western and Eastern European countries (60%–80%) than in the Mediterranean region (20%–60%). Other rather frequent mutations in Central Europe with an incidence of more than 1% are the missense mutations R347P, G551D, and N1303 K, the nonsense mutations G542X and R553X, and the cryptic splice site mutation 3849+10 kb C-T. Some dozen mutations were identified in several countries, but most mutations are sporadic or were described in only a single family (Welsh et al. 1995; Zielenski and Tsui 1995).

CF follows an autosomal recessive trait with a single *CFTR* mutation on each CF chromosome. However, a few exceptions were noted in our laboratory. De novo mutations in the parental germline are rare, but they exist and may pose problems for genetic counseling. Complex alleles with more than one *CFTR* mutation on one CF chromosome may result in atypical manifestations of symptoms such as overweight or close-to-normal sweat electrolytes (Dörk et al. 1991). Moreover, we characterized the basic defect in a carrier of a rare *CFTR* mutation who suffered from severe CF-like pulmonary disease (Bronsveld et al. 1999). CFTR function was normal in sweat glands, pancreas, and gut but impaired in the respiratory epithelium. This index case suggests that one CF allele may be sufficient to cause disease if the genetic background predisposes to CF. Pseudohypoaldosteronism is another clinical entity which may mimic the clinical manifestations of CF, but other rare inherited conditions must exist in addition which cause CF-like disease without *CFTR* being affected. At our CF clinic we have cared for a male pancreas-sufficient individual with a positive sweat test who has been suffering from the typical manifestations of CF lung disease (Mekus et al. 1998). No *CFTR* mutation has yet been identified. The index case shares the same intragenic *CFTR* haplotypes with his asymptomatic sister, which provides strong evidence that a gene other than *CFTR* is causing CF in this individual. Since we have, in the meantime, detected a *CFTR* mutation on 97% of the CF chromosomes in our local patient population (Dörk et al. 1994), a gene other than *CFTR* can be responsible for CF in only very few patients. Genetic heterogeneity is the rule rather than the exception for inherited disease in man. Although non-*CFTR* disease alleles must be rare, they sensitively impair the accuracy of *CFTR*-based tests for genetic counseling and screening programs.

Molecular Pathology of CFTR Mutants

CFTR mutations are differentiated by their effects on CFTR mRNA transcript and protein into six classes, as first suggested by A. Smith and M. Welsh (Welsh and Smith 1993; Zielenski and Tsui 1995):

I Diminished or undetectable synthesis of protein
II Defective intracellular maturation and trafficking
III Altered regulation of the CFTR ion channel
IV Altered conductance properties of CFTR ion channel
V Perturbed interaction with other proteins (allosteric mutant)
VI Reduced concentration of wild-type CFTR protein

Most mutations have so far been classified on the basis of the heterologous expression of mutated *CFTR* in *Xenopus* oocytes, CF mice, or cell lines, but our own work indicates that assays on CF patients' specimens will often be discordant with the outcome of experiments in model systems.

Frameshifts, nonsense mutations, and splice site mutations that affect obligatorily conserved nucleotides in donor or acceptor splice sites cause a premature stop codon and usually belong to class I. When we studied frameshift and nonsense mutations in patient material, aberrant splicing and reduction of transcript were the most common effects (Will et al. 1995). Tissues from CF patients who are homozygous for G542X or R553X showed no or strongly reduced immunoreactive CFTR signals, indicating that these mutations are null alleles.

Heterologous expression of the most common and the third most frequent mutations ΔF508 and N1303K in mammalian cells demonstrated temperature-sensitive defects in post-translational maturation and trafficking (class II). However, the phenotype of ΔF508 CFTR in patient tissues is variable and may range from reduced amounts of mislocalized protein in sweat glands to an apparently normal distribution in pseudostratified airway epithelium. ΔF508 CFTR exhibits a broad spectrum of tissue-dependent class II, III, and IV characteristics.

Missense mutations in the NBDs (G551D) often cause a class III and those in the TMs (R117H, R334 W, R347P) a class IV phenotype. An example of an allosteric mutant (class V) is A455E CFTR, which has wild-type chloride channel properties but is impaired in its interaction with other proteins. Class VI is represented by splice site mutations (3849+10 kb C-T) which give rise to residual amounts of correctly spliced CFTR mRNA transcripts.

Genotype–Phenotype Associations

The clinical presentation of CF is complex because the disease can involve pancreatic, hepatobiliary, pulmonary, and reproductive complications (Welsh et al. 1995). Gastrointestinal and, in particular, pulmonary disease is highly variable in the CF patient population. The relationship between *CFTR* mutation genotype and clinical phenotype has been analyzed in order to gain a better understanding of the function of CFTR and to improve diagnosis, prognosis, and management of patients. The associations between *CFTR* mutation genotype and clinical manifestation of disease in the individual organ systems depend on (a) the susceptibility of the organ to *CFTR* mutations and (b) the impact of environmental and other genetic factors on manifestation of disease (Summers 1996).

The associations between *CFTR* genotype and phenotypic features can be divided into three categories (Welsh et al. 1995). The first category includes the symptoms that are common to most CF patients. The male reproductive tract most sensitively responds to molecular lesions in the *CFTR* gene. Almost all CF males are infertile because of an obliteration of the vas deferens. CBAVD may be the only clinical manifestation in males carrying class IV, V, or VI mutations. An abnormal electrolyte composition of sweat is observed in almost all patients, and the Gibson-Cooke pilocarpine iontophoresis sweat test is correspondingly still the accepted standard for diagnosing CF. Only a few class III (G551S) or class IV (R117H) and most class V and class VI mutations were found to be associated with normal or close-to-normal sodium and chloride concentrations in the sweat.

The second category of phenotypic features in CF includes symptoms that can be differentiated by the *CFTR* mutation genotype. This category is best represented by exocrine pancreatic function (Kristidis et al. 1992). Pancreatic status is highly concordant among affected siblings. *CFTR* mutations are classified as being either PS or PI alleles. PI mutations are associated with exocrine pancreatic insufficiency since infancy or toddler age, whereas PS mutations manifest in exocrine pancreatic insufficiency not before late school age or adolescence. CF patients are exocrine pancreatic insufficient from the first year of life only if they harbor two PI mutations. All class I and II and most class III mutations are PI alleles, whereas most class IV and all class V and VI mutations are PS alleles. The only rather frequent *CFTR* mutation which, depending on the genetic background, can confer either a PI or a PS phenotype is the class IV mutation R347P.

The third category of phenotypic features includes the symptoms that are variable in patients with the same *CFTR* mutation genotype. Diabetes mellitus, pulmonary status, and gastrointestinal and hepatobiliary disease fall into this category and are the most important conditions that determine the course and prognosis of CF.

Although the clinical manifestations are variable, the underlying basic defect can be reliably demonstrated in both respiratory and gastrointestinal epithelia. The impermeability of the nasal respiratory epithelium to chloride is a sensitive and specific feature which enables reliable diagnosis of CF by the nasal potential difference (NPD) (Rosenstein and Cutting 1998), and the failure of secretagogues to evoke luminal chloride secretion has been established as an aid to diagnosing CF by intestinal current measurements (ICM) in rectal suction biopsies (Veeze et al. 1994). NPD and ICM measurements in clinically highly discordant or concordant ΔF508 homozygous siblings revealed that ion conductances conferred by alternative channels modulate the severity of CF disease.

Growth (weight predicted for height, WfH) and lung function (FVC, FEV1) are the most sensitive determinants of the clinical status in CF. The distribution of WfH, FVC, and FEV1 is as variable among ΔF508 homozygotes as among all other patients with CF, indicating that genes other than *CFTR* and environmental factors are highly relevant for the phenotypic diversity of CF. The major impact of genetic factors is substantiated by our observation that monozygous CF twins are significantly more concordant in growth and lung function than dizygous CF twins or ΔF508 homozygous siblings. Polymorphic genes encoding elements of ion transport, the host defense system, or the metabolism of xenobiotics have already been identified as genetic modifiers in CF.

Perspectives of Gene Therapy

Isolation of the CF gene has led to the development of gene transfer vectors to replace the defective gene (Boucher 1996; Wagner and Gardner 1997; Wilson 1995). Since chronic pulmonary disease determines the prognosis of most patients with CF, investigators have focused on the lungs as the first organ of gene replacement, although recent work in CF mice indicates that intratracheal administration of the *CFTR* gene may also restore defective bicarbonate secretion in the gallbladder (Curtis et al. 1998).

Preclinical Evaluation of *CFTR* Gene Transfer

Several in vitro studies have demonstrated that delivery of a normal *CFTR* gene to CF epithelial cells restores cAMP-mediated chloride conductance. With respect to the superficial epithelium that lines the airway lumen, only 6%–10% of the CF epithelial columnar cells need to be corrected in order to restore normal chloride secretion (Johnson et al. 1992).

The vectors used in published gene transfer studies were recombinant adenoviruses, adenovirus-associated virus (AAV), lentivirus, artificial chromosomes, liposomes, and molecular conjugates.

Adenovirus Vectors

Numerous studies revealed substantial cell-type and species variation in in vivo adenoviral gene transfer efficiency. Regenerating poorly differentiated cells of human airway epithelium represent preferential cell targets for recombinant adenoviral gene vectors, but the transduction of uninjured airway is low (Dupuit et al. 1997). Further substantial problems of adenoviral vectors are unfavorable inductions of host defense mechanisms. The major barrier to successful gene therapy is the immune system. Cytotoxic T lymphocytes, NK cells, and T_{H1} helper cells, together with cytokines, collaborate in the destruction of the genetically modified cell. Moreover, neutralizing antibodies impede the success of repetitive treatment with adenoviral vector. To overcome the immune barrier, a transient immune blockade at the time of virus administration has been suggested.

Lentiviral Vectors

A replication-defective vector based on human immundeficiency virus (HIV) effectively transduced *CFTR* into CF-derived cells of a human bronchial xenograft and corrected the CF defect as long as the epithelium was undifferentiated (Goldman et al. 1998). However, after differentiation the entry of lentivirus was blocked.

AAV Vectors

AAV vectors are based on the single-strand DNA nonenveloped parvovirus (Flotte and Carter 1997). Recombinant AAV has been shown to transduce nondividing cells and to provide CFTR transgene expression for several months in rabbits. Wild-type AAV has been shown to integrate into a defined region of chromosome 19; the CFTR-AAV transgene, however, integrates into human cell lines at random. Further current problems of this vector are the rather small capacity of 4.5–5 kb and the difficulty of producing pure AAV in high titer in bulk amounts.

Yeast Artificial Chromosomes

Yeast artificial chromosomes with *CFTR* insert have been constructed which contain selection markers for propagation in mammalian cells, a putative human origin of replication, a synthetic matrix attachment region, and two loxP sites for recombination (Ripoll et al. 1998).

Liposomes and Molecular Conjugates

Most in vivo work with liposomes has been performed in CF mice. Liposome-mediated gene transfer restored chloride transport in the nasal epithelium and trachea, but transfection activity was low with nonmitotic, highly polarized, and differentiated airway epithelial cells – the natural targets of CFTR expression (Jiang et al. 1998).

The combined delivery of *CFTR* by adenovirus and liposomes seems to be advantageous, as vector-specific complementation profiles have been elucidated in a human bronchial xenograft model of the CF airway (Zhang et al. 1998). Recombinant adenovirus efficiently restored defective cAMP-activatable chloride currents in epithelial cells, whereas cationic liposomes preferentially corrected excessive mucous sulfation in CF goblet cells.

Human Trials

To date there are more than a dozen human protocols either ongoing or approved for CF. The published studies have demonstrated that it is feasible to transfer CFTR cDNA to the respiratory epithelium and to partially correct defective airway epithelial chloride transport in some subjects.

Delivery of recombinant adenovirus vector to the nose or to the lungs did not, in most cases, induce any adverse effects (Crystal et al. 1994; Knowles et al. 1995; Zabner et al. 1996). However, a few individuals who received high doses of recombinant adenovirus developed both local (a pulmonary infiltrate and decrease of pulmonary function) and systemic (fever and hypotension) toxicity. Since adenovirus-mediated gene transfer is transient, repeat administration to the nose was tested in phase I trials. Less correction of the chloride transport defect was observed with subsequent administration, perhaps because the immune response limited gene transfer.

Transfer of CFTR cDNA to the nasal epithelium of patients with CF with DNA-lipid complexes has been evaluated in double-blind placebo-controlled clinical trials (Caplen et al. 1995; Porteous et al. 1997). Transgene DNA was detected in most transduced tissues, but sustained correction of CFTR-related functional changes toward normal values was observed in only a minority of subjects during the first week after administration. The level of gene transfer and functional correction were comparable in these first clinical trials using adenoviral vectors or DNA-liposome complex.

Unresolved Issues

The course and prognosis of CF are determined in most patients by chronic infection with opportunistic viral and bacterial pathogens. It is still necessary to establish how the CFTR-mediated basic defect translates to the abnormal airway secretions and the predilection for infection with *Staphylococcus aureus* and *Pseudomonas aeruginosa*, but current gene therapy approaches are based on the hypothesis that the loss of function of CFTR perturbs the salt and water composition of secretions, leads to aberrant glycosylation of mucins, slows the clearance of airways, and predisposes to infection. "The failure to elucidate CF lung disease pathogenesis reflects an absence of information in two areas: (1) the full spectrum of CFTR functions and malfunctions; and (2) the anatomic sites(s) within the airways where CFTR function is most important" (Boucher 1996).

Gene transfer of *CFTR* to organs other than the respiratory tract was studied mainly in CF mice, with some encouraging results. Recent experiments indicate that treatment of the airways may also target the biliary tract (Curtis et al. 1998). Intratracheal instillation of *CFTR*-liposome complex restored the phenotype of CF gallbladders to that of the wild type. In these null CF mice the unusual intratracheal route was more effective than oral, intravenous, intramuscular, subcutaneous, or intraperitoneal administration of recombinant vector. Complementation of null CF mice with a human *CFTR* YAC transgene induced chloride secretory responses in the gastrointestinal tract as large as or larger than those in wild-type tissues (Manson et al. 1997). The coming years will show whether artificial chromosomes can promise somatic gene therapy in man.

References

Akabas MH, Cheung M, Guinamard R (1997) Probing the structural and functional domains of the CFTR chloride channel. J Bioenerg Biomembr 29:453–463

Bear CE, Li C, Galley K, Wang Y, Garami E, Ramjeesingh M (1997) Coupling of ATP hydrolysis with channel gating by purified, reconstituted CFTR. J Bioenerg Biomembr 29:465–473

Boucher RC (1996) Current status of CF gene therapy. Trends Genet 12:81–84

Bremer S, Hoof T, Wilke M, Busche R, Scholte B, Riordan JR, Maass G, Tümmler B (1992) Quantitative expression patterns of multidrug-resistance P-glycoprotein (MDR1) and differentially spliced cystic-fibrosis transmembrane-conductance regulator mRNA transcripts in human epithelia. Eur J Biochem 206:137–149

Bronsveld I, Bijman J, Mekus F, Ballmann M, Veeze H, Tümmler B (1999) Clinical presentation of exclusive cystic fibrosis lung disease. Thorax (in press)

Brown CR, Hong-Brown LQ, Welch WJ (1997) Strategies for correcting the delta F508 CFTR protein-folding defect. J Bioenerg Biomembr 29:491–502

Caplen NJ, Alton EWFW, Middleton PG, Dorin JR, Stevenson BJ, Gao X, Durham SR, Jeffery PK, Hodson ME, Coutelle C, Huang L, Porteous DJ, Williamson R, Geddes DM (1995) Liposome-mediated CFTR gene transfer to the nasal epithelium of patients with cystic fibrosis. Nat Med 1:39–46

Crystal RG, McElvaney NG, Rosenfeld MA, Chu CS, Mastrangeli A, Hay JG, Brody SL, Jaffe HA, Eissa NT, Danel C (1994) Administration of an adenovirus containing the human CFTR cDNA to the respiratory tract in individuals with cystic fibrosis. Nat Genet 8:42–51

Curtis CM, Martin LC, Higgins CF, Colledge WH, Hickman ME, Evans MJ, MacVinish LJ, Cuthbert AW (1998) Restoration by intratracheal gene transfer of bicarbonate secretion in cystic fibrosis mouse gallbladder. Am J Physiol 274:G1053–G1060

Devidas S, Guggino WB (1997) CFTR: domains, structure, and function. J Bioenerg Biomembr 29:443–451

Dörk T, Wulbrand U, Richter T, Neumann T, Wolfes H, Wulf B, Maass G, Tümmler B (1991) Cystic fibrosis with three mutations in the cystic fibrosis transmembrane conductance regulator gene. Hum Genet 87:441–446

Dörk T, Mekus F, Schmidt K, Boßhammer J, Fislage R, Heuer T, Dziadek V, Neumann T, Kälin N, Wulbrand U, Wulf B, von der Hardt H, Maaß G, Tümmler B (1994) Detection of more than 50 different CFTR mutations in a large group of German cystic fibrosis patients. Hum Genet 94:533–542

Dupuit F, Kälin N, Brezillon S, Hinnrasky J, Tümmler B, Puchelle E (1995) CFTR and differentiation markers expression in non-CF and ΔF508 homozygous CF nasal epithelium. J Clin Invest 96:1601–1611

Dupuit F, Chinet T, Zahm JM, Pierrot D, Hinnrasky J, Kaplan H, Bonnet N, Puchelle E (1997) Induction of a cAMP-stimulated chloride secretion in regenerating poorly differentiated airway epithelial cells by adenovirus-mediated gene transfer. Hum Gene Ther 8:1439–1450

Flotte TR, Carter BJ (1997) In vivo gene therapy with adeno-associated virus vectors for cystic fibrosis. Adv Pharmacol 40:85–101

Foskett JK (1998) ClC and CFTR chloride channel gating. Annu Rev Physiol 60:689–717

Goldman MJ, Lee PS, Yang JS, Wilson JM (1998) Lentiviral vectors for gene therapy of cystic fibrosis. Hum Gene Ther 8:2261–2268

Hall RA, Ostedgaard LS, Premont RT, Blitzer JT, Rahman N, Welsh MJ, Lefkowitz RJ (1998) A C-terminal motif found in the beta2-adrenergic receptor, P2Y1 receptor and cystic fibrosis transmembrane conductance regulator determines binding to the Na^+/H^+ exchanger regulatory factor family of PDZ proteins. Proc Natl Acad Sci U S A 95:8496–8501

Jiang C, O'Connor SP, Fang SL, Wang KX, Marshall J, Williams JL, Wilburn B, Echelard Y, Cheng SH (1998) Efficiency of cationic lipid-mediated transfection of polarized and differentiated airway epithelial cells in vitro and in vivo. Hum Gene Ther 9:1531–1542

Johnson LG, Olsen JC, Sarkadi B, Moore KL, Swanstrom R, Boucher RC (1992) Efficiency of gene transfer for restoration of normal airway epithelial function in cystic fibrosis. Nat Genet 2:21–25

Kerem B, Rommens JM, Buchanan JA, Markiewicz D, Cox TK, Chakravarti A, Buchwald M, Tsui LC (1998) Identification of the cystic fibrosis gene: genetic analysis. Science 245: 1073–1080

Knowles MR, Hohenker KW, Zhou Z, Olsen JC, Noah TL, Hu PC, Leigh MW, Engelhardt JF, Edwards LJ, Jones KR, Grossman M, Wilson JM, Johnson LG, Boucher RC (1995) A controlled study of adenoviral-vector-mediated gene transfer in the nasal epithelium of patients with cystic fibrosis. N Engl J Med 333:823–831

Kristidis P, Bozon D, Corey M, Markiewicz D, Rommens J, Tsui L-C, Durie P (1992) Genetic determinants of exocrine pancreatic function in cystic fibrosis. Am J Hum Genet 50:1178–1184

Linsdell P, Hanrahan JW (1998) Glutathione permeability of CFTR. Am J Physiol 275:C323–C326

Mall M, Bleich M, Greger R, Schreiber R, Kunzelmann K (1998) The amiloride-inhibitable sodium conductance is reduced by the cystic fibrosis transmembrane conductance regulator in normal but not in cystic fibrosis airways. J Clin Invest 102:15–21

Manson AL, Trezise AE, MacVinish LJ, Kasschau KD, Birchall N, Episkopou V, Vassaux G, Evans MJ, Colledge WH, Cuthbert AW, Huxley C (1997) Complementation of null CF mice with a human CFTR YAC transgene. EMBO J 16:4238–4249

Mekus F, Ballmann M, Bronsveld I, Dörk T, Bijman J, Tümmler B, Veeze HJ (1998) Cystic fibrosis-like disease unrelated to the cystic fibrosis transmembrane conductance regulator. Hum Genet 102:582–586

Naren AP, Nelson DJ, Xie W, Jovov B, Pevsner J, Bennett MK, Benos DJ, Quick MW, Kirk KL (1997) Regulation of CFTR chloride channels by syntaxin and Munc18 isoforms. Nature 390:302–305

Pier GB, Grout M, Zaidi T, Meluleni G, Mueschenborn SS, Banting G, Ratcliff R, Evans MJ, Colledge WH (1998) Salmonella typhi uses CFTR to enter intestinal epithelial cells. Nature 393:79–82

Porteous DJ, Dorin JR, McLachlan G, Davidson-Smith H, Davidson H, Stevenson BJ, Carothers AD, Wallace WA, Moralee S, Hoenes C, Kallmeyer G, Michaelis U, Naujoks K, Ho LP, Samways JM, Imrie M, Greening AP, Innes JA (1997) Evidence for safety and efficacy of DOTAP cationic liposome mediated CFTR gene transfer to the nasal epithelium of patients with cystic fibrosis. Hum Gene Ther 4:210–218

Qu BH, Strickland E, Thomas PJ (1997) Cystic fibrosis: a disease of altered protein folding. J Bioenerg Biomembr 29:483–490

Quinton PM (1990) Cystic fibrosis: a disease in electrolyte transport. FASEB J 4:2709–2717

Riordan JR, Rommens JM, Kerem B, Alon N, Rozmahel R, Grzelczak Z, Zielenski J, Lok S, Plavsic N, Chou JL, Drumm ML, Iannuzzi ML, Collins FS, Tsui L-C (1989) Identification of the cystic fibrosis gene: cloning and characterization of complementary DNA. Science 245:1066–1073

Ripoll PJ, Cowper A, Salmeron S, Dickinson P, Porteous D, Arveiler B (1998) A new yeast artificial chromosome vector designed for gene transfer into mammalian cells. Gene 210:163–172

Rommens JM, Iannuzzi MC, Kerem B, Drumm ML, Melmer G, Dean M, Rozmahel R, Cole JL, Kennedy D, Hidaka N, Zsiga M, Buchwald M, Riordan JR, Tsui L-C, Collins FS (1989) Identification of the cystic fibrosis gene: chromosome walking and jumping. Science 245:1059–1065

Rosenstein BJ, Cutting GR (1998) The diagnosis of cystic fibrosis: a consensus statement. Cystic Fibrosis Foundation Consensus Panel. J Pediatr 132:589–595

Rozmahel R, Heng HH, Duncan AM, Shi XM, Rommens JM, Tsui LC (1997) Amplification of CFTR exon 9 sequences to multiple locations in the human genome. Genomics 45:554–561

Schneider E, Hunke S (1998) ATP-binding-cassette (ABC) transport systems: functional and structural aspects of the ATP-hydrolyzing subunits/domains. FEMS Microbiol Rev 22:1–20

Schwiebert EM, Benos DJ, Fuller CM (1998) Cystic fibrosis: a multiple exocrinopathy caused by dysfunctions in a multifunctional transport protein. Am J Med 104:576–590

Seibert FS, Loo TW, Clarke DM, Riordan JR (1997) Cystic fibrosis: channel, catalytic, and folding properties of the CFTR protein. J Bioenerg Biomembr 29:429–442

Short DB, Trotter KW, Reczek D, Kreda SM, Bretscher A, Boucher RC, Stutts MJ, Milgram SL (1998) An apical PDZ protein anchors the cystic fibrosis transmembrane conductance regulator to the cytoskeleton. J Biol Chem 273:19797–19801

Sugita M, Yue Y, Foskett JK (1998) CFTR chloride channel and CFTR-associated ATP channel: distinct pores regulated by common gates. EMBO J 17:898–908

Summers KM (1996) Relationship between genotype and phenotype in monogenic diseases: relevance to polygenic diseases. Hum Mutat 7:283–293

Tümmler B, Puchelle E (1997) CFTR: a multifaceted molecule. Trends Cell Biol 7:250–251

Veeze HJ, Halley DJJ, Bijman J, de Jongste JC, de Jonge HR, Sinaasappel M (1994) Determinants of mild symptoms in cystic fibrosis patients – residual chloride secretion measured in rectal biopsies in relation to the genotype. J Clin Invest 93:461–466

Wagner JA, Gardner P (1997) Toward cystic fibrosis gene therapy. Annu Rev Med 48:203–216

Welsh MJ, Smith AE (1993) Molecular mechanisms of CFTR chloride channel dysfunction in cystic fibrosis. Cell 73:1251–1254

Welsh MJ, Tsui LC, Boat TF, Beaudet AL (1995) Cystic fibrosis. In: Scriver CR, Beaudet AL, Sly WS, Valle D (eds) The metabolic and molecular bases of inherited disease. McGraw Hill, New York, pp 3799–3876

Will K, Dörk T, Stuhrmann M, von der Hardt H, Ellemunter H, Tümmler B, Schmidtke J (1995) Transcript analysis of CFTR nonsense mutations in lymphocytes and nasal epithelial cells from cystic fibrosis patients. Hum Mutat 5:210–220

Wilson JM (1995) Gene therapy for cystic fibrosis: challenges and future directions. J Clin Invest 96:2547–2554

Zabner J, Ramsey BW, Meeker DP, Aitken ML, Balfour RP, Gibson RL, Launspach J, Moscicki RA, Richards SM, Standaert TA, et al (1996) Repeat administration of an adenovirus vector encoding cystic fibrosis transmembrane conductance regulator to the nasal epithelium of patients with cystic fibrosis. J Clin Invest 97:1504–1511

Zhang Y, Jiang Q, Dudus L, Yankaskas JR, Engelhardt JF (1998) Vector-specific complementation profiles of two independent defects in cystic fibrosis airways. Hum Gene Ther 9:635–648

Zielenski J, Tsui L-C (1995) Cystic fibrosis: genotypic and phenotypic variations. Annu Rev Genet 29:777–807

CHAPTER 18

Treatment of Gastrointestinal Manifestations in Cystic Fibrosis

M. Stern

Old and New Gastrointestinal Problems in Cystic Fibrosis

Cystic fibrosis (CF) is a disease still to be discovered by clinical adult gastroenterologists, particularly in European countries, where most adult patients are currently treated in pediatric centers. Gastrointestinal manifestations of CF are very much age related: meconium ileus occurring in the newborn, consequences of exocrine pancreatic insufficiency becoming obvious during the infant period, CF liver disease appearing at school age, diabetes mellitus and adenocarcinoma being observed in adulthood (Park and Grand 1981; Shalon and Adelson 1996) (Table 1).

When the classical review by Shwachman (1975) is compared with the recent overview by Shalon and Adelson (1996), it becomes evident that many old gastrointestinal problems still exist, and that some new ones have

Table 1. Clinical gastroenterology of cystic fibrosis

Site	Condition
Esophagus, stomach	Gastroesophageal reflux disease
Small bowel	Meconium ileus
	Distal intestinal obstruction
	Intussusception
	Adenocarcinoma
Large bowel	Submucosal wall thickening
	Fibrosing colonopathy
	Constipation
	Rectal prolapse
Pancreas	Exocrine insufficiency (PI)
	Pancreatitis (PS)
	Diabetes mellitus
Liver	Steatosis
	Focal biliary cirrhosis
	Multilobular cirrhosis
	Portal hypertension
Biliary	Neonatal cholestasis
	Microgallbladder
	Cholelithiasis
	Bile duct stenosis

PI, pancreatic insufficiency; PS, pancreatic sufficiency.

evolved. While the term "pancreatic infantilism" (Shwachman 1975) no longer appears timely, its underlying problems of maldigestion and malnutrition are still major factors in CF today, limiting quality of life and survival (Sinaasappel 1995). Thus, it is important to assess exocrine pancreatic function and to monitor pancreatic enzyme therapy. This is the basis of adequate nutritional management of CF patients (Ramsey et al. 1992). Fibrosing colonopathy, a new gastrointestinal manifestation of cystic fibrosis has shed some light on pancreatic enzyme overdose and on large bowel involvement recently. Finally, the full extent of CF liver disease becomes obvious only now, with increased life expectancy. There is a strong discrepancy between the severe therapeutic problems of end-stage CF liver disease and the still not well-defined but apparently good potential of early treatment with ursodeoxycholic acid (UDCA). This chapter reviews clinical gastroenterology of cystic fibrosis with respect to these topics (Sinaasappel 1995; Figarella 1996; Grand 1996; Shalon and Adelson 1996).

Exocrine Pancreatic Insufficiency: Assessment and Enzymatic Treatment

Exocrine pancreatic insufficiency, bile acid loss, and intestinal dysfunction are instrumental in maldigestion, contributing to malnutrition and growth failure in CF. Cystic fibrosis is the most frequent cause of exocrine pancreatic insufficiency in childhood. The genetic basis of this inherited autosomal recessive disease are mutations of the cystic fibrosis transmembrane conductance regulator gene (CFTR). More than 700 mutations have now been registered. The most important one, delta F 508, accounts for 70% of mutations in Western Europe and is associated with pancreatic insufficiency. Other less frequent mutations (e.g., R117H) are associated with pancreatic sufficiency, which occurs in approximately 15% of CF patients and is connected with a more favorable prognosis. Thus, exocrine pancreatic insufficiency is a good example of genotype-phenotype correlations in CF (Shalon and Adelson 1996; Koletzko 1997).

Pancreatic pathology includes progressive ductular obstruction, acinar disruption, and replacement of pancreatic lobules by fibrous tissue and by cyst formation. Fat and protein digestion are severely affected by decreased secretion of lipase and colipase and by decreased bicarbonate production, which renders small intestinal contents more acidic (Gregory 1996). Since pancreatic enzyme replacement and nutritional therapy are based on the evidence of pancreatic insufficiency, this condition has to be assessed at the initial diagnostic workup of each CF patient. Introducing pancreatic enzymes just on the basis of a pathological sweat test, without evidence of pancreatic dysfunction, not only is a waste of resources but may also lead to unnecessary side effects.

For assessment of pancreatic function, direct tests require duodenal intubation and quantification of pancreatic enzymes as well as bicarbonate. This invasive technique makes marker perfusion studies possible and serves as a gold standard. More practical and feasible in children are indirect methods,

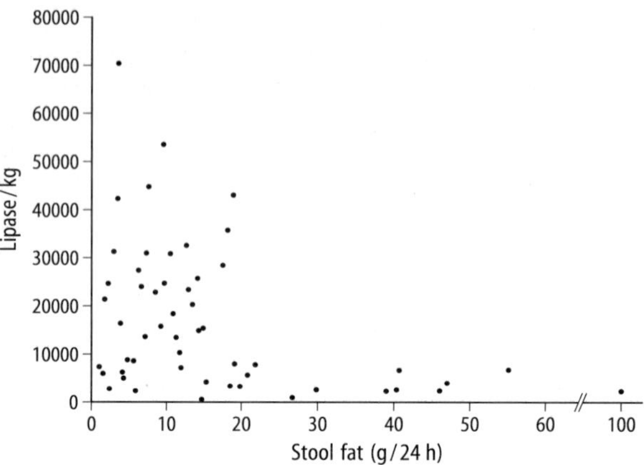

Fig. 1. Dosage of pancreatic enzyme treatment: Lipase (IU/kg body wt. and day) vs 24-h stool fat excretion in 55 Tübingen CF patients from pediatric to adult age (Fitzke et al. 1994, unpublished data)

namely 72-h fat balance study, determination of pancreatic elastase in the stool, and, recently, breath tests using 13 C mixed triglycerides. Stool elastase is a reliable noninvasive diagnostic tool independent of pancreatic enzyme treatment (Löser et al. 1996; Soldan et al. 1997) showing good correlation with secretin-pancreozymin testing and giving high sensitivity and good specificity. For therapy monitoring, measurement of stool fat by the van de Kamer method or by near infrared spectroscopy is suitable. Stool microscopy is still a valuable simple method for orientation. It has to be noted that particularly the indirect pancreatic function tests cover only a limited aspect. It is well known, for instance, that decreased bicarbonate secretion precedes impaired enzyme excretion and that fat absorption might be normal in spite of decreased lipase production. Finally, pancreatic reserve is high, and maldigestion occurs only when 98% of pancreatic tissue is destroyed. It is useful to establish pancreatic sufficiency of CF patients at the initial diagnostic workup. However, pancreatic failure may develop at a later age (Couper et al. 1992). Thus, assessment of pancreatic function should be repeated for a minority of pancreatic-sufficient individuals.

The aim of pancreatic enzyme replacement therapy is to restore digestion. In CF patients, this aim has been reached only incompletely even with modern pancreatin preparations due to such multiple concomitant gastrointestinal factors as disturbed motility, acid-base balance, loss of bile salts, and hepatobiliary pathology. Thus, relatively high doses of lipase may be necessary in CF to obtain stool fat values near normal and fat absorption coefficients over 85% (Fig. 1). It has been a clear historical error to reduce the fat intake by CF patients in order to reduce steatorrhea. Negative energy balance and malnutrition have been simple consequences. Today hypercaloric nutrition rich in fat is advocated. This calls for more efficient pancreatic enzyme treatment.

For this purpose, acid-resistant microsphere preparations of porcine pancreatin were introduced in the late 1980s. Even with acid protection of pancreatin by enteric coating, duodenal enzyme levels were relatively low, indicating inefficient utilization of ingested lipase (Guarner et al. 1993, non-CF patients). Recently, multiple randomized studies have shown that steatorrhea can be effectively reduced in CF patients using new pancreatic preparations (Brady et al. 1991; Lancellotti et al. 1996; Regele et al. 1996). However, results were highly variable, and the question was raised as to what harm the high pancreatic enzyme concentrations induced by the new preparations in the ileum and large intestine could possibly exert (Guarner et al. 1993; Lancellotti et al. 1996). A tendency towards overdosing pancreatic enzymes is enforced by the fact that, due to limited shelf-life, most preparations contain lipase activities in excess of what is stated on the packets (O'Hare et al. 1995). In view of the development of fibrosing colonopathy in young patients treated with excessively high doses of lipase, overdosage should be avoided (Smyth et al. 1995).

It is obvious that the situation of pancreatic enzyme therapy in CF is today far from ideal. Development of new preparations that better comply with the difficult gastrointestinal pathophysiology of CF is a necessity. Side effects of enzyme treatment are mouth ulcers caused by incompletely swallowed particles and perianal irritation caused by particles reaching the anus. Allergic reactions are a rare event, but hyperuricemia has been reported, particularly with older preparations, and fibrosing colonopathy has recently been reported. These side effects clearly show that it was an error to consider pancreatic enzyme preparations relatively harmless substances which could be used without dose limitations.

In a 1995 consensus paper, Borowitz et al. (1995) drew clear conclusions from the dilemma in pancreatic enzyme therapy in CF. They defined factors contributing to a poor response such as enzyme storage, inadequate nutrition, poor adherence to prescription, and acidity of the small intestine. In addition, concurrent gastrointestinal disorders were listed, such as lactose intolerance, enteric bacterial overgrowth, giardiasis, celiac disease, short bowel syndrome, Crohn's disease, and colitis. These conditions call for additional diagnostic efforts in order to avoid indiscriminate increase of pancreatic enzyme dosage in CF patients showing poor response. A recommended maximum dosage of 500–2500 lipase units per kilogram per meal was set by the consensus committee. Dose reduction was recommended for patients under 12 years of age taking more than 6000 lipase units per kilogram per meal. That this dose reduction can be safe in terms of maintenance of growth was later shown by Lowdon et al. (1998) and Stevens et al. (1998). It is clear from these papers that pancreatic enzyme replacement in CF should be carefully monitored by stool fat balance studies, particularly if doses over 6000 lipase units per kilogram per meal have been reached, and that multiple individual factors have to be taken into account, requiring a full diagnostic workup in cases showing a "poor response" to pancreatic supplements.

Large Bowel Manifestations of CF: Submucosal Wall Thickening and Fibrosing Colonopathy

There are several clinical manifestations of CF in the colon: rectal prolapse, distal intestinal obstruction syndrome, intussusception, appendiceal abscess, and constipation. Shwachman described large intestinal wall thickening as early as 1975. Fibrosing colonopathy has been reported (Smyth et al. 1995) as a severe colonic manifestation with surgical consequences. First observations were made in Liverpool in five young boys who had been switched to high-dose pancreatin several months before they developed colonic obstruction requiring surgery. Two major case-control studies have since been carried out: 14 cases were identified in the United Kingdom (Smyth et al. 1995), and 29 patients were described in a careful epidemiological study in the USA (FitzSimmons et al. 1997). The disease is generally a rare event, occurring exclusively in children below 12 years of age. A clear correlation was found with high-dose pancreatin: The risk factor to develop fibrosing colonopathy was 200-fold that of controls in patients who were treated with more than 50,000 units of lipase per kilogram and day. There were no correlations found with individual preparations or manufacturers, enteric coating, and strength of preparations. Pre-existing gastrointestinal problems such as gastrointestinal surgery, distal intestinal obstruction syndrome, abdominal pain, bloody stools, colitis, and the use of H_2-receptor blockers, corticosteroids, laxatives, and recombinant human DNase were associated with a higher incidence of fibrosing colonopathy (FitzSimmons et al. 1997). Although dose-response correlation was strong, single cases were also reported in children on low-strength pancreatic enzymes (Littlewood and Hind 1996). It should also be noted that in such Western European countries as France and Germany the condition of fibrosing colonopathy is an extremely rare, singular event. Since 1996 only sporadic new cases have been described. It remains unclear whether the new policy in pancreatic enzyme dosage could be a reason for this (Borowitz et al. 1995; Lowdon et al. 1998; Stevens et al. 1998).

Pathologically, fibrosing colonopathy was described as a form of long-segment colonic disease with stenosis resulting from submucosal fibrosis (Littlewood and Hind 1996). Originally, there was no evidence of inflammation. The lesion had to be differentiated from Crohn's disease, from pseudomembranous colitis, and from colonic diaphragm disease as a consequence of potassium chloride or nonsteroidal anti-inflammatory drugs. Although experimental studies with rats and pigs have shown pathology comparable to that of fibrosing colonopathy after gavage feeding of methacrylate monomers forming the copolymer eudragit L30D55 used for enteric coating, the clinical correlation between eudragit and fibrosing colonopathy was not made in man. Histological description was suggestive of ischemia. However, neither a vascular pathogenetic theory nor a luminal nutritive theory was substantiated in the development of fibrosing colonopathy (Dodge and Macpherson 1996; Littlewood and Hind 1996).

The diagnostic value of contrast enema in fibrosing colonopathy has been a matter of conflict (Crisci et al. 1997; Littlewood and Hind 1996; Reichard et

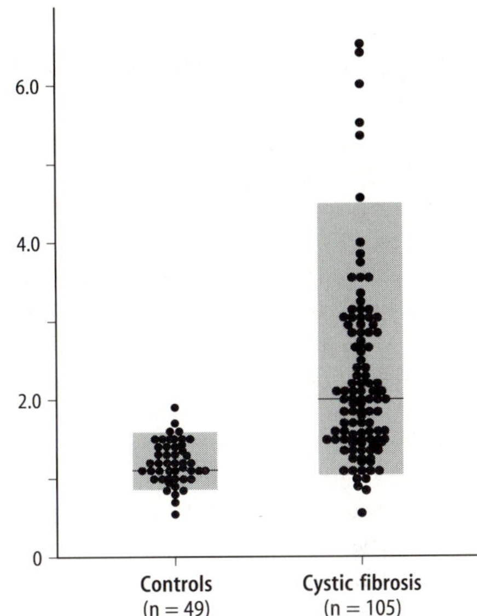

Fig. 2. Wall thickness (ultrasonography) of ascending colon in patients with cystic fibrosis (*n*=49) and in controls (*n*=105). Values are expressed as median and 5–95 percentiles (Haber et al., unpublished data)

al. 1997). Still, definitive diagnosis by histology is mandatory after resection. Only recently was the role of active or chronic eosinophilic inflammation emphasized by pathological studies (Pawel et al. 1997). Computer tomographic (CT) findings showed a mean of 6.5 mm colonic wall thickening in fibrosing colonopathy vs controls who never exceeded a wall thickness of 2 mm (Pickhardt et al. 1998).

There are now several ultrasonographic studies of small and large intestine in CF which might bear on the detection of early stages of fibrosing colonopathy (Mac Sweeney et al. 1995; Haber et al. 1997; Pohl et al. 1997). In all of these studies, maximal colonic wall thickening was found at the ascending colon. Haber et al. 1997 described a clear-cut distinction of colonic wall thickness in CF patients vs controls (Fig. 2). The value of 2 mm was never exceeded in controls, while 81% of CF patients showed colonic wall thickness of 2 mm or more. The maximum found was 6.5 mm, a value that was close to observations made with ultrasonography in the original Liverpool series with fibrosing colonopathy (R.L. Smyth, personal communication).

No difference in colonic wall thickness was found between patients with and those without pancreatic insufficiency. There was no correlation of wall measurements and pancreatic enzyme dose. This result, however, was disputed by others (Pohl et al. 1997). It should be kept in mind that none of these ultrasound studies included any patients with fibrosing colonopathy. Ultrasonographic re-examination after 1–3 years did not show much change in colonic wall thickness of CF patients besides a slight reduction, particularly in the ones who had relatively high values in the beginning. There was no progression, even with high-dose pancreatic enzyme supplementation over 15,000 units lipase per kilogram per day. Possibly, colonic wall thickening seen on ultrasonography shows genuine large bowel involvement in CF with a potential to develop into fibrosing colonopathy if special eliciting factors are present (e.g., excessive pancreatin doses, which were never used in the studies cited). Generally, the entity of fibrosing colonopathy has increased our awareness of the complex relation between gastrointestinal CF manifestations and therapeutic attempts to overcome pancreatic insufficiency.

CF Liver Disease and Ursodeoxycholic Acid

The frequency of CF hepatobiliary manifestations is increasing with age. There is no known genotype-phenotype correlation for these. Hepatobiliary involvement does not depend directly upon pancreatic insufficiency. In fact, different pathophysiological factors induce several clinical presentations (Park and Grand 1981; Scott-Jupp et al. 1991; Feigelson et al. 1993; Colombo et al. 1994; Shalon and Adelson 1996).

CFTR is expressed in bile canalicular cells but not in hepatocytes. In CF, viscous bile obstructs the bile canaliculi. Portal obstruction is followed by fibrosis. Only in a small but clinically significant group portal hypertension due to multilobular biliary cirrhosis is a final consequence. Biliary obstruction is accompanied by metabolic, toxic, and inflammatory mechanisms (e.g., antitoxins and free radicals have been shown to contribute to liver damage). Secondarily, malnutrition, particularly deficiency in essential fatty acids and vitamins A and E in CF, has a further damaging influence.

Hepatobiliary manifestations include steatosis, fibrosis, focal biliary cirrhosis, and multilobular biliary cirrhosis. Neonatal cholestasis, which does not predict severe CF liver disease, microgallbladder, cholelithiasis, and bile duct stenosis add to the clinical picture (compare Table 1). Depending upon age-group, steatosis occurs in up to two thirds of patients. Mostly, liver function is preserved over a long period. In 5%–25%, however, multilobular cirrhosis and portal hypertension and hypersplenism lead to severe end-stage liver disease, increasing mortality.

Since early treatment with UDCA possibly prevents severe courses, it is necessary to define early stages of hepatobiliary CF involvement. However, this is made difficult by short-term changes of liver enzymes, by variable biliary obstruction, and by methodological problems. For many years now, liver biopsy has not been widely carried out in CF for various reasons. Doppler ultrasonography studies have demonstrated pathological portal vein diameters, diminished flow, or even flow reversal due to portal hypertension in CF. However, interobserver reproducibility of these results was low. Colombo et al. (1994) tried to establish diagnostic criteria of CF liver disease: hepatomegaly more than 2.5 cm below the right costal margin, persistent (longer than 1 year) and significant (more than 1.5 times the upper limit of normal values) increase of at least two serum liver enzyme levels (alanine aminotransferase, aspartate aminotransferase, gamma glutamyl transpeptidase, alkaline phosphatase), hyperechogenic liver with formation of cirrhotic nodules, dilated collateral veins, and splenomegaly (ultrasound). This definition became the basis for therapeutic studies (see below). Attempts to arrive at more definite sonographic scores, to better describe biliary dysfunction by hepatobiliary scintigraphy, and to better define tissue changes by histology have added to the discussion. Still, an international consensus concerning clinical definition of CF liver disease is not available.

The natural history of CF liver disease is often mild, and histological changes might not correlate well with the clinical course. Thus, it is difficult to foresee which direction CF liver disease will take, even after a complete diagnostic workup. Meconium ileus and distal intestinal obstruction syndrome were found as risk factors for the development of CF liver disease (Colombo et al. 1994). Therapy of CF liver disease includes hypercaloric nutrition with essential fatty acids and fat-soluble vitamins. Treatment of end-stage liver disease in CF is a separate problem, very often leaving patients in unsatisfactory condition. For some of these patients, especially those with minor lung disease, liver transplantation (Mack et al. 1995) is an encouraging option. On the other hand, successful lung transplantation in spite of CF liver disease in four patients has been described (Klima et al. 1997). All of these patients, however, had good synthetic function, normal serum bilirubin, minimal esophageal varices, and no ascites or encephalopathy. Prophylactic portocaval shunting is no longer recommended (Shwachman 1975). Only in a few cases with severe portal hypertension and hypersplenism is shunting carried out as a definitive therapy, possibly aided by partial splenectomy (Feigelson et al. 1993).

Apart from the difficult situation of treating end-stage liver disease in CF, it is worthwhile to discuss several studies on the use of UDCA in treating early hepatobiliary disease (Balistreri 1997) (Table 2). UDCA is a $3\alpha,7\beta$-dihydroxy cholic acid occurring in bear bile and normally constituting 1%–2% of human bile acids. Pharmacologically, UDCA accumulates by enterohepatic circulation. There are no known side effects. It has a well-described choleretic effect, exerts favorable modulatory effects on immune functions, and shows cytoprotective effects on hepatocytes, e.g., at the mitochondrial level (Balistreri 1997).

Although the UDCA dosage in CF was started at 10 mg/kg per day, an increase to 20 mg/kg per day has proven more effective (Van de Meeberg et al. 1997). Initial studies (Colombo et al. 1990) did not differentiate well between the effect of UDCA and that of taurine supplementation. In consequential studies, however, it became clear that taurine was not essential and that the action of UDCA on liver enzymes was highly reproducible (Cotting et al. 1990; Galabert et al. 1992; Feigelson et al. 1993). Not only were elevated aminotransferase, gamma glutamyl transpeptidase, and alkaline phosphatase levels effectively and persistently diminished by oral UDCA, but also hepatobiliary excretion function was improved, as shown by scintigraphy. Scintigraphic findings, however, were disputed by O'Brien et al. in 1992. In a single study (Cotting et al. 1990) liver function improved, as indicated by sulfobromophthalein and by ^{14}C-aminopyrine breath testing. At the same time, the patients gained weight and their muscle mass increased. A very recent open study was carried out over 24 months using liver morphology as a main criterion (Lindblad et al. 1998). In seven of ten patients liver histology scores

Table 2. UDCA therapy studies in CF liver disease

Design	Author	Year	*n*	Time (months)	Results
Open	Colombo et al.	1990	9	6	Lab ↓
	Cotting et al.	1990	9	6	Lab ↓
					Weight +
	Galabert et al.	1992	22	12	Lab ↓
	Arvanitakis et al.	1993	30	24	Lab ↓
	Feigelson et al.	1993	15	24	Lab ↓
	van de Meeberg et al.	1997	30	12	Lab ↓
	Lindblad et al.	1998	10	24	Lab ↓
					Histol +
Double-blind	Bittner et al.	1990	38	6	Lab ↓
	O'Brien et al.	1992	12	16	Lab ↓
					Scinti =
	Colombo et al.	1996	55	12	Lab ↓
	Lepage et al.	1997	19	12	Lab ↓

UDCA, ursodeoxycholic acid; CF, cystic fibrosis; m months; Lab, liver laboratory tests (transaminases, alkaline phosphatase); Scinti, liver scintigraphy; Histol, liver histology.

improved; one patient showed progression in spite of UDCA therapy. Liver enzymes and serum IgG values decreased. The latter finding appeared important in terms of immunomodulatory functions of UDCA and in terms of inflammatory contribution to CF liver disease. If histological improvement could be confirmed by more long-term studies, its favorable prognostic effect would be substantiated.

Four double-blind controlled studies were carried out on the use of UDCA in CF liver disease (Bittner et al. 1990; O'Brien et al. 1992; Colombo et al. 1996, cited in Balistreri 1997; Lepage et al. 1997). A consistent decrease of liver enzymes towards normal was observed in all of these studies. In addition, UDCA therapy led to an improvement in essential fatty acids and retinol (Lepage et al. 1997). Based on these studies, it is clear that UDCA is safe and effective in CF liver disease before it has reached severe forms. Before a general recommendation for UDCA treatment can be made, however, a long-term well-controlled multicenter study should be carried out, giving clear evidence that it prevents progression to cirrhosis.

Clinical and Molecular Perspectives in Gastroenterology of CF

In spite of the general progress that has been made in the comprehensive treatment of CF, many problems remain incompletely solved with respect to gastrointestinal manifestations:

- Adult gastroenterology has to be addressed for gastrointestinal problems in adult CF patients.
- Assessment of pancreatic function at the initial diagnostic workup is an absolute necessity for all patients; follow-up is necessary for pancreatic-sufficient patients.
- Drugs for pancreatic enzyme replacement therapy are far from ideal; new formulations with improved pH optimum, the appropriate size of microgranules, and lack of side effects are subjects for further practical research.
- Restriction of pancreatic enzyme dosage and careful therapy monitoring including stool fat analysis have to be carried out at all CF centers; "poor responders" require additional diagnostic evaluation.
- Colonic wall thickening and fibrosing colonopathy are colonic manifestations that are incompletely understood, both in their natural course and in their etiology, and further clinical research is mandatory.
- A clinical definition of CF liver disease at its early stage has to be set by an international consensus panel.
- Definitive long-term studies on the effect of UDCA in hepatobiliary manifestations are necessary.

This list of topics for future research is not complete; e.g., disorders of gastrointestinal motility, gastroesophageal reflux disease, and distal intestinal obstruction syndrome are still incompletely understood and frequently insufficiently treated. Furthermore, the question of bile salt supplementation has not been definitely answered. The use of percutaneous endoscopic gastrostomy for aggressive effective nutritional treatment has to be defined. Clinical gastroenterology, particularly as it concerns adult CF patients, has to contribute much more to improving quality of life and life expectancy.

Genetic engineering has produced interesting new sources of pancreatic enzymes, particularly of lipase. In this context, acid resistance of fungal lipase, decreased denaturation by intraluminal conditions of bacterial lipase vs porcine lipase, and cloning of human gastric lipase and its expression in yeast are steps towards improved pancreatic enzyme replacement in CF (Bodmer et al. 1987; Zentler-Munro et al. 1992; Raimondo and DiMagno 1994; Suzuki et al. 1997). However, clinical use of these enzymes, which can be given in liquid form, has not yet fulfilled its high promise (Zentler-Munro et al. 1992). Better galenic formulations and more appropriate composition of lipolytic and proteolytic enzyme activities are being investigated at present.

Somatic gene therapy has been introduced experimentally in sheep, with the transfer of human lipase DNA in vitro and ex vivo to gallbladder epithelium (Maeda et al. 1994). An adenovirus vector was used, and lipase expression continued for 14 days. The study has opened new perspectives for future research. Still, many practical problems remain unsolved. The hepatobiliary system has been the target of another highly promising study involving gene therapy: Human intrahepatic biliary epithelial cell lines were infected by adenovirus, and the defective CFTR was complemented (Grubman et al. 1995). Normalization of chloride efflux was observed in CF-derived biliary epithelium for 31 days. Together with the former study concentrating on lipase transfer, this work indicates the accessibility of the hepatobiliary system to somatic gene therapy.

CFTR expression is found throughout the gastrointestinal tract, from the stomach to the colon (Strong et al. 1994). Thus, attempts to correct the defect either by somatic gene therapy or by pharmacologically influencing CFTR (Delaney and Wainwright 1996) are significant options also on the gastrointestinal level, however limited by accessibility, rapid turnover of epithelial cells, and practical feasibility. Future research will show how the high potential of genetic engineering and gene therapy can be utilized in the treatment of gastrointestinal manifestations of CF.

References

Balistreri WF (1997) Bile acid therapy in pediatric hepatobiliary disease: the role of ursodeoxycholic acid. J Pediatr Gastroenterol Nutr 24:573–589

Bittner P, Sailer T, Posselt H-G, Bender SW, Bertele-Harms RM, Arleth S, Magdorf K, Wolf A, Krawinkel M, Ott H (1990) Behandlung der Mukoviszidose mit Ursodeoxycholsäure: Ergebnisse einer kontrollierten Doppelblindstudie. Internationales Mukoviszidose-Symposium, Titisee (Germany), October 19–21, 1990, pp 1–2

Bodmer MW, Angal S, Yarranton GT, Harris TJR, Lyons A, King DJ, Pieroni G, Riviere C, Verger R, Lowe PA (1987) Molecular cloning of a human gastric lipase and expression of the enzyme in yeast. Biochim Biophys Acta 909:237–244

Borowitz DS, Grand RJ, Durie PR, Consensus Committee (1995) Use of pancreatic enzyme supplements for patients with cystic fibrosis in the context of fibrosing colonopathy. J Pediatr 127:681–684

Brady MS, Rickard K, Yu P-L, Eigen H (1991) Effectiveness and safety of small vs. large doses of enteric coated pancreatic enzymes in reducing steatorrhea in children with cystic fibrosis: a prospective randomized study. Pediatr Pulmonol 10:79–85

Colombo C, Setchell KDR, Podda M, Crosignani A, Roda A, Curcio L, Ronchi M, Giunta A (1990) Effects of ursodeoxycholic acid therapy for liver disease associated with cystic fibrosis. J Pediatr 117:482–489

Colombo C, Apostolo MG, Ferrari M, Seia M, Genoni S, Giunta A, Sereni LP (1994) Analysis of risk factors for the development of liver disease associated with cystic fibrosis. J Pediatr 124:393–399

Cotting J, Lentze MJ, Reichen J (1990) Effects of ursodeoxycholic acid treatment on nutrition and liver function in patients with cystic fibrosis and long-standing cholestasis. Gut 31:918–921

Couper RTL, Corey M, Moore DJ, Fisher LJ, Forstner GG, Durie PR (1992) Decline of exocrine pancreatic function in cystic fibrosis patients with pancreatic sufficiency. Pediatr Res 32:179–182

Crisci KL, Greenberg SB, Wolfson BJ, Geller E, Vinocur CD (1997) Contrast enema findings of fibrosing colonopathy. Pediatr Radiol 27:315–316

Delaney SJ, Wainwright BJ (1996) New pharmaceutical approaches to the treatment of cystic fibrosis. Nat Med 2:392–393

Dodge JA, Macpherson C (1996) Colonic strictures in cystic fibrosis. J R Soc Med 88 [Suppl 25]:3–8

Feigelson J, Anagnostopoulos C, Poquet M, Pecau Y, Munck A, Navarro J (1993) Liver cirrhosis in cystic fibrosis – therapeutic implications and long-term follow-up. Arch Dis Child 68:653–657

Figarella C (ed) (1996) Advances in cystic fibrosis: gastrointestinal and nutritional aspects. Eur J Gastroenterol Hepatol 8:729

FitzSimmons SC, Burkhart GA, Borowitz D, Grand RJ, Hammerstrom T, Durie PR, Lloyd-Still JD, Lowenfels AB (1997) High-dose pancreatic-enzyme supplements and fibrosing colonopathy in children with cystic fibrosis. N Engl J Med 336:1283–1289

Galabert C, Montet JC, Lengrand D, Lecuire A, Sotta C, Figarella C, Chazalette JP (1992) Effects of ursodeoxycholic acid on liver function in patients with cystic fibrosis and chronic cholestasis. J Pediatr 121:138–141

Grand RJ (1996) Gastrointestinal manifestations of cystic fibrosis. Gastrointestinal Dis Today 5:8–13

Gregory PC (1996) Gastrointestinal pH, motility/transit and permeability in cystic fibrosis. J Pediatr Gastroenterol Nutr 23:513–523

Grubman SA, Fang SL, Mulberg AE, Perrone RD, Rogers LC, Lee DW, Armentano D, Murray SL, Dorkin HL, Cheng SH, Smith AE, Jefferson DM (1995) Correction of the cystic fibrosis defect by gene complementation in human intrahepatic biliary epithelial cell lines. Gastroenterology 108:584–592

Guarner L, Rodríguez R, Guarner F, Malagelada J-R (1993) Fate of oral enzymes in pancreatic insufficiency. Gut 34:708–712

Haber HP, Benda N, Fitzke G, Lang A, Langenberg M, Riethmüller J, Stern M (1997) Colonic wall thickness measured by ultrasound: striking differences in patients with cystic fibrosis versus healthy controls. Gut 40:406–411

Klima LD, Kowdley KV, Lewis SL, Wood DE, Aitken ML (1997) Successful lung transplantation in spite of cystic fibrosis-associated liver disease: a case series. J Heart Lung Transplant 16:934–938

Koletzko S (1997) Pankreasbeteiligung bei Cystischer Fibrose. Z Gastroenterol [Suppl 1]:143–159

Lancellotti L, Cabrini G, Zanolla L, Mastella G (1996) High- versus low-lipase acid-resistant enzyme preparations in cystic fibrosis: a crossover randomized clinical trial. J Pediatr Gastroenterol Nutr 22:73–78

Lepage G, Paradis K, Lacaille F, Senechal L, Ronco N, Champagne J, Lenaerts C, Roy CC, Rasquin-Weber A (1997) Ursodeoxycholic acid improves the hepatic metabolism of essential fatty acids and retinol in children with cystic fibrosis. J Pediatr 130:52–58

Lindblad A, Glaumann H, Strandvik B (1998) A two-year prospective study of the effect of ursodeoxycholic acid on urinary bile acid excretion and liver morphology in cystic fibrosis-associated liver disease. Hepatology 27:166–174

Littlewood JM, Hind CRK (eds) (1996) Fibrosing colonopathy in children with cystic fibrosis. Postgrad Med J 72 [Suppl 2]:S2–S64

Löser C, Möllgaard A, Fölsch UR (1996) Faecal elastase 1: a novel, highly sensitive, and specific tubeless pancreatic function test. Gut 39:580–586

Lowdon J, Goodchild MC, Ryley HC, Doull IJM (1998) Maintenance of growth in cystic fibrosis despite reduction in pancreatic enzyme supplementation. Arch Dis Child 78:377–378

Mack DR, Traystman MD, Colombo JL, Sammut PH, Kaufman SS, Vanderhoof JA, Antonson DL, Markin RS, Shaw BW, Langnas AN (1995) Clinical denouement and mutation analysis of patients with cystic fibrosis undergoing liver transplantation for biliary cirrhosis. J Pediatr 127:881–887

Mac Sweeney EJ, Oades PJ, Buchdahl R, Rosenthal M, Bush A (1995) Relation of thickening of colon wall to pancreatic-enzyme treatment in cystic fibrosis. Lancet 345:752–756

Maeda H, Danel C, Crystal RG (1994) Adenovirus-mediated transfer of human lipase complementary DNA to the gallbladder. Gastroenterology 106:1638–1644

O'Brien S, Fitzgerald MX, Hegarty JE (1992) A controlled trial of ursodeoxycholic acid treatment in cystic fibrosis-related liver disease. Eur J Gastroenterol Hepatol 4:857–863

O'Hare MMT, McMaster C, Dodge JA (1995) Stated versus actual lipase activity in pancreatic enzyme supplements: implications for clinical use. J Pediatr Gastroenterol Nutr 21:59–63

Park RW, Grand, RJ (1981) Gastrointestinal manifestations of cystic fibrosis: a review. Gastroenterology 81:1143–1161

Pawel BR, de Chadarevian JP, Franco ME (1997) The pathology of fibrosing colonopathy of cystic fibrosis: a study of 12 cases and review of the literature. Hum Pathol 28:395–399

Pickhardt PJ, Yagan N, Siegel MJ, Balfe DM, Rothbaum RJ (1998) Cystic fibrosis: CT findings of colonic disease. Radiology 206:725–730

Pohl M, Krackhardt B, Posselt HG, Lembcke B (1997) Ultrasound studies of the intestinal wall in patients with cystic fibrosis. J Pediatr Gastroenterol Nutr 25:317–320

Raimondo M, DiMagno EP (1994) Lipolytic activity of bacterial lipase survives better than that of porcine lipase in human gastric and duodenal content. Gastroenterology 107:231–235

Ramsey BW, Farrell PM, Pencharz P, Consensus Committee (1992) Nutritional assessment and management in cystic fibrosis: a consensus report. Am J Clin Nutr 55:108–116

Regele S, Henker J, Münch R, Barbier Y, Stern M (1996) Indirect parameters of pancreatic function in cystic fibrosis (CF) during a controlled double-blind trial of pancreatic supplementation. J Pediatr Gastroenterol Nutr 22:68–72

Reichard KW, Vinocur CD, Franco M, Crisci KL, Flick JA, Billmire DF, Schidlow DV, Weintraub WH (1997) Fibrosing colonopathy in children with cystic fibrosis. J Pediatr Surg 32:237–241

Scott-Jupp R, Lama M, Tanner MS (1991) Prevalence of liver disease in cystic fibrosis. Arch Dis Child 66:698–701

Shalon LB, Adelson JW (1996) Cystic fibrosis: gastrointestinal complications and gene therapy. Pediatr Clin North Am 43:157–196

Shwachman H (1975) Gastrointestinal manifestations of cystic fibrosis. Pediatr Clin North Am 22:787–805

Sinaasappel M (1995) Present and future treatment modalities for gastrointestinal diseases in cystic fibrosis. Neth J Med 46:275–279

Smyth RL, Ashby D, O'Hea U, Burrows E, Lewis P, van Velzen D, Dodge JA (1995) Fibrosing colonopathy in cystic fibrosis: results of a case-control study. Lancet 346:1247–1251

Soldan W, Henker J, Sprössig C (1997) Sensitivity and specificity of quantitative determination of pancreatic elastase 1 in feces of children. J Pediatr Gastroenterol Nutr 24:53–55

Stevens JC, Maguiness KM, Hollingsworth J, Heilman DK, Chong SK (1998) Pancreatic enzyme supplementation in cystic fibrosis patients before and after fibrosing colonopathy. J Pediatr Gastroenterol Nutr 26:80–84

Strong TV, Boehm K, Collins FS (1994) Localization of cystic fibrosis transmembrane conductance regulator mRNA in the human gastrointestinal tract by in situ hybridization. J Clin Invest 93:347–354

Suzuki A, Mizumoto A, Sarr MG, DiMagno P (1997) Bacterial lipase and high-fat diets in canine exocrine pancreatic insufficiency: a new therapy of steatorrhea? Gastroenterology 112:2048–2055

Van de Meeberg PC, Houwen RHJ, Sinaasappel M, Heijerman HGM, Bijleveld CMA, van Berge Henegouwen GP (1997) Low-dose versus high-dose ursodeoxycholic acid in cystic fibrosis-related cholestatic liver disease. Scand J Gastroenterol 32:369–373

Zentler-Munro PL, Assoufi BA, Balasubramanian K, Cornell S, Benoliel D, Northfield TC, Hodson ME (1992) Therapeutic potential and clinical efficacy of acid-resistant fungal lipase in the treatment of pancreatic steatorrhoea due to cystic fibrosis. Pancreas 7:311–319

CHAPTER 19

Is Idiopathic Chronic Pancreatitis Cystic Fibrosis?

J. A. Cohn

Introduction

Chronic pancreatitis is a prevalent and commonly life-threatening condition. The two leading causes of chronic pancreatitis are alcoholic pancreatitis (AP) and idiopathic chronic pancreatitis (ICP). Among alcoholics, the risk of developing pancreatitis is small (<5%) and correlates poorly with the amount of alcohol consumed. This suggests that individual alcoholics vary in their susceptibility to pancreatitis. It is unknown whether genetic factors influence the risk of chronic pancreatitis in either alcoholics or nondrinkers [1, 2].

This chapter will review evidence that ICP is associated with abnormalities of the gene encoding a pancreatic duct cell protein, the cystic fibrosis transmembrane conductance regulator (CFTR). Certain mutations of the CFTR gene cause cystic fibrosis (CF), a disease in which 85%–90% of patients develop pancreatic insufficiency and in which almost all patients develop debilitating lung disease, abnormalities of sweat secretion, and male infertility due to abnormalities of the vas deferens [3, 4] The newly recognized association between ICP and certain types of abnormal CFTR genotypes has many implications regarding the pathogenesis and classification of ICP, and possibly also regarding prevention.

Background on Pathogenesis of Chronic Pancreatitis

The pathogenesis of chronic pancreatitis is incompletely understood. In both AP and ICP, plugging of the smaller pancreatic ducts is a prominent early event [5–7]. These plugs consist of precipitates containing the proteins, glycoproteins, and mucins normally present in pancreatic juice. Even though two specific proteins have been associated with these plugs [8, 9], the cause of ductal protein plugging in AP and in ICP remains unknown.

For ICP, no information exists concerning any potential predisposing factors. By contrast, the relationship between alcohol consumption and AP has been studied in detail. Even though high levels of alcohol consumption are required for AP, only a minority of alcoholics develop AP. This suggests that individuals vary widely in their susceptibility to AP. This variability could result from genetic factors, and early support for this concept came from reports of familial clustering in AP [10, 11]. Since then, conflicting data about the role of heredity in AP has emerged from studies testing AP patients for a variety of genetic markers, including HLA antigens, α_1-antitrypsin phenotypes, blood groups, and ADH polymorphisms. A crucial limitation of these data (and of the familial clustering data) is that almost all these studies failed to compare AP patients with alcoholic controls. Because heredity correlates closely with alcoholism, this limitation renders the data from these studies inconclusive with respect to the question of whether genetic factors determine which alcoholics will develop pancreatitis [2]. To date, this question remains unanswered.

Background on CFTR

CFTR plays an important role during exocrine secretion by the normal human pancreas [12, 13]. The predominant site of CFTR in human pancreas is the apical plasma membrane of the epithelial cells lining the intralobular ducts; individuals with insufficient CFTR at this site are thought to have difficulty alkalinizing and diluting their pancreatic secretions [13]. This concept provides a physiologic explanation for the occurrence of plugging of the small pancreatic ducts as a prominent early finding in CF [14]. Because similar plugging occurs in many forms of chronic pancreatitis [5–7], this suggests that abnormalities in CFTR function might contribute to the pathogenesis of pancreatic diseases other than CF.

Two additional findings support the suggestion that abnormalities in CFTR function might play a role in chronic pancreatitis. First, abnormal sweat electrolyte values similar to those seen in cystic fibrosis occur in many patients with chronic pancreatitis [15, 16]. Second, pancreatitis occurs in 1%–2% of individuals with cystic fibrosis, indicating that it is possible for mutations of the CFTR gene to cause pancreatic dysfunction, leading to pancreatitis [3, 17].

Background on CFTR Genotype-Phenotype Correlation

The association of CFTR mutations with ICP will be reviewed by building on emerging concepts related to the cell biology and clinical genetics of CFTR. During the 9 years that have elapsed since the discovery of CFTR, 50 000 mutant chromosomes have been tested for CFTR mutations and 700+ different CFTR mutations have been associated with CF [3, 18]. (Throughout this chapter, genetic data have been updated from cited references based on data from the CF Genetic Analysis Consortium available at http://www.genet.sickkids.on.ca/cftr/.) As first reported in 1989, a single mutation, ΔF508, accounts for roughly 70% of CF-causing alleles in most Caucasian populations [19]. Roughly 50% of CF patients are ΔF508 homozygotes, and an additional 40% are compound heterozygotes with one ΔF508 allele and one other CF-causing allele. The protein product of the CFTR gene normally occurs at the cell membrane of epithelial cells, where it functions as a Cl^- channel and as a regulator of other ion channels [3, 13, 20–22].

Because so many different CFTR mutations have been identified, a wealth of data exists related to genotype-phenotype correlation. One emerging concept is that different types of CFTR genotypes are associated with different clinical presentations of CF. The presence or absence of pancreatic insufficiency (PI) was the first clinical feature found to correlate with the CFTR genotype, and this has therefore been emphasized in efforts to distinguish mild from severe forms of CF [19, 23]. Subsequently, it was recognized that an additional group of abnormal CFTR genotypes can cause vas deferens dysfunction in the absence of CF lung disease. This vas deferens disease, termed congenital bilateral absence of the vas deferens (CBAVD), is associated with CFTR genotypes causing partial (~90%) loss of CFTR function [24, 25]. By contrast, CF lung disease with PI results from genotypes causing very severe loss of CFTR (~99%), while pancreatic-sufficient CF lung disease results from genotypes causing only moderately severe loss of CFTR (~95%) [4]. Thus, even though CF and CBAVD are each caused by CFTR genotypes consisting of two abnormal alleles, CBAVD patients do not develop CF lung disease because one of their mutant alleles impairs CFTR function to a lesser degree than mutations causing CF lung disease [24].

The most common example of a CFTR allele which causes CBAVD without CF lung disease is the intron 8 5T splicing variant ("5T"). Three variants occur at this splicing site, termed 5T, 7T, and 9T (depending on the number of pyrimidines). The 5T variant occurs on 5% of chromosomes in the general population and differs from the 7T and 9T variants because it reduces the efficiency of exon 9 splicing and thereby causes CBAVD by reducing the abundance of functional CFTR. Patients with ΔF508 allele and one 5T allele (ΔF508/5T) do not develop CF because they produce enough functional (properly spliced) CFTR to prevent lung disease, but they do not produce enough functional CFTR to protect the vas deferens [24].

CFTR Mutations Are Associated with ICP

Our group recently reported a study examining the relationship between CFTR mutations and ICP [26]. Briefly, this study was designed to address four questions: Are CFTR mutations associated with ICP? Do CBAVD-causing CFTR genotypes predispose to ICP? Do ICP patients with abnormal CFTR genotypes actually have unrecognized CF lung disease? Is CFTR function defective in ICP patients who have abnormal CFTR genotypes?

We addressed these questions by testing DNA from 27 Caucasian ICP patients who had been selected based on a review of the clinical records of all patients referred to Duke University Medical Center for ERCP from 1991 to 1996. Stringent inclusion and exclusion criteria were defined to identify patients in whom there was a suspicion of any of the known causes for pancreatitis. Most patients had severe pain, and patients with equivocal or

Table 1. CFTR genotypes of seven ICP patients with CFTR mutations

Patient no.	Sex	Mutations	Intron 8	Age at onset (years)	ICP hospitalization (number)	(days)	ERCP class
1	M	ΔF508/R117H	9T/7T	45	11	46	Moderate
2	F	ΔF508/wt	9T/5T	32	7	52	Moderate
3	F	ΔF508/wt	9T/5T	48	20	100+	Moderate
4	F	ΔF508/wt	9T/7T	40	25	100+	Moderate
5	F	ΔF508/wt	9T/7T	15	16	62	Mild
6	F	R117H/wt	7T/7T	32	6	60	Moderate
7	M	N1303 K/wt	7T/9T	43	1	6	Moderate

uncertain clinical histories were excluded (e.g., patients reporting moderate levels of alcohol consumption). The DNA samples were tested for 17 common CF-causing mutations and for the 5T allele, a common CBAVD-causing allele (see above). Thirteen abnormal alleles were detected in ten patients of these 27 ICP patients. None of these ten patients had typical CF lung disease based on clinical history or a recent chest X-ray. As a group, these patients had severe pancreatitis (four required surgery), and the mean age at diagnosis was 33 years. Clinical data for the seven ICP patients with CFTR mutations are shown in Table 1. Six of the seven had moderately severe pancreatic duct abnormalities at ERCP [27], supporting the clinical impression that these patients have ICP, rather than relapsing acute pancreatitis.

In the 27 ICP patients tested we detected eight CF-causing mutations (11-fold expected frequency, $p<0.000001$) and five patients with the 5T allele (1.9-fold, nonsignificant). Three of the ICP patients tested had genotypes in which both CFTR alleles were affected, and this represents an 80-fold increase over the expected frequency for these rare genotypes ($p<0.00001$). The two genotypes observed in these three patients (ΔF508/R117H; 9T/7T and ΔF508/WT; 9T/5T) are the most common CBAVD genotypes [24, 28–32], and each is known not to cause CF [33].

Clinical and Physiological Testing of ICP Patients with CFTR Mutations

The three patients with an abnormality of both CFTR alleles were further evaluated to test whether they might have unrecognized CF lung disease. None of these patients had a diagnostic sweat test result, although two had borderline values. The baseline nasal potential difference (PD) values for these patients ranged from –24 to –21 mV and were equivalent to those in normal adults [34]. Two patients reported no chronic respiratory symptoms, and spirometry was normal in each. In the third patient, the FEV_1 was reduced (58% predicted), and this seemed most consistent with a diagnosis of chronic obstructive pulmonary disease due to cigarette use (two packs/day). Sputum from this patient contained normal flora. Urological evaluation of the only man in the group revealed CBAVD. Thus, none of the three tested ICP patients has typical CF lung disease [3, 35].

To test CFTR-mediated ion transport more directly, nasal bioelectric responses were measured in these ICP patients. In this protocol, the combined effect of Cl^--substitution and isoproterenol (ΔPD) reflects CFTR-mediated Cl^- transport [34]. Each of the tested ICP patients showed a ΔPD value equivalent to those seen in CF. The values in ICP were consistently lower ($p<0.001$) than those in normal individuals. Thus, CFTR-mediated Cl^- transport is impaired in the nasal epithelia of these ICP patients. This suggests that in ICP patients with two abnormal CFTR alleles, CFTR function may be similarly impaired in the ductal epithelium of the exocrine pancreas.

Synopsis of Other Studies Testing for CFTR Mutations in Pancreatitis

During 1998, four other groups reported data concerning the frequency of CFTR mutations in pancreatitis. Two of these studies were reported as full publications [36, 37] and two were reported only as abstracts [38, 39].

Three of these additional studies tested patients with nonalcoholic chronic pancreatitis for CFTR mutations [37–39]. Among a total of 187 Caucasian patients tested in the three studies, 35 had mutations (19%). One of these studies reported whether individual patients with mutations also had the 5T allele [37]. In this study, three patients had CBAVD-causing genotypes among the 60 nonalcoholic chronic pancreatitis who were tested. Finally, three studies examined the frequency of CFTR mutations in patients with pancreatitis due to alcohol [36–38]. If the data from these studies are pooled, eight patients had mutations among the 126 (6%) AP patients tested. Even though this is not a statistically significant increase above the expected value, these data suggest a trend towards a small (roughly 60%) increase in the frequency of mutations.

Summary of Existing Data Regarding CFTR Mutations in Pancreatitis

CFTR mutations are strongly associated with ICP. Among 216 patients with nonalcoholic chronic pancreatitis tested in all studies reported to date (most of whom have ICP), 42 (20%) have CFTR mutations [26, 37–39]. Thus, mutations are increased approximately sixfold in these patients. The association of CBAVD-causing CFTR genotypes with nonalcoholic chronic pancreatitis is even stronger: Among 87 patients tested in the two studies reported to date, six (7%) have these very rare genotypes [26, 37]. Thus, these CFTR genotypes are increased about 50-fold in this group. Finally, in ICP patients with CBAVD-causing genotypes, nasal CFTR-mediated Cl^- transport is defective. To date, this conclusion is based on data from one study only [26].

Implications for the Pathogenesis of ICP

The main point of this chapter is that many patients carrying a diagnosis of unexplained chronic pancreatitis have a disease in which genetics plays a major and previously unsuspected role. This is most clearly illustrated by the group of ICP patients found to have abnormalities of both copies of the CFTR gene. For them it seems likely that there will be major parallels between CBAVD and ICP with respect to genotype-phenotype correlation and molecular pathogenesis (Table 2). Specifically, the genotypes causing CBAVD or ICP apparently reduce CFTR function to roughly 5%–10% of normal levels in many epithelial tissues. This reduction of CFTR function is severe enough to affect the vas deferens and pancreas but not severe enough to cause classic CF (including CF lung disease and abnormal sweat electrolytes). CBAVD can be viewed as an autosomal recessive variant or atypical form of CF, and the same concept applies to this group of ICP patients. One implication of this concept is that when ICP occurs in patients with CBAVD-causing genotypes, it is anticipated that there will be an association of ICP with other conditions, including CBAVD and possibly sinusitis. These conditions were not previously linked with ICP.

A second important conclusion is that individuals with one CFTR mutation are at increased risk for ICP. In spite of being at increased risk, the vast majority of CF carriers are not expected to develop ICP, because there are at least 50 times as many CF carriers in the general population as there are patients with ICP. This suggests that other factors must also play a role in determining which predisposed individuals develop pancreatitis. One possibility is that mutations of another gene determine which CF carriers develop ICP. Alternatively, extragenic (environmental) factors may be decisive in some cases. Finally, it remains possible that some of the ICP patients now thought to be CF carriers may eventually be recognized as compound heterozygotes in whom both copies of the CFTR gene are abnormal (but in whom a second mutation was not detected by the initial genetic testing procedure).

Table 2. Different CFTR genotypes cause different phenotypes

CFTR genotype	Severe/severe	Severe/mild	Mild/mild, any/5T
Functional CFTR	0%–2%	2%–5%	5%–10%
Pancreatitis	No	Yes	Yes
CBAVD	Yes	Yes	Yes
CF lung disease	Yes	Yes	No
Abnormal sweat test	Yes	Yes	No
Pancreatic insufficiency (PI)	Yes	No	No
Clinical diagnosis	CF with PI	CF without PI	CBAVD or ICP

Implications for Diagnosis of ICP

The strong association of CFTR mutations with ICP raises the issue of genetic testing for patients with ICP. At this time, I advise testing ICP patients for CFTR mutations only if this is being done for research purposes. No guidelines exist for genetic counseling based on the results of these tests. At present, commercial labs do not routinely test for the 5T allele, and testing for this allele is necessary to detect the more common genotypes that most strongly predispose to ICP. Finally, the results of genetic testing should not affect clinical management in any way.

In my opinion, it would be premature for practicing gastroenterologists to routinely test their ICP patients for CFTR mutations at this time. However, I anticipate that, as basic research further clarifies the relationship between CFTR and ICP, guidelines will be developed for the use of this type of genetic testing in patients with this and other pancreatitic diseases.

Directions for Future Research

Several issues present important topics for further study in this area. One priority concerns testing whether CFTR mutations are also associated with pancreatic diseases other than ICP. If CFTR mutations prove to be associated with pancreatitis attributed to conditions such as alcohol use [37] or pancreas divisum [38], then this could provide important clues about early events in the pathogenesis of these disorders.

From the standpoint of ICP, one high priority concerns understanding how CFTR function is affected in different epithelial tissues in genotyped individuals with ICP. Based on studies of a limited number of ICP patients [26], it seems likely that defective CFTR function will be evident in some epithelial tissues from ICP patients with certain types of abnormal CFTR genotypes. However, additional studies are needed to determine whether this occurs in multiple tissues and whether this occurs in individuals with other types of abnormal genotypes (e.g., CF carriers vs. individuals with two abnormal copies of the gene).

A related question concerns whether the ICP patients identified as CF carriers based on initial genetic testing truly have one normal copy of the CFTR gene. Since 700+ different mutations are known to occur in this gene, it is possible that many of these individuals actually have a second mutation on their "normal" copy of the gene. Comprehensive genetic testing of DNA samples from these individuals will clarify this question and will also determine whether any rare mutations in the CFTR gene are specifically associated with ICP.

Finally, the association of CFTR mutations with ICP calls attention to the central role played by the duct cell in the pathophysiology of the exocrine pancreas. Current concepts regarding the role of CFTR in the pancreas suggest that it may be possible to delay the progression of ICP by using drugs to augment ductal bicarbonate secretion. If safe, it is conceivable that such drugs might eventually enable us to prevent ICP in individuals who are genetically predisposed to this condition.

References

1. Steer ML, Waxman I, Freedman S (1995) Chronic pancreatitis. N Engl J Med 332:1482–1490
2. Haber P, Wilson J, Apte M, Korsten M, Pirola R (1995) Individual susceptibility to alcoholic pancreatitis: still an enigma. J Lab Clin Med 125:305–312
3. Welsh MJ, Tsui LC, Boat TF, Beaudet AL (1995) Cystic fibrosis. In: Scriver CR, Beaudet AL, Sly WS, Valle D (eds) The metabolic basis of inherited disease, 7th edn. McGraw-Hill, New York, pp 3799–3876
4. Davis PB, Drumm M, Konstan MW (1996) Cystic fibrosis. Am J Respir Crit Care Med 154:1229–1256
5. Nakamura K, Sarles H, Payan H (1972) Three-dimensional reconstruction of the pancreatic ducts in chronic pancreatitis. Gastroenterology 62:942–949
6. Longnecker DS (1982) Pathology and pathogenesis of diseases of the pancreas. Am J Pathol 107:103–121
7. De Angelis C, Valente G, Spaccapietra M, Angonese C, Del Favero G, Naccarato R, et al (1992) Histological study of alcoholic, nonalcoholic, and obstructive chronic pancreatitis. Pancreas 7:193–196
8. Giorgi D, Bernard JP, Rouquier S, Iovanna J, Sarles H, Dagorn JC (1989) Secretory pancreatic stone protein messenger RNA. Nucleotide sequence and expression in chronic calcifying pancreatitis. J Clin Invest 84:100–106
9. Freedman SD, Sakamoto K, Venu RP (1993) GP2, the homologue to the renal cast protein uromodulin, is a major component of intraductal plugs in chronic pancreatitis. J Clin Invest 92:83–90
10. Marks IN, Bank S, Louw JH (1973) Chronic pancreatitis in the Western Cape. Digestion 9:447–453
11. Sarles H, Bernard JP, Gullo L (1990) Pathogenesis of chronic pancreatitis. Gut 31:629–632
12. Kopelman H, Forstner GG, Durie PR, Corey M (1989) Origins of chloride and bicarbonate secretory defects in the cystic fibrosis pancreas as suggested by pancreatic function studies on control and CF subjects with preserved pancreatic function. Clin Invest Med 12:207–211
13. Marino CR, Matovcik LM, Gorelick FS, Cohn JA (1991) Localization of the cystic fibrosis transmembrane conductance regulator in pancreas. J Clin Invest 88:712–716
14. Oppenheimer EH, Esterly JR (1975) Pathology of cystic fibrosis: review of the literature and comparison with 146 autopsied cases. Perspect Pediatr Pathol 2:241–278
15. Bank S, Marks IN, Novis B (1978) Sweat electrolytes in chronic pancreatitis. Am J Dig Dis 23:178–181
16. Hanawa M, Takebe T, Takahashi S, Koizumi M, Endo K (1978) The significance of the sweat test in chronic pancreatitis. Tohoku J Exp Med 125:59–69
17. Shwachman H, Lebenthal E, Khaw KT (1975) Recurrent acute pancreatitis in patients with cystic fibrosis with normal pancreatic enzymes. Pediatrics 55:86–95
18. Zielenski J, Tsui LC (1995) Cystic fibrosis: genotypic and phenotypic variations. Annu Rev Genet 29:777–807
19. Kerem BS, Rommens JM, Buchanan JA, Markiewicz D, Cox TK, Chakravarti A, et al (1989) Identification of the cystic fibrosis gene: genetic analysis. Science 245:1073–1080
20. Riordan JR, Rommens JM, Kerem BS, Alon N, Rozmahel R, Grzelczak Z, et al (1989) Identification of the cystic fibrosis gene: cloning and characterization of complementary DNA. Science 245:1066–1073
21. Bear CE, Li CH, Kartner N, Bridges RJ, Jensen TJ, Ramjeesingh M, et al (1992) Purification and functional reconstitution of the cystic fibrosis transmembrane conductance regulator (CFTR). Cell 68:809–818
22. Stutts MJ, Canessa CM, Olsen JC, Hamrick M, Cohn JA, Rossier BC, et al (1995) CFTR as a cAMP-dependent regulator of sodium channels. Science 269:847–850
23. Anonymous (1993) Correlation between genotype and phenotype in patients with cystic fibrosis. The Cystic Fibrosis Genotype-Phenotype Consortium. N Engl J Med 329:1308–1313

24. Chillon M, Casals T, Mercier B, Bassas L, Lissens W, Silber S, et al (1995) Mutations in the cystic fibrosis gene in patients with congenital absence of the vas deferens. N Engl J Med 332:1475–1480
25. Anguiano A, Oates RD, Amos JA, Dean M, Gerrard B, Stewart C, et al (1992) Congenital bilateral absence of the vas deferens. A primarily genital form of cystic fibrosis. JAMA 267:1794–1797
26. Cohn JA, Friedman KJ, Noone PG, Knowles MR, Silverman LM, Jowell PJ (1998) Relation between mutations of the cystic fibrosis gene and idiopathic pancreatitis. N Engl J Med 339:653–658
27. Axon AT, Classen M, Cotton PB, Cremer M, Freeny PC, Lees WR (1984) Pancreatography in chronic pancreatitis: international definitions. Gut 25:1107–1112
28. Mercier B, Verlingue C, Lissens W, Silber SJ, Novelli G, Bonduelle M, et al (1995) Is congenital bilateral absence of vas deferens a primary form of cystic fibrosis? Analyses of the CFTR gene in 67 patients. Am J Hum Genet 56:272–277
29. Costes B, Girodon E, Ghanem N, Flori E, Jardin A, Soufir JC, et al (1995) Frequent occurrence of the CFTR intron 8 (TG)n 5T allele in men with congenital bilateral absence of the vas deferens. Eur J Hum Genet 3:285–293
30. Dumur V, Gervais R, Rigot JM, Delomel-Vinner E, Decaestecker B, Lafitte JJ, et al (1996) Congenital bilateral absence of the vas deferens (CBAVD) and cystic fibrosis transmembrane regulator (CFTR): correlation between genotype and phenotype. Hum Genet 97:7–10
31. Colin AA, Sawyer SM, Mickle JE, Oates RD, Milunsky A, Amos JA (1996) Pulmonary function and clinical observations in men with congenital bilateral absence of the vas deferens. Chest 110:440–445
32. Jezequel P, Dorval I, Fergelot P, Chauvel B, Le Treut A, Le Gall JY, et al (1995) Structural analysis of CFTR gene in congenital bilateral absence of vas deferens. Clin Chem 41:833–835
33. Kiesewetter S, Macek M, Jr, Davis C, Curristin SM, Chu CS, Graham C, et al (1993) A mutation in CFTR produces different phenotypes depending on chromosomal background. Nat Genet 5:274–278
34. Knowles MR, Paradiso AM, Boucher RC (1995) In vivo nasal potential difference: techniques and protocols for assessing efficacy of gene transfer in cystic fibrosis. Hum Gene Ther 6:445–455
35. Stern RC (1997) The diagnosis of cystic fibrosis. N Engl J Med 336:487–491
36. Norton ID, Apte M, Dixson H, Trent RJ, Haber PS, Pirola RC, et al (1998) Cystic fibrosis genotypes and alcoholic pancreatitis. J Gastroenterol Hepatol 13:496–499
37. Sharer N, Schwarz M, Malone G, Howarth A, Painter J, Super M, et al (1998) Mutations of the cystic fibrosis gene in patients with chronic pancreatitis. N Engl J Med 339:645–652
38. Choudari CP, Yu AC, Imperiale TF, Fogel EL, Sherman S, Lehman GA (1998) Significance of heterozygous cystic fibrosis gene in idiopathic pancreatitis. Gastroenterology 114:A447 (Abstr)
39. Castellani C, Sgarbi D, Cavallini G, DiFrancesco V, Bovo P, Frulloni L, et al (1998) CFTR mutations and IVS8-5T prevalence in idiopathic chronic and acute recurrent pancreatitis. Gastroenterology 114:A445 (Abstr)

Part IV
Pancreatic Cancer

CHAPTER 20

Growth Factors and Transcription Factors in Pancreatic Cancer

H. FRIESS, Z.W. ZHU, L. WANG, and M.W. BÜCHLER

Introduction

Pancreatic cancers originate from both exocrine and endocrine components of the pancreas. However, about 90% derive from the exocrine portion, and about 80% of all pancreatic cancers are ductal adenocarcinomas (Zimmermann 1994). The emphasis of this review is on ductal pancreatic adenocarcinoma, and the term *pancreatic cancer* refers in this article to this kind of carcinoma.

Pancreatic cancer is currently the fourth or fifth leading cause of cancer-related death in Western countries (Warshaw and Fernandez-Del Castillo 1992; Parker et al. 1997). An increase in the number registered annually worldwide in recent years is most probably based on improvements in diagnostic measures (Warshaw and Fernandez-Del Castillo 1992; Parker et al. 1997). Cigarette smoking, intake of coffee and alcohol, a diet rich in fat and meat, diabetes mellitus, chronic pancreatitis, and stomach operations have been proposed to be risk factors for the development of pancreatic carcinomas (Harnack et al. 1997). However, more recent data indicate that alcohol consumption has largely no relationship, and coffee consumption shows only little association with the occurrence of pancreatic cancer (Gold and Goldin 1998), whereas a protective effect of dietary fiber and consumption of fruits and vegetables on pancreatic cancer development was reported (Gold and Goldin 1998).

It is difficult to detect pancreatic cancer in early tumor stages due to the frequently nonspecific symptoms (Lee and Williams 1994). More than 80% of patients with cancer of the pancreas are therefore diagnosed in advanced tumor stages (stage III or IV) (Gudjonsson 1987; Warshaw and Fernandez-Del Castillo 1992; Parker et al. 1997). Consequently, at the time of diagnosis between 75% and 85% of pancreatic cancer patients have unresectable or metastatic tumors, and these patients can be offered only palliative surgical options, such as biliary or enteral bypass operations or interventional stenting (Gudjonsson 1987; Büchler et al. 1993; Friess et al. 1993a). More recent studies demonstrate that the 5-year survival following the resection of pancreatic tumors is about 15%–40% (Ozaki et al. 1990; Trede et al. 1990; Cameron et al. 1991). Pancreatic cancer is extremely unresponsive to traditional cancer therapies, and therefore new possibilities such as gene therapy, immunotherapy, and hormonal therapy, are presently under evaluation (Nio and Tamura 1997).

The reasons for the aggressive growth and metastatic behavior of pancreatic cancer are poorly understood. Based on recent molecular analysis, we now know that pancreatic cancer is associated with a variety of genetic alterations. Many disturbances in oncogenes and tumor suppressor genes have been demonstrated to be closely related to the aggressive growth behavior of pancreatic tumors. Point mutations of the K-ras proto-oncogene are present in 85%–95% of pancreatic cancers but are rarely found in chronic pancreatitis (Grünewald et al. 1989; Hsiang et al. 1997; Kasuya et al. 1997). In addition, p53, a tumor suppressor gene which is located on the short arm of chromosome 17 and encodes a 53-kDa nuclear phosphoprotein (Levine et al. 1991), is mutated in 40%–60% of the tumors (Ruggeri et al. 1992; Casey et al. 1993). Furthermore, accumulating evidence indicates that growth factors and their receptors, such as epidermal growth factor (EGF) and transforming growth factors (TGFs) and their receptors, play an important role in the growth regulation of pancreatic cancer through autocrine and paracrine actions (Korc and Magun 1985; Korc et al. 1986; Friess et al. 1993 a; Korc 1998). Analyses of growth factor and growth factor receptor alterations in pancreatic cancer supplement our understanding of tumor biology and provide new molecular markers for earlier diagnosis and better markers for the estimation of prognosis and treatment of pancreatic cancer patients (Friess et al. 1997). Recently, the role of another group of molecular factors – transcription factors (TFs) – has received attention, and growing knowledge of transcriptional control mechanisms might provide the basis for innovative cancer therapies (Hurst 1996).

In the present review, we primarily summarize the recent advances in research on some important growth factors, growth factor receptors, and transcription factors whose activation generally enhances cell proliferation in pancreatic cancer.

Growth Factors and Their Corresponding Receptors in Pancreatic Cancer

Growth factors are produced by a variety of different cells, and they function via autocrine and/or paracrine mechanisms, either near their site of expression or systemically. Enhanced expression of growth factors and their receptors has been implicated in the uncontrolled growth of cancer cells (Aaronson 1991). At the same time, an inhibitory effect on the growth of cancer cells has also been observed for some of these growth factors (Kingsley 1994). In pancreatic cancer, the important growth factors and growth factor receptors are (a) the epidermal growth factor (EGF) family and their receptors (EGFR), (b) transforming growth factor-betas (TGF-βs) and their receptors (TβRs), (c) fibroblast growth factors (FGFs) and their receptors (FGFRs), (d) insulin-like growth factors (IGFs) and their receptors (IGFRs), (e) hepatocyte growth factor (HGF) and its receptor c-met, and (f) platelet-derived growth factor (PDGF) and its receptor (PDGFR).

The Epidermal Growth Factor Family and Its Receptors

In addition to epidermal growth factor (EGF) itself, the EGF family also includes transforming growth factor-alpha (TGF-alpha), heparin-binding EGF-like growth factor (HB-EGF), betacellulin, and amphiregulin (Plowman et al. 1990; Abraham et al. 1993; Shing et al. 1993). These five growth factors all possess six cysteine residues in the same relative position, which results in the formation of disulfide bonds that confer similar three-dimensional configurations on these polypeptides. All six can bind to the epidermal growth factor receptor (EGFR). The EGFR is a 170-kilodalton (kDa) glycosylated phosphoprotein which is encoded by a gene located on the short arm of chromosome 7 (Shimizu et al. 1984; Ullrich et al. 1984). There are three additional receptors which are closely related to the EGFR. They have been variably named as the human EGF receptor type 2 (HER-2) or c-erbB-2, the human EGF receptor type 3 (HER-3) or c-erbB-3, and the human EGF receptor type 4 (HER-4) or c-erbB-4 (Plowman et al. 1993a). They are composed of an extracellular ligand-binding domain with two cysteine-rich regions, a transmembrane domain, and an intracellular domain with tyrosine kinase activity residues within a continuous region of amino acids (Peles et al. 1992; Plowman et al. 1993b). Binding of ligands to the extracellular domain leads to receptor activation by dimerization of the receptor with auto- and transphosphorylation on tyrosine residues (Schlessinger and Ullrich 1992). Several ligands which interact with the EGFR family have been described in the past (Marchionni et al. 1993; Yamanaka et al. 1993a): c-erbB-2 is activated by binding of specific ligands such as Neu differentiation factor (NDF), glial growth factors, and heregulin (Holmes et al. 1992; Marchionni et al. 1993; Peles et al. 1993); c-erbB-3 and c-erbB-4 bind NDFs and possibly other ligands.

Early studies on cancer cells showed that overexpression of the EGFR leads to malignant transformation, and that the presence of TGF-alpha additionally stimulates the proliferation of transformed cells (Libermann et al. 1985; Neal et al. 1985). These in vitro studies initially indicated that alterations within the EGFR family and their ligands might also be important for the course and prognosis of cancers in vivo. The overexpression of EGFR and its ligands has been demonstrated in many human pancreatic cancer cell lines (Korc and Magun 1985; Korc et al. 1986; Smith et al. 1987; Korc and Finman 1989; Oikawa et al. 1995). Following binding of EGF or TGF-alpha to the EGFR, the receptor-ligand complex is internalized. EGF is often recycled, whereas TGF-alpha is rapidly degraded (Korc and Magun 1985; Derynck 1988; Korc and Finman 1989). However, TGF-alpha was found to be 10 to 100-times more potent than EGF in enhancing the anchorage-independent growth of pancreatic cancer cell lines (Korc and Magun 1985). Binding of EGF and TGF-alpha to the EGFR induces its down-regulation (Korc and Magun 1985); EGF is more efficient than TGF-alpha in this regard (Korc and Finman 1989). These findings suggest that overexpression of EGFR in conjunction with production of TGF-alpha and the recycling of EGF may give pancreatic cancer cells a major growth advantage. This hypothesis can be demonstrated by transfecting an expression plasmid encoding a kinase-deficient EGFR cDNA (HER653) into cultured human pancreatic cancer cells (PANC-1) by a retroviral vector transfer (Wagner et al. 1996). The EGF- and TGF-alpha-mediated EGFR tyrosine phosphorylation is markedly attenuated and pancreatic cancer cell growth is inhibited (Wagner et al. 1996). Therefore, it is suggested that dominant negative inhibition of the EGFR pathway may have therapeutic potential in pancreatic cancer patients. Overexpression of EGF, TGF-alpha, and EGFR has been described in human pancreatic cancer tissues (Barton et al. 1991a; Korc et al. 1992; Yamanaka et al. 1993 a), and the concomitant overexpression of EGFR and its activating ligands in most pancreatic cancer cells suggests that they function via autocrine and/or paracrine mechanisms. An important observation is that the prognosis of pancreatic cancer patients overexpressing the EGFR and EGF and/or TGF-alpha or amphiregulin concomitantly is poorer than that of patients not overexpressing either the receptor or one of the ligands (Yamanaka et al. 1993 a; Ebert et al. 1994a; Yokoyama et al. 1995). These data were recently confirmed by analysis of EGF and EGFR in 60 primary and 26 metastatic pancreatic cancer lesions (Uegaki et al. 1997). Furthermore, it was demonstrated that up-regulation of EGF and EGFR occurs more frequently in metastasis than in primary lesions of pancreatic cancer. Therefore, concomitant analysis of EGFR with its activating ligands seems to be a beneficial prognostic factor in pancreatic cancer patients (Yamanaka et al. 1993a; Uegaki et al. 1997).

Betacellulin, HB-EGF, and amphiregulin also belong to the epidermal growth factor family, and all three growth factors are expressed in pancreatic cancer cells in vitro and in vivo. Betacellulin expression was found in five of six human pancreatic cancer cell lines (Yokoyama et al. 1995), and HB-EGF immunoreactivity was demonstrated in 50% of human pancreatic cancer samples (Yokoyama et al. 1996). However, the exact effects of betacellulin and HB-EGF on pancreatic cancer pathogenesis are poorly understood, and further investigation is needed to define their potential functions in cancer cell biology in vivo.

The c-erbB-2 receptor also has a potential role in the tumor pathogenesis of pancreatic cancer (Hall et al. 1990; Yamanaka et al. 1993 b). Overexpression of c-erbB-2 in cultured cells leads to malignant cell transformation (Di Fiore et al. 1987; Hudziak et al. 1987). In pancreatic cancer, c-erbB-2 was overexpressed in 34 of 76 cancer samples (45%), and its overexpression was associated with better tumor differentiation (Yamanaka et al. 1993 b). In contrast to other growth factors and growth factor receptors, the presence of c-erbB2 in the pancreatic cancer cells is not associated with advanced tumor stage or shorter postoperative survival (Yamanaka et al. 1993 b). These findings in human pancreatic cancer agree with those from studies of cultured cancer cell lines whereby c-erbB-2 activation leads to better tumor differentiation (Peles et al. 1993).

c-erbB-3, the third member of the EGFR family, is increased up to sixfold in pancreatic cancer samples compared with the normal pancreas, and its presence in the tumor samples is associated with advanced tumor stage and significantly shorter postoperative survival after tumor resection (Friess et al. 1995).

The c-erbB-4 gene encodes a 180-kDa transmembrane protein (HER4/p180erbB-4) that is structurally most closely related to the 185-kDa product (HER2/p180erbB-2) of the HER2/erbB-2 proto-oncogene. Heregulin, NDF, and neuregulin-2 are potential ligands which bind and activate c-erbB-4 (Plowman et al. 1993b; Carraway et al. 1997). However, we still know too little about c-erbB-4 in pancreatic cancer. First findings indicate that c-erbB-4 is of limited importance in pancreatic cancer pathogenesis (Graber et al. 1999), but further research is required to determine the interaction of the EGFRs with each other in the pathogenesis of pancreatic cancer.

Transforming Growth Factor-betas and Their Receptors

Transforming growth factor betas (TGF-βs) constitute a family of bifunctional polypeptide growth factors that either inhibit or stimulate cell proliferation depending on cell type, TGF-β concentration, culture condition, etc. (Sporn and Roberts 1992). The mammalian TGF-β family includes three isoforms: TGF-β1, TGF-β2, and TGF-β3. In most cases, TGF-βs inhibit the growth in many epithelial cells, influence the structure of the extracellular matrix, stimulate angiogenesis, and might function as immunosuppressive agents (Massague 1990; Massague et al. 1992; Sporn and Roberts 1992). All three TGF-β isoforms are overexpressed in many pancreatic cancer samples, and their overexpression is associated with more aggressive tumor growth and a significantly shorter postoperative survival (Friess et al. 1993a). These findings indicate that TGF-βs might act as growth stimulators in human pancreatic cancer in vivo, thus contributing to the neoplastic process. However, in vitro studies indicate that TGF-β1 inhibits the growth of the pancreatic cancer cell lines COLO 357 and PANC-1 by 50% and 25%, respectively (Baldwin and Korc 1993). In COLO 357 cells, TGF-β1 exposure induces up-regulation of its signaling receptors, which then exert growth inhibitory effects by up-regulating cyclin-dependent kinase inhibitors $p15^{INK4B}$, $p21^{cip1}$, and $p27^{kip1}$ which suppress cell cycle progression (Kleeff and Korc 1998). However, it is not known whether the inhibitory effect of TGF-β in vitro is influenced by cell culture conditions or whether it is one of the inherited characteristics of TGF-β1. Therefore, further investigation is needed to characterize the exact functions of TGF-βs in physiological and pathophysiological studies.

TGF-βs act through specific cell surface receptors – transforming growth factor-β type I, type II, and type III receptors (TβRI, II, and III) (Friess et al. 1996). TβRI needs the presence of TβRII to bind the ligands. In turn, TβRII activates signal transmission by an intracellular serine-threonine kinase, and the signaling is dependent on the presence of TβRI (Lin et al. 1992; Wrana et al. 1992). TβRIII is a proteoglycan also known as betaglycan and is not directly involved in signal transmission (Lopez-Casillas et al. 1991). All three TGF-β receptors are found in the normal human pancreas; however, only TβRI and TβRII are overexpressed in pancreatic cancer tissues (Friess et al. 1993b; Lu et al. 1997). In situ hybridization has revealed that TβRI and

TβRII mRNA are present both in cancer cells and in the desmoplastic tissues adjacent to the tumor (Friess et al. 1993 b; Lu et al. 1997). Furthermore, the overexpression of TβRI and TβRII is associated with advanced tumor stage (Friess et al. 1993b; Lu et al. 1997).

Fibroblast Growth Factors and Their Receptors

Fibroblast growth factors (FGFs) transmit mitogenic signaling and influence various biological functions such as cell differentiation and angiogenesis. Acidic fibroblast growth factor (aFGF, or FGF-1) and basic fibroblast growth factor (bFGF, or FGF-2) are the prototypes of this growth factor family. This family also includes int-2 (FGF-3), hst (Kaposi FGF or FGF-4), FGF-5, FGF-6, keratinocyte growth factor (KGF or FGF-7), androgen-induced growth factor (FGF-8), and glia-activating factor (FGF-9) (Friess et al. 1997). The stimulation of cellular metabolism by the nine fibroblast growth factors is mediated by a dual-receptor system. This comprises a family of four receptor tyrosine kinases (FGFR) and heparin sulfate proteoglycans (HSPG). The four high-affinity FGFRs were designated as FGFR-1, FGFR-2, FGFR-3, and FGFR-4. They possess intracellular tyrosine kinase activity, and consist of an extracellular domain containing two or three immunoglobulin-like regions (Klagsbrun 1989; Givol and Yayon 1992). The stimulation of cell division by FGFs has an obligate requirement for both partners of the dual-receptor system: FGFR and HSPG (Fernig and Gallagher 1994). It appears that HSPGs act as low-affinity receptors to which FGFs must bind in order to successfully activate the high-affinity FGFRs (Coutts and Gallagher 1995). The four FGFR genes can result in more than 100 possible receptor protein sequences by alternative splicing (Lappi 1995).

aFGF, bFGF, and their four high-affinity FGF receptors have already been reported in the normal human pancreas (Friess et al. 1992). It has since been demonstrated that aFGF and bFGF are overexpressed in a significant number of human pancreatic cancers and that their expression in cancer patients is associated with advanced tumor stage (Yamanaka et al. 1993 c). Furthermore, the presence of bFGF but not of aFGF was associated in 78 pancreatic tumors with shorter postoperative survival after tumor resection. In a later clinical study, bFGF and FGFR were analyzed in a small number of human pancreatic ductal adenocarcinomas (Ohta et al. 1995). Positive bFGF immunoactivity in 54% and positive FGFR immunoreactivity in 93% of 32 examined tumors were demonstrated. The levels of bFGF expression were not associated with tumor size, differentiation, stage, or postoperative survival, whereas the presence of FGFR showed a significant association with tumor invasion and tumor stage and a reverse relationship with postoperative survival. The divergence in histopathological and survival findings for bFGF might result from the different races of the chosen patients and from limited patient numbers in the later study. However, experimental data support the observation that bFGF increases pancreatic cancer growth in vivo. In a rat pancreatic cancer cell line, bFGF exhibits mitogenic effects. In addition, recent investigations demonstrated that suppression of FGFR signaling by transfection of a truncated FGFR-1 complementary DNA (FGF405) into PANC-1 cells can inhibit pancreatic cancer growth in vitro and in vivo (Wagner et al. 1998). These findings suggest that FGFR-dependent signaling is crucial for pancreatic cancer growth and raise the possibility that inhibition of the FGFR signaling pathways may ultimately provide a useful new therapeutic approach.

In addition to aFGF and bFGF, FGF-4, 5, and 7 have also been reported to be involved in growth regulation of pancreatic cancer. It was demonstrated that low molecular forms of FGF-4 have a higher receptor affinity and biological activity than FGF-4 itself, and may also have biological activity in human pancreatic cancer tissues (Bellosta et al. 1993). FGF-5 is overexpressed in human pancreatic cancer samples, is present in cells of the human pancreatic cancer cell line COLO-357, and is released in the conditioned medium. Exogeneously applied FGF-5 stimulates the growth of COLO-357 cells, suggesting that FGF-5 may participate in autocrine and paracrine pathways promoting pancreatic cancer cell growth in vivo (Kornmann et al. 1997). Furthermore, keratinocyte growth factor (KGF), also named FGF-7, is an important mitogen for a variety of epithelial cells and is often expressed in fibroblasts and other mesenchymal cells (Finch et al. 1989). Its expression is up-regulated in many human pancreatic cancer tissue samples and in most cultured pancreatic cancer cell lines, and it promotes cancer cell growth via autocrine and paracrine mechanisms (Siddiqi et al. 1995).

Insulin-like Growth Factors and Their Receptors

This growth factor family mainly includes insulin-like growth factors (IGF-I and IGF-II), their receptors (IGF-IR and IGF-IIR), and their binding proteins (IGFBP-1, 2, 3, 4, 5, and 6) (Roberts and Leroth 1988; el-Roeiy et al. 1994). The IGFs constitute a family of proteins with insulin-like growth-stimulating properties. The IGFBPs are thought to be important in positively or negatively modulating the actions of IGFs. They have been implicated as regulators of cell differentiation and of cell proliferation in a number of cell systems, and have also been shown to play an important role in growth regulation of human tumors (Bergmann et al. 1995; Lee and Yee 1995). Recently, they have been widely investigated in human pancreatic cancers.

Overexpression of IGF-I and IGF-I receptor was reported in human pancreatic cancer tissues (Bergmann et al. 1995). By in situ hybridization, IGF-I mRNA signals were found to be present both in cancer cells and in the surrounding stroma, suggesting that IGF-I may participate in aberrant autocrine and paracrine activation of IGF-IR in pancreatic cancer in vivo. However, subsequent in vitro studies did not show the presence of IGF-I in several pancreatic cancer cell lines, but revealed the presence of IGF-IR in the cancer cells (Bergmann et al. 1995). Inasmuch as IGF-I enhances the growth of cultured human pancreatic cancer cell lines, it can be significantly inhibited by alpha-IR3, a specific anti-IGF-I antibody (Bergmann et al. 1995) and by IGF antisense oligonucleotides that specifically block IGF receptor synthesis (Bergmann et al. 1995). Therefore, the IGF/IGF-IR signaling pathway may play an important role in mediating growth-stimulatory signals in pancreatic cancer cells.

Recently, IGF-IIR expression was examined in normal and cancerous human pancreatic tissues (Ishiwata et al. 1997). In the normal pancreas, moderate to strong IGF-IIR immunoreactivity was present in the cytoplasm of islet cells, and mild cytoplasmic immunoreactivity was also occasionally evident in ductal and acinar cells. Furthermore, some of the normal pancreas ductal cells also exhibited nuclear IGF-IIR immunoreactivity. In pancreatic cancer, strong IGF-IIR immunoreactivity was present in the duct-like cancer cells, often exhibiting nuclear localization. These results were further confirmed by in situ hybridization and Northern blot analysis, with seven of 12 pancreatic cancers exhibiting a 5.6-fold increase in IGF-IIR mRNA levels and IGF-IIR immunoreactivity. Based on these data, it was concluded that IGFs and their receptors may contribute only locally to the pathobiology of pancreatic cancer, because no elevation of serum levels of IGFs was found in pancreatic cancer patients (Evans et al. 1997).

Other Growth Factors and Their Receptors

The platelet-derived growth factor (PDGF) A and B chains and PDGF receptor beta (PDGFR β) were first detected in PANC-1 and HPAF human pancreatic cancer cells (Ebert et al. 1995). PDGFR α and β were found to be more highly expressed in human pancreatic cancer tissues than in the normal pancreas, giving first hints that PDGF and its receptor may also be involved in the pathogenesis of pancreatic cancer (Ebert et al. 1995). Also, hepatocyte growth factor (HGF), a widely expressed growth factor secreted by cells of mesenchymal origin, and the HGF receptor, the product of the c-met proto-oncogene, are expressed in increased amounts in various malignant human tumors. Recently, the HGF receptor (c-met) was found to be more highly expressed in human pancreatic cancer tissues (Ebert et al. 1994b), and also stimulating effects of HGF on pancreatic cancer cells were observed in vitro (Kiehne et al. 1997). Therefore, it is suggested that HGF can function as a growth-promoting factor in pancreatic cancer via stimulation of its overexpressed tyrosine kinase receptor.

Transcription Factors in Pancreatic Cancer

There are many processes involved when premature mRNA becomes mature and enters into the cytoplasm of the cells for protein synthesis. These processes include transcription initiation, elongation, termination, splicing, polyadenylation, and nuclear export. The most important step of this cascade is transcription initiation, in which the DNA sequences around the start of the gene are recognized by a number of nuclear proteins termed *transcription factors* (TFs). Transcription factors can be divided operationally into two groups. The first group includes a series of 20–30 proteins, found in all cells, which will combine with RNA polymerase II (a multiprotein complex termed the holoenzyme itself) to form a complex at the transcription start site. The role of these transcription factors is to recognize and bind to gene promotors and subsequently to position the polymerase II holoenzyme accurately at the beginning of the gene. These factors are collectively called the "basal machinery" or "general transcription factors" (GTF), and they are required for the initiation of transcription of all protein-encoding genes (Zawel and Reinberg 1995). The second group of TFs are more gene and cell-type specific. Some of them may be active only at particular points within the cell cycle (Muller 1995), and some are synthesized only within defined cell types at certain stages in cellular development (Lobe 1992). These proteins usually have two main functional domains. One domain specifically recognizes and binds to DNA sequences within the gene regulatory elements, while the second interacts with the GTFs to regulate the efficiency of transcription initiation. Thus, these factors are also called *upstream transcription factors.* DNA binding of these factors can either enhance (activators) or discourage (repressors) the binding of GTFs through protein–protein interactions via their transcription modulation domains.

Evidence is now accumulating that transcriptional deregulation is important in the process of neoplasia, and a number of possible mechanisms can be envisaged (Cox and Goding 1991): (a) Transcription factors regulating genes involved in cell growth and division might be inappropriately expressed; (b) mutations in the protein coding sequence of such factors might alter their ability to activate transcription, or might affect their interaction with other parts of the transcriptional machinery; (c) mutations in the DNA-binding domains between unrelated factors could change which targeted genes are activated, resulting in stimulation of cell division; and (d) transcription factors which normally mediate differentiation or which repress cell growth might be deleted or inactivated. Therefore, further investigation of TFs will contribute to our understanding of the development and progression of cancer and might suggest new concepts for treatment (Hurst 1996; Wiman 1997).

Our knowledge of TFs in human malignancies is limited. The presence of transcription factor ETS-2 and the overexpression of PEA3 have been reported in prostate (Liu et al. 1997) and breast cancer (Benz et al. 1997), respectively. In human pancreatic cancer, some growth factors and receptors, such as TGF-α and EGFR, have been demonstrated to be overexpressed, but this appears to be a consequence not of gene amplification but of enhanced transcriptional activation (Barton et al. 1991 a; Korc et al. 1992; Lemoine et al. 1992 a, Yamanaka et al. 1993 b; Friess et al. 1995). Moreover, some growth factors such as TGF-α can increase their own transcription (Hudson et al. 1989). Classical TFs have not been investigated in pancreatic cancer, although the protein products of some oncogenes (myc, jun, fos) and tumor suppressor genes (p53 and Rb) have been thought for a long time to function as transcription factors, which have an important role in the regulation of cancer cell growth. On the other hand, K-ras, c-myc, c-fos, c-jun, and p53 have been studied widely in pancreatic cancer, and the transformation effect of activated K-ras by point mutations in codons 12, 13, and 61 has also been thought to be associated with the further activation of transcription factors located in the nucleus (Schmid et al. 1994). We concentrate below on a discussion of their detected alterations.

ras Mutations

The ras family includes three 21-kDa ras proteins, named H-ras, N-ras, and K-ras, which exist in both active and inactive states. The active ras protein contains a bound guanosine triphosphate (GTP) molecule, and the inactive one contains guanosine diphosphate (GDP). Activation of ras occurs by the replacement of bound GDP with GTP. The activation of ras genes by point mutations occurs with varying frequency in most human cancers. Point mutations of ras usually occur in either codon 12, 13, or 61, leading to an amino acid substitution and conformational change in the encoded p21 protein. This change will result in a decrease in GTP hydrolysis to GDP, which thereby keeps the ras protein longer in an active state.

K-ras point mutations of codon 12 are present in up to 85%–95% of pancreatic cancer (Almoguera et al. 1988; Lemoine et al. 1992b; Kasuya et al. 1997). The spectrum of K-ras mutations, with G to A transition as the most frequent substitutions in pancreatic cancer, reveals significant similarities with colorectal carcinomas and adenomas (Pellegata et al. 1994) and differs from those found in lung carcinomas, where G to T transitions are more frequent (Capella et al. 1991). A number of transcription factors have been implicated in the ras-mediated activation of transcription, including AP-1 (c-jun, c-fos), SRF ($p67^{SRE}$, $p62^{TCF}$), ETS (Elk1, pointed 1 and 2), NF-IL-6, c-myc, and NF-kB/Rel (Schmid et al. 1994). However, the signal transduction pathways downstream of ras are poorly understood and need further evaluation.

c-myc, c-fos, and c-jun

c-myc is a cellular counterpart of v-myc, which is one of the earliest discovered viral transforming genes carried by the avian retrovirus MC29. c-myc and its related L-myc and N-myc genes are expressed in the nucleus (Abrams et al. 1982) and have an evident effect on growth stimulation (Kelly et al. 1983). The myc proteins possess the basic/helix-loop-helix (bHLH) motif, a domain which is also found in many known and putative transcription factors and which is involved in differentiation and tissue-specific gene expression (Murre et al. 1989; Davis et al. 1990). This observation strongly suggests that myc functions, at least in part, as a transcription factor. In human pancreatic cancer, c-myc is weakly expressed in the nucleus of the cancer cells, but only in a limited number of tumors (Sakorafas et al. 1995). However, whether c-myc plays an important role in the progression of pancreatic cancer still requires further study, because one older study indicated a 50-fold amplification of the c-myc gene in primary pancreatic cancer and in the lymph metastasis (Yamada et al. 1986).

c-jun and c-fos also function as oncogenic transcription factors (Angel et al. 1988; Vogt and Bos 1990; Distel and Spiegelman 1990). Both c-jun and c-fos have a leucine zipper, which enables protein-protein interactions necessary for DNA binding. Fos is unable to form homodimers, and thus it cannot bind to DNA on its own. Similarly, jun-jun homodimers bind only weakly to the AP1 recognition site. In contrast, fos-jun heterodimers are stable, bind strongly to AP1 sites, and activate gene transcription (Smeal et al. 1989). In human pancreatic cancer tissues, overexpression of c-fos was thought to be implicated in the development of the disease (Wakita et al. 1992; Lee and Charalambous 1994). On the other hand, a study of pancreatic cancer cell lines showed that pituitary adenylate-cyclase-activating polypeptide (PACAP) can stimulate the expression of c-fos and c-jun and can strongly increase the DNA-binding activity of the c-fos/c-jun heterodimer transcription factor AP1, and also stimulate AP1 transcriptional activity up to 20-fold in AR4–2J cells (Schafer et al. 1996). Therefore, it seems that c-fos/c-jun as transcription factors might play a critical role in the development and progression of pancreatic cancer.

p53

p53, a so-called tumor suppressor gene, is located on the short arm of chromosome 17 and encodes a 53-kDa nuclear phosphoprotein (Lane and Bechimol 1990; Levine et al. 1991). Mutations of the p53 gene are the most common somatic genetic alterations in human cancers (Friess et al. 1996) and are present in 40%–50% of all tumors. In pancreatic cancer, the prevalence of p53 mutations is about 40%–60% (Barton et al. 1991b; Casey et al. 1993; Nakamori et al. 1995). Mutant p53 protein overexpression was found in 23% of ductectatic carcinomas and 61% of solid pancreatic malignancies (Kasuya et al. 1997). p53 overexpression was correlated with tumor stage, tumor size, grading, and lymph node metastases (Harada et al. 1997) and associated with shorter survival of pancreatic cancer patients following tumor resection (Nakamori et al. 1995).

p53 functions as a transcription factor that triggers cell cycle arrest and programmed cell death (apoptosis) in response to certain types of cellular stress, including DNA damage (Diller et al. 1990; Horikoshi 1997; Wiman 1997). The normal p53 gene may contain a potential transcription activation element and may function as a transcriptional activating factor (TAF). This means that p53 might be a positive regulator of transcription, which might mediate its suppressor role by inducing expression of a set of genes with a negative effect on cellular growth (Fields and Jang 1990; Raycroft et al. 1990). The insertion of an intact p53 gene in tumor cells carrying mutant p53 has been shown to result in tumor regression in lung cancer patients (Wiman 1997), and this seems to be an interesting approach in pancreatic cancer patients as well.

Conclusion

Pancreatic cancer is a devastating disease, in general with a poor prognosis. Clinically, pancreatic cancer is characterized by its aggressive growth and early metastatic growth behavior. A variety of growth factors (EGF, TGF-α, amphiregulin, FGFs, TGF-βs) and their receptors (EGFR, c-erbB-2, c-erbB-3, FGFRs, TβRs) seem to play an important role in this process, as do proteins involved in transcription control (myc, fos, jun, p53, ras). This implies that alterations in growth factors and transcription factors may result in a major growth advantage of pancreatic cancer, leading to rapid tumor progression and insensitivity to chemotherapy, radiotherapy, immunotherapy, and hormone therapy. Although the present molecular studies cannot give definitive solutions for the prevention and treatment of pancreatic cancer, they offer the possibility of new diagnostic and prognostic markers and new therapeutic directions in the future. Certainly, further detailed studies of growth factors and transcription factors are urgently needed to improve our pathophysiological understanding of this disease and to develop better and more effective adjuvant and palliative treatment possibilities.

References

Aaronson SA (1991) Growth factors and cancer. Science 254:1146–1153

Abraham JA, Damm D, Bajardi A, Miller J, Klagsbrun M, Ezekowitz RA (1993) Heparin-binding EGF-like growth factor: characterization of rat and mouse cDNA clones, protein domain conservation across species, and transcript expression in tissues. Biochem Biophys Res Comm 190:125–133

Abrams HD, Rohrschneider LR, Eisenman RN (1982) Nuclear location of the putative transforming protein of avian myelocytomatosis virus. Cell 29:427–439

Almoguera C, Shibata D, Forrester K, Martin J, Arnheim N, Perucho M (1988) Most human carcinomas of the human exocrine pancreas contain mutant c-K-ras genes. Cell 53:549–554

Angel P, Allegretto EA, Okino ST, Hattori K, Boyle WJ, Hunter T, Karin M (1988) Oncogene jun encodes a sequence-specific trans-activator similar to AP-1. Nature 332:166–171

Baldwin RL, Korc M (1993) Growth inhibition of human pancreatic carcinoma cells by transforming growth factor beta-1. Growth Factors 8:23–34

Barton CM, Hall PA, Hughes CM, Gullick WJ, Lemines NR (1991a) Transforming growth factor alpha and epidermal growth factor in human pancreatic cancer. J Pathol 163:111–116

Barton CM, Staddo SL, Hughes CM, Hall PA, O'Sullivan C, Klöppel G, Theis B, Russell RC, Neoptolemos J, Williamson RC (1991b) Abnormalities of the p53 tumor suppressor gene in human pancreatic cancer. Br J Cancer 64:1076–1082

Bellosta P, Talarico D, Rogers D, Basilico C (1993) Cleavage logical activity and receptor binding affinity. J Cell Biol 121:705–713

Benz CC, Ohagan RC, Richter B, Scott GK, Chang CH, Xiong X, Chew K, Ljung BM, Edgerton S, Thor A, Hassell JA (1997) HER2/Neu and the Ets transcription activator PEA3 are coordinately upregulated in human breast cancer. Oncogene 15:1513–1525

Bergmann U, Funatomi H, Yokoyama M, Beger HG, Korc M (1995) Insulin-like growth factor I overexpression in human pancreatic cancer: evidence for autocrine and paracrine roles. Cancer Res 55:2007–2011

Büchler M, Ebert M, Beger HG (1993) Grenzen chirurgischen Handelns beim Pankreaskarzinoma. Langenbecks Arch Chir [Suppl]:460–464

Cameron JL, Crist DW, Sitzmann JV, Hruban RH, Boitnott JK, Seidler AJ, Coleman J (1991) Factors influencing survival after pancreaticoduodenectomy for pancreatic cancer. Am J Surg 161:120–124

Capella G, Cronauer-Mitra S, Peinado MA, Perucho M (1991) Frequency and spectrum of mutations at codons 12 and 13 of the K-ras gene in human tumors. Environ Health Perspect 93:125–131
Carraway KL 3rd, Weber JL, Ledesma J, Yu N, Gassman M, Lai C (1997) Neuregulin-2, a new ligand of ErbB3/ErbB4-receptor tyrosine kinases. Nature 387:512–516
Casey G, Yamanaka Y, Friess H, Kobrin MS, Lopez ME, Büchler M, Beger HG, Korc M (1993) p53 mutations are common in pancreatic cancer and are absent in chronic pancreatitis. Cancer Lett 69:151–160
Coutts JC, Gallagher JT (1995) Receptors for fibroblast growth factors. Immunol Cell Biol 73:584–589
Cox PM, Goding CR (1991) Transcription and cancer. Br J Cancer 63:651–662
Davis RL, Cheng PF, Lassar AB, Weintraub H (1990) The MyoD DNA-binding domain contains a recognition code for muscle-specific gene activation. Cell 60:733–746
Derynck R (1988) Transforming growth factor-alpha. Cell 54:593–595
Di Fiore PP, Pierce JH, Kraus MH, Segatto O, King CR, Aaronson SA (1987) erbB-2 is a potent oncogene when overexpressed in NIH/3T3 cells. Science 237:178–182
Diller L, Kassel J, Nelsonn CE, Gryka MA, Litwak G, Gebhardt M, Bressac B, Ozturk M, Baker SJ, Vogelstein B (1990) p53 functions as a cell cycle control protein in osteosarcoma. Mol Cell Biol 10:5772–5781
Distel RJ, Spiegelman BM (1990) Protooncogene c-fos as a transcription factor. Adv Cancer Res 55:37–55
Ebert M, Yokoyama M, Kobrin MS, Friess H, Lopez ME, Büchler MW, Johnson GR, Korc M (1994a) Induction and expression of amphiregulin in human pancreatic cancer. Cancer Res 54:3959–3962
Ebert M, Yokoyama M, Friess H, Büchler MW, Korc M (1994b) Coexpression of the c-met protooncogene and hepatocyte growth factor in human pancreatic cancer. Cancer Res 54:5775–5778
Ebert M, Yokoyama M, Friess H, Kobrin MS, Büchler MW, Korc M (1995) Induction of platelet-derived growth factor A and B chains and overexpression of their receptors in human pancreatic cancer. Int J Cancer 62:529–535
el-Roeiy A, Chen X, Roberts VJ, Shimasakai S, Ling N, Le Roith D, Roberts CT Jr, Yen SS (1994) Expression of the genes encoding the insulin-like growth factors (IGF-I and IGF-II), the IGF and insulin receptors, and IGF-binding proteins 1–6 and the localization of their gene products in normal and polycystic ovary syndrome ovaries. J Clin Endocrinol Metab 78:1488–1496
Evans JD, Eggo MC, Donovan IA, Bramhall SR, Neoptolemos JP (1997) Serum levels of insulin-like growth factors (IGF-I and IGF-II) and their binding protein (IGFBP-3) are not elevated in pancreatic cancer. Int J Pancreatol 22:95–100
Fernig DG, Gallagher JT (1994) Fibroblast growth factors and their receptors: an information network controlling tissue growth, morphogenesis and repair. Prog Growth Factor Res 5:353–377
Finch PW, Rubin JS, Miki T, Ron D, Aaronson SA (1989) Human KGF is FGF-related with properties of a paracrine effector of epithelial cell growth. Science 245:752–755
Fields S, Jang SK (1990) Presence of a potent transcription activating sequence in the p53 protein. Science 249:1046–1049
Friess H, Kobrin MS, Korc M (1992) Acidic and basic fibroblast growth factors and their receptors are expressed in human pancreas (abstr). Pancreas 7:737
Friess H, Yamanaka Y, Büchler MW, Ebert M, Beger HG, Gold LI, Korc M (1993a) Enhanced expression of transforming growth factor beta isoforms in pancreatic cancer correlates with decreased survival. Gastroenterology 105:1846–1856
Friess H, Yamanaka Y, Büchler MW, Berger HG, Kobrin MS, Baldwin RL, Korc M (1993b) Enhanced expression of the type II transforming growth factor beta receptor in human pancreatic cancer cells without alteration of type III receptor expression. Cancer Res 53:2704–2707
Friess H, Yamanaka Y, Kobrin MS (1995) Enhanced erbB3 expression in human pancreatic cancer correlates with tumor progression. Clin Cancer Res 1:1413–1420
Friess H, Berberat P, Schilling M, Kunz J, Korc M, Büchler MW (1996) Pancreatic cancer: the potential clinical relevance of alterations in growth factors and their receptors. J Mol Med 74:35–42
Friess H, Kleeff J, Gumbs A, Büchler MW (1997) Molecular versus conventional markers in pancreatic cancer. Digestion 58:557–563
Givol D, Yayon A (1992) Complexity of FGF receptors: genetic basis for structural diversity and functional specificity. FASEB J 6:3362–3369

Gold EB, Goldin SB (1998) Epidemiology and risk factors for pancreatic cancer. Surg Oncol Clin N Am 7:67–91
Graber HU, Friess H, Kaufmann B, Willi D, Zimmermann A, Korc M, Büchler MW (1999) ErbB-4 mRNA expression is decreased in non-metastatic pancreatic cancer. Int J Cancer 84:24–27
Grünewald K, Lyons J, Fröhlich A, Feichtiger H, Weger RA, Schwab G, Janssen JWG, Bartram CR (1989) High frequency of K-ras codon 12 mutations in pancreatic adenocarcinomas. Int J Cancer 43:1037–1041
Gudjonsson B (1987) Cancer of the pancreas. 50 years of surgery. Cancer 60:2284–2303
Hall PA, Hughes CM, Staddon SL, Richman PI, Gullic WJ, Lemoine NR (1990) The c-erbB-2 protooncogene in human pancreatic cancer. J Pathol 161:1995–2000
Harada N, Gansauge S, Gansauge F, Gause H, Shimoyama S, Imaizumi T, Mattfeld T, Schoenberg MH, Beger HG (1997) Nuclear accumulation of p53 correlates significantly with clinical features and inversely with the expression of the cyclin-dependent kinase inhibitor p21(WAF1/CIP1) in pancreatic cancer. Br J Cancer 76:299–305
Harnack LJ, Anderson KE, Zheng W, Folsom AR, Sellers TA, Kushi LH (1997) Smoking, alcohol, coffee, and tea intake and incidence of cancer of the exocrine pancreas: the Iowa Women's Health Study. Cancer Epidemiol Biomarkers Prev 6:1081–1086
Holmes WE, Sliwkowski MX, Akita RW (1992) Identification of heregulin, a specific activator of p185erbB2. Science 256:1205–1210
Horikoshi N (1997) Regulation of cell growth by the transcriptional factor p53, a tumor suppressor gene product. Tanpakushitsu Kakusan Koso 42:1585–1593
Hsiang D, Friess H, Büchler MW, Ebert M, Butler J, Korc M (1997) Absence of K-ras mutations in the pancreatic parenchyma of patients with chronic pancreatitis. Am J Surg 174:242–246
Hudson LG, Santon JB, Gill GN (1989) Regulation of epidermal growth factor receptor gene expression. Mol Endocrinol 3:400–408
Hudziak RM, Schlessinger J, Ullrich A (1987) Increased expression of the putative growth factor receptor p185HER2 causes transformation and tumorigenesis of NIH 3T3 cells. Proc Natl Acad Sci U S A 84:7159–7163
Hurst HC (1996) Transcription factors as drug targets in cancer. Eur J Cancer 32A:1857–1863
Ishiwata T, Bergmann U, Kornmann M, Lopez M, Beger HG, Korc M (1997) Altered expression of insulin-like growth factor II receptor in human pancreatic cancer. Pancreas 15:367–373
Kasuya K, Watanabe H, Nakasako T, Ajioka Y, Koyanagi Y (1997) p53 protein overexpression and K-ras codon 12 mutation in pancreatic ductal carcinoma: correlation with histologic factors. Pathol Int 47:531–539
Kelly K, Cochran BH, Stiles CD, Leder P (1983) Cell-specific regulation of the c-myc gene by lymphocyte mitogens and platelet-derived growth factor. Cell 35:603–610
Kiehne K, Herzig KH, Fölsch UR (1997) c-met expression in pancreatic cancer and effects of hepatocyte growth factor on pancreatic cancer growth. Pancreas 15:35–40
Kingsley DM (1994) The TGF-beta superfamily: New members, new receptors, and new genetic tests of function in different organisms. Genes Dev 8:133–146
Klagsbrun M (1989) The fibroblast growth factor family: structural and biological properties. Prog Growth Factor Res 1:207–235
Kleeff J, Korc M (1998) Up-regulation of transforming growth factor (TGF)-β receptors by TGF-β1 in COLO-357 cells. J Bio Chem 273:7495–7500
Korc M (1998) Role of growth factors in pancreatic cancer. Surg Oncol Clin N Am 7:25–41
Korc M, Finman JE (1989) Attenuated processing of epidermal growth factor in the face of marked degradation of transforming growth factor alpha. J Bio Chem 264:14990–14999
Korc M, Magun B (1985) Recycling of epidermal growth factor in a human pancreatic carcinoma cell line. Proc Natl Acad Sci U S A 82:6172–6175
Korc M, Meltzer P, Trent J (1986) Enhanced expression of epidermal growth factor receptor correlates with alterations of chromosome 7 in human pancreatic cancer. Proc Natl Acad Sci U S A 83:5141–5144
Korc M, Chandrasekar B, Yamanaka Y, Friess H, Büchler M, Beger HG (1992) Overexpression of the epidermal growth factor receptor in human pancreatic cancer is associated with concomitant increase in the levels of epidermal growth factor and transforming growth factor alpha. J Clin Invest 90:1352–1360
Kornmann M, Ishiwata T, Beger HG, Korc M (1997) Fibroblast growth factor-5 stimulates mitogenic signaling and is overexpressed in human pancreatic cancer: evidence for autocrine and paracrine actions. Oncogene 15:1417–1424

Lane DP, Bechimol S (1990) p53: oncogene or anti-oncogene? Gene Dev 4:1–8
Lappi DA (1995) Tumor targeting through fibroblast growth factor receptors. Semin Cancer Biol 6:279–288
Lee AV, Yee D (1995) Insulin-like growth factors and breast cancer. Biomed Pharmacother 49:415–421
Lee CS, Charalambous D (1994) Immunohistochemical localization of the c-fos oncoprotein in pancreatic cancers. Zentralbl Pathol 140:271–275
Lee YT, Williams M (1994) Clinical and laboratory findings of carcinoma of the pancreas and periampullary structures. J Surg Oncol 25:1–7
Lemoine NR, Hughes CM, Barton CM, Poulsom R, Jeffery RE, Kloppel G, Hall PA, Gullick WJ (1992a) The epidermal growth factor receptor in human pancreatic cancer. J Pathol 166:7–12
Lemoine NR, Jain S, Hughes CM, Staddon SL, Maillet B, Hall PA, Kloppel G (1992b) Ki ras oncogene activation in preinvasive pancreatic cancer. Gastroenterology 102:230–236
Levine AJ, Momand J, Finaly CA (1991) The p53 tumor suppressor gene. Nature 351:453–456
Libermann TA, Nusbaum HR, Razon N, Kris R, Lax I, Soreq H, Whittle N, Waterfield MD, Ullrich A, Schlessinger J (1985) Amplification, enhanced expression, and possible rearrangement of the EGF receptor gene in primary human brain tumors of glial origin. Nature 313:144–147
Lin HY, Wang X-F, Ng-Eaton E, Weinberg RA, Lodish HF (1992) Expression cloning of the TGF-beta type II receptor, a functional transmembrane serine/threonine kinase. Cell 68:775–785
Liu AY, Corey E, Vessella RL, Lange PH, True LD, Huang GM, Nelson PS, Hood L (1997) Identification of differentially expressed prostate genes: increased expression of transcription factor ETS-2 in prostate cancer. Prostate 30:145–153
Lobe CG (1992) Transcription factors and mammalian development. Curr Top Dev Biol 27:351–383
Lopez-Casillas F, Cheifetz S, Doody J, Andres JL, Lane WS, Massague J (1991) Structure and expression of the membrane proteoglycan betaglycan, a component of the TGF-beta receptor system. Cell 67:785–795
Lu Z, Friess H, Graber HU, Gou XZ, Schilling M, Zimmermann A, Korc M, Büchler MW (1997) Presence of two signaling TGF-beta receptors in human pancreatic cancer correlates with advanced tumor stage. Dig Dis Sci 42:2054–2063
Marchionni MA, Goodear ADJ, Chen MS, Bermingham-McDonogh O, Kirk C, Hendrick SM, Danehy F, Misumi D, Sudhalter J, Kobayashi K (1993) Glial growth factors are alternatively spliced erbB2 ligands expressed in the nerve system. Nature 362:312–318
Massague J (1990) The transforming growth factor-beta family. Annu Rev Cell Biol 6:597–641
Massague J, Cheifetz S, Laiho M, Ralph DA, Weiss FMB, Zentella A (1992) The transforming growth factor beta. Cancer Surv 12:81–103
Muller R (1995) Transcription factors and mammalian development. Trends Genet 11:173–178
Murre C, McCaw PS, Baltimore D (1989) A new DNA-binding and dimerisation motif in immunoglobulin enhancer-binding, daughterless, MyoD and myc proteins. Cell 56 777–783
Nakamori S, Yashima K, Murakami Y, Ishikawa O, Ohigashi H, Imaoka S, Yaegashi S, Konishi Y, Sekiya T (1995) Association of p53 gene mutation with short survival in pancreatic carcinoma. Jpn J Cancer Res 86:174–181
Neal DE, Marsh C, Bennett MK, Abel PD, Hall RR, Sainsbury JR, Harris AL (1985) Epidermal growth factor receptors in human bladder cancer: comparison of invasive and superficial tumors. Lancet 1:366–368
Nio Y, Tamura K (1997) Newly-developing therapies of pancreatic cancer – immunotherapy, gene therapy, differentiation therapy, endocrine therapy and others. Nippon Geka Gakkai Zasshi 98:639–645
Ohta T, Yamamoto M, Numata M, Iseki S, Tsukioka Y, Miyashita T, Kayahara M, Nagakawa T, Miyazaki I, Nishikawa K, Yoshtake Y (1995) Expression of basic fibroblast growth factor and its receptor in human pancreatic carcinomas. Br J Cancer 72:824–831
Oikawa T, Hitomi J, Kono A, Kaneko E, Yamaguchi K (1995) Frequent expression of genes for receptor tyrosine kinases and their ligands in human pancreatic cancer cells. Int J Pancreatol 18:15–23
Ozaki H, Kinoshita T, Kosuge T, Egawa S, Kishi K (1990) Effectiveness of multimodality treatment for resectable pancreatic cancer. Int J Pancreatol 7:195–200
Parker SL, Tong T, Bolden S, Wingo PA (1997) Cancer statistics. CA Cancer J Clin 47:5–27

Peles E, Bacus SS, Koski RA, Lu HS, Wen D, Ogden SG, Levy RB, Yarden Y (1992) Isolation of the Neu/HER-2 stimulatory ligand: a 44 kD glycoprotein that induces differentiation of mammary tumor cells. Cell 62:205–216
Peles E, Ben-Levy R, Tzahar E, Liu N, Wen D, Yarden Y (1993) Cell-type specific interaction of Neu differentiation factor (NDF/heregulin) with Neu/Her-2 suggests complex ligand receptor relationships. EMBO J 12:961–971
Pellegata NS, Sessa F, Renault B, Bonato M, Leone BE, Solcia E, Ranzani GN (1994) K-ras and p53 gene mutations in pancreatic cancer: ductal and nonductal tumors progress through different genetic lesions. Cancer Res 54:1556–1560
Plowman GD, Green JM, McDonald VL Neubauer MG, Disteche CM, Todaro GJ, Shoyab M (1990) The amphiregulin gene encodes a novel epidermal growth factor-related protein with tumor-inhibitory activity. Mol Cell Biol 10:1969–1981
Plowman GD, Culouscou J-M, Whitney GS, Green JM, Carton GW, Foy L, Neubauer MG, Shoyab M (1993a) Ligand-specific activation of HER4/180^{erbB4}, a fourth member of the epidermal growth factor receptor family. Proc Natl Acad Sci U S A 90:1746–1750
Plowman GD, Green JM, Culouscou JM, Carlton GW, Rothwell VM, Buckley S (1993b) Heregulin induces tyrosine phosphorylation of HER4/p180erbB4. Nature 366:473–475
Raycroft L, Wu HY, Lozano G (1990) Transcriptional activation by wild-type but not transforming mutants of the p53 antioncogene. Science 249:1049–1051
Roberts CT jr, Leroth D (1988) Molecular aspects of insulin-like growth factors, their binding proteins and receptors. Baillieres Clin Endocrinol Metab 2:1069–1085
Ruggeri B, Zhang SY, Caamano J, Dirado M, Flynn SD, Kleinszanto AJP (1992) Human pancreatic carcinomas and cell lines reveal frequent and multiple alterations in the p53 and Rb-1 tumor suppressor genes. Oncogene 7:1503–1511
Sakorafas GH, Lazris A, Tsiotuo AG, Koullias G, Glinatsis MT, Golematis BC (1995) Oncogenes in cancer of the pancreas. Eur J Surg Oncol 21:251–253
Schäfer H, Zheng J, Gundlach F, Günther R, Schmidt WE (1996) PACAP stimulates transcription of c-fos and c-jun and activates the AP1 transcription factor in rat pancreatic carcinoma cells. Biochem Biophys Res Commun 221:111–116
Schlessinger J, Ullrich A (1992) Growth factor signaling by receptor tyrosine kinases. Neuron 9:383–391
Schmid RM, Liptay S, Weidenbach H, Adler G (1994) Transcription factors in pancreatic cancer. Dig Surg 11:160–163
Shimizu N, Kondo I, Gamon S, Behzadian M, Shimizu Y (1984) Genetic analysis of hyperproduction of epidermal growth factor receptors in human epidermoid carcinoma A431 cells. Somat Cell Mol Genet 10:45–53
Shing Y, Christofori G, Hanahan D, Ono Y, Sasada R, Igarashi K, Folkman J (1993) Betacellulin: a mitogen from pancreatic beta cell tumors. Science 259:1604–1607
Siddiqi I, Funatomi H, Kobrin MS, Friess H, Büchler M, Korc M (1995) Increased expression of keratinocyte growth factor in human pancreatic cancer. Biochem Biophys Res Commun 215:309–315
Smeal T, Angel P, Meek J, Karin M (1989) Different requirements for formation of jun:jun and jun:fos complexes. Genes Dev 3:2091–2100
Smith JJ, Derynck R, Korc M (1987) Production of transforming growth factor in human pancreatic cancer cells: evidence for a superagonist autocrine cycle. Proc Natl Acad Sci U S A 84:7567–7570
Sporn MB, Roberts AB (1992) Transforming growth factor-beta: recent progress and new challenges. J Cell Biol 119:1017–1021
Trede M, Schwall G, Saeger HD (1990) Survival after pancreatoduodenectomy. Ann Surg 211:447–458
Uegaki K, Nio Y, Inoue Y, Minari Y, Sato Y, Song MM, Dong M, Tamaura K (1997) Clinicopathological significance of epidermal growth factor and its receptor in human pancreatic cancer. Anticancer Res 17:3841–3847
Ullrich A, Coussens L, Hayflick JS, Dull TJ, Gray A, Tam AW, Lee J, Yarden Y, Libermann TA, Schlessinger J (1984) Human epidermal growth factor receptor cDNA sequence and aberrant expression of the amplified gene in A431 epidermoid carcinoma cells. Nature 309:418–425
Vogt PK, Bos TJ (1990) Jun: oncogene and transcription factor. Adv Cancer Res 55:1–35
Wagner M, Cao T, Lopez ME, Hope C, van Nostrand K, Kobrin MS, Fan HU, Büchler MW, Korc M (1996) Expression of a truncated EGFR is associated with inhibition of pancreatic cancer cell growth and enhanced sensitivity to cisplatinum. Int J Cancer 68:782–787

Wagner M, Lopez ME, Cahn M, Korc M (1998) Suppression of fibroblast growth factor receptor signaling inhibits pancreatic cancer growth in vitro and in vivo. Gastroentrology 114:798–807

Wakita K, Ohyanagi H, Yamamoto K, Tokuhisa T, Saitoh Y (1992) Overexpression of c-Ki-ras and c-fos in human pancreatic carcinoma. Int J Pancreatol 11:43–47

Warshaw AL, Fernandez-Del Castillo C (1992) Pancreatic carcinoma. N Engl J Med 326:455–465

Wiman KG (1997) New transcription factor-based cancer therapy. Gene therapy, cell lysis, reactivation of p53 are the new approaches. Lakartidningen 94:3268–3272

Wrana JL, Attisano L, Carcamo J, Zentella A, Doody J, Laiho M, Wang X-F, Massague J (1992) TGF-beta signals through a heteromeric protein kinase receptor complex. Cell 71:1003–1014

Yamada H, Sakamato H, Taira M, Nishimura S, Shimosato Y, Terada M, Sugimura T (1986) Amplifications of both c-Ki-ras with a point mutation and c-myc in a primary pancreatic cancer and its metastatic tumors in lymph nodes. Jpn J Cancer Res 77:370–375

Yamanaka Y, Friess H, Kobrin MS, Büchler M, Beger HG, Korc M (1993a) Co-expression of epidermal growth factor receptor and ligands in human pancreatic cancer is associated with enhanced tumor aggressiveness. Anticancer Res 13:565–570

Yamanaka Y, Friess H, Kobrin MS, Büchler M, Kunz J, Beger HG, Korc M (1993b) Overexpression of HER-2 /neu oncogene in human pancreatic carcinoma. Hum Pathol 24:1127–1134

Yamanaka Y, Friess H, Büchler M, Beger HG, Uchida E, Onda M, Kobrin MS, Korc M (1993c) Overexpression of acidic and basic fibroblast growth factors in human pancreatic cancer correlates with advanced tumor stage. Cancer Res 53:5289–5296

Yokoyama M, Funatomi H, Kobrin MS, Ebert M, Friess H, Büchler MW, Korc M (1995) Betacellulin, a member of the epidermal growth factor family, is overexpressed in human pancreatic cancer. Int J Oncol 7:825–829

Yokoyama M, Funatomi H, Hope C, Damm D, Friess H, Büchler MW, Abraham J, Korc M (1996) Heparin-binding EGF-like growth factor expression and biological action in human pancreatic cancer cells. Int J Oncol 8:289–295

Zawel L, Reinberg D (1995) Common themes in assembly and function of eucaryotic transcription complexes. Ann Rev Biochem 64:533–561

Zimmermann A (1994) Carcinoma of pancreas: morphology. Dig Surg 11:338–341

CHAPTER 21

Biological Approaches to the Therapy of Pancreatic Cancer

M. A. Tempero

Introduction

Treatment of adenocarcinoma of the pancreas remains a challenging task. Some improvements have occurred in surgical management. Although a relatively small proportion of patients who present with pancreatic adenocarcinoma are candidates for surgery, it is now clear that in experienced centers, the perioperative mortality can be less than 5% [1]. Furthermore, the addition of adjuvant 5-fluorouracil (5-FU)-based chemoradiation may have a role in prolonging the median survival following surgery [2]. Despite these advances, the 5-year survival for pancreatic adenocarcinoma in the United States has improved only slightly and remains low at 4% [3].

Some progress has also been made in the management of patients with locally unresectable or metastatic adenocarcinoma of the pancreas. Chemoradiation for disease that is truly limited to the locoregional area may almost double the median survival [4]. Chemotherapy for metastatic disease is of modest effectiveness. Drugs known to reproducibly result in a median survival of 5 months or more include gemcitabine [5], 5-FU [6], tamoxifen [7], and groserelin [8]. It is becoming increasingly apparent that chemotherapy can alter the natural history of this disease. 5-FU-based chemotherapy regimens have produced an improved median survival compared with supportive care in three of four trials [9–12] attempting to address this question. The only chemotherapy drug which may have an advantage over 5-FU is gemcitabine [5], which has been demonstrated to be more effective in relieving pancreatic cancer-associated symptoms and results in a modest (approximately 5 weeks) improvement in median survival. Despite some advances, there are many opportunities for improvement of the systemic management of pancreatic adenocarcinoma. This chapter will provide an overview of emerging therapies in four areas: (a) unique biochemical targets, (b) gene therapy, (c) targeted therapy, and (d) immunobiological therapy.

Unique Biochemical Targets

One of the histologic hallmarks of pancreatic adenocarcinoma involves mutations of K-ras, which are most common in the 12th, 13th, or 61st codon and are present in up to 100% of lesions studied [13, 14]. Knowledge of this very common ras mutation has lead to consideration of the role of ras protein function in pancreatic as well as other cancers. The gene product of K-ras is a membrane-associated nucleotide-binding protein which is probably involved in signal transduction of growth-promoting effectors. Post-translational processing (farnesylation) is necessary to locate ras proteins to the plasma cell membrane. Specific small molecules have been developed that inhibit farnesyl transferase, and preclinical studies have suggested a potential for cancer therapy [15, 16]. At least three farnesyl transferase inhibitors are currently being investigated in phase-I clinical trials.

An alternate approach to affecting farnesylated ras protein levels involves the use of monoterpenes such as limonene or perillyl alcohol [17, 18]. Although the mechanism leading to this decrease in farnesylated ras levels is not entirely clear with the monoterpenes, preclinical studies have been very encouraging. Perillyl alcohol has completed phase-I testing at the University of Wisconsin [19], demonstrating very good tolerance and some antitumor activity. Phase-II trials are in the planning stages.

Another unique biochemical approach has involved inhibition of matrix metalloproteinases (MMP). These are a family of proteolytic enzymes that have a role in tumor invasion and metastasis and possibly in angiogenesis [20, 21]. Selected MMP enzymes are expressed in human pancreatic cancers but not in normal pancreas. At least one MMP inhibitor (BB25160, Marimastat) has been developed as a therapeutic agent and has completed phase-II and -III testing in patients with advanced metastatic pancreatic cancer [22]. The results of the phase-III trial have not yet been published. Another phase-III trial in the adjuvant setting is in progress, comparing Marimastat and 5-FU-based chemoradiation with chemoradiation alone.

Gene Therapy

A broad definition of gene therapy is used in this paper. Specifically, consideration is given to the use of antisense oligonucleotides or ribozymes that can neutralize activated oncogenes or reverse the effect of inactivated tumor suppressor genes, and to genetic drug or prodrug activation therapy.

In addition to the molecular hallmark of K-ras mutations, the p53 tumor suppressor gene is commonly inactivated in pancreatic adenocarcinoma. Roughly 70% of primary pancreatic adenocarcinomas have p53 mutations [23]. Thus, both mutated ras and p53 have been common targets of preclinical studies involving gene therapy. While none of these approaches have reached clinical trials, some preclinical studies are worth mentioning. Shichinohe et al. [24] have shown reversal of the malignant phenotype with a transfection of an h-ras mutant (N116Y). A ribozyme specific for K-ras mRNA has also been designed, and in vitro studies have shown effective transfer to the molecular target [25].

Multiple studies have now demonstrated that in vivo introduction of a wild-type p53 gene into tumor cells expressing mutant p53 suppresses malignant growth. This has been shown both in vivo and in vitro. Replication-incompetent adenoviruses have been used to deliver the p53 gene in human tumors such as head and neck squamous cell carcinoma [26]. A similar approach with intratumoral administration of wild-type p53 could be taken in adenocarcinoma of the pancreas.

Not specifically categorized as gene therapy, but clearly dependent on the presence of abnormal p53, is the use of a cytolytic adenovirus which multiplies preferentially in mutant p53 cells [27]. This approach has been used in both head and neck cancers and in pancreatic adenocarcinoma. A phase-I trial in adenocarcinoma of the pancreas has been completed at the University of California at San Francisco [28]. Some minor regressions were observed with this approach, and a phase-II trial is in progress.

Another gene therapy approach involving mutant p53 has focused on p21WAF1, a p53-inducible gene which acts as a downstream effector of p53 function and mediates G_1 cycle arrest by inhibiting cyclin-dependent kinases. Introduction of p21 using a recombinant adenoviral vector system has been shown to inhibit pancreatic tumor cell growth in vitro [29]. Finally, antisense oligonucleotides designed against p53 have been shown to have antiproliferative effects; however, these effects occur regardless of the p53 status of the pancreatic cancer cell line studied [30]. Thus, much work needs to be done on exploring the mechanism of action prior to introduction of these agents into the clinic.

Preclinical approaches with gene therapy using prodrug systems have taken two general pathways. One approach has been to use a lipofection-based suicidal gene strategy. In this approach the herpes simplex virus thymidine kinase (HSV-TK) gene is prepared as an expression plasmid under the potent hybrid promoter CAG and incorporated into a lipopolyamine complex [31]. This reagent has been injected intraperitoneally into mice bearing human pancreatic cancer cells. Following successful transfection, ganciclovir was administered, and slightly greater than 50% of the mice were found to be tumor free. A similar approach has been used with an adenovirus carrying the HSV-TK gene under the control of a carcinoembryonic antigen (CEA) promoter. Preclinical studies have suggested antitumor efficacy with ganciclovir in transfected CEA producing pancreatic cancer in vivo [32]. Another prodrug approach calls for the targeted delivery of tumoricidal drugs. One model involves cytosine deaminase, a bacterial enzyme that converts 5-fluorocytosine, a nontoxic agent, to 5-FU. Neoplastic cells can be induced to express the cytosine deaminase gene. Treatment with 5-fluorocytosine generates locally high concentrations of 5-FU with minimal systemic toxicity. Preclinical studies using an adenoviral vector for the cytosine deaminase gene have shown some efficacy [33]. A similar strategy involves the use of CB1954, a weak monofunctional alkylating agent, which is activated by *Escherichia coli* nitroreductase to a potent dysfunctional alkylating agent which cross-links DNA [34]. Efficient transfer of the nitroreductase gene has been accomplished in a variety of pancreatic cancer cell lines, and in vitro studies have shown appropriate sensitivity to CB1954.

All of the aforementioned approaches with gene therapy carry a common pitfall. While introduction of new genes in vivo may be possible with local intratumoral administration, strategies must be devised to allow effective gene introduction into tumor cells at metastatic cites.

Targeted Therapy

This section will focus on targeting tumor-associated antigen with radiolabeled monoclonal antibodies. Several antigens have been used as targets for radioimmunoconjugate therapy using monoclonal antibodies (MAbs) in patients with pancreatic adenocarcinoma and other gastrointestinal cancers. These antigens have included TAG-72 [35], 17-1A [36], CEA [37], A33 [38], and PAMM [39]. Our group has focused on TAG-72, an antigen that is preferentially expressed in adenocarcinomas; there is little expression in normal tissue with the exception of secretory endometrium [35]. We have completed phase-I trials with the parental murine MAb B72.3 and with the second generation MAb CC49. MAb CC49 is a very high affinity antibody which recognizes an epitope on TAG-72 different from that recognized by B72.3 [40]. Using beta-emitting radionuclide such as iodine 131(^{131}I) and ^{90}Y, we have demonstrated absorbed radiation doses of up to 3300 cGy in metastatic sites [41, 42]. Unfortunately, the murine antibodies produce a human MAb response which precludes multiple administration of the product to achieve a higher accumulative radiation dose to the tumor. Current strategies are focusing on less immunogenic antibodies as well as on strategies to improve the sensitivity of the tumor to the radiation delivered. MAb CC49 has been humanized and further engineered to delete the CH_2 portion of the Fc fragment [43]. This has resulted in the creation of a nonimmunogenic molecule when tested in primates with a favorable half-life for human therapeutic studies (unpublished data). Another approach has been to combine single-chain (Fv) fragments covalently. Studies by Colcher et al. [44] have shown favorable tumor-to-blood and tumor deposition with covalently bound dimers. Studies with trimers and tetramers may approximate the tumor deposition seen with intact IgG molecules. Sensitivity of the tumor to radiation may be improved using radiosensitizing drugs such as gemcitabine. We have shown that a modest dose of gemcitabine combined with an ineffective dose of ^{131}I-labeled MAb B72.3 has synergistic efficacy in a preclinical model [45]. Other strategies in development involve selective alteration of vascular permeability to allow a higher deposition of radiolabeled antibody in the tumor target.

MAb PAM4 represents another monoclonal antibody under development for therapeutic use as a radioimmunoconjugate in patients with pancreatic cancer. This murine IgG_1 antibody recognizes a pancreatic cancer-associated mucin. Preclinical studies in athymic nude mice have shown therapeutic efficacy with this antibody conjugated to ^{131}I [39]. Clinical biodistribution studies have demonstrated good localization of ^{131}I-labeled PAM4 in patients with pancreatic cancer [46].

Immunobiological Strategies

The most common immunobiological approach in pancreatic cancer has involved vaccination. In general, vaccine strategies have focused on either synthetic peptides or gene-modified tumor cells. All vaccine strategies for cancer therapy are based on the presumption that certain cancer-associated antigens can provoke a cytolytic T-cell (CTL) response. Induction of a naive CD8-positive T cell (cytotoxic T cell) requires presentation of antigen in association with MHC class I molecules to a T-cell precursor, as well as activation of a CD4-positive T cell (helper T cell), which serves to manufacture cytokines that can fully activate the CD8-positive precursor and stimulate its properties. Since most tumor cells do not express MHC class II molecules, the target antigen is presumably taken up and processed by professional antigen-presenting cells (APCs) such as macrophages or dendritic cells. These cells then present antigen to the CD8-positive T cell.

Regarding synthetic antigen vaccines, three approaches are being developed. Based on the observation that MUC-1, the peptide core of a pancreatic cancer-associated mucin antigen, invoked a cytolytic response in patients with breast and pancreatic cancer [47], clinical trials (primarily phase I) have been conducted with mannan-conjugated MUC-1 [48]. This trial demonstrated both humoral and CTL response to the immunogen. Another approach involves the use of synthetic ras peptides corresponding to individual ras mutations. Gjertsen et al [49] have initiated studies with this approach using an ex vivo presentation of the peptide to APCs harvested from peripheral blood. Following exposure to antigen, the APCs were reinjected and the patients continued on vaccination with the ras peptides. Appropriate immunologic responses occurred in five patients treated. Finally, sialyl-Tn, a carbohydrate antigen similar to TAG-72, has been widely tested in patients with breast, colon, and pancreatic cancer. Although cytolytic T-cell responses have not been studied in these patients, it has been noted that those patients with a robust antibody response appear to have prolonged survival [50].

Two vaccine approaches using gene-modified allogeneic tumor cells are in progress. Preclincal studies have shown in vivo regression of tumors following vaccination with cells from a murine ductal pancreatic adenocarcinoma cell line, PANC-02, that were genetically engineered to secrete human IL-2 [51]. Jaffee and colleagues [52] have taken a somewhat different approach with the development of a human allogeneic pancreatic cancer cell vaccine genetically engineered to produce GM-CSF. This approach is now being tested in a phase-I trial in patients following resection of pancreatic adenocarcinoma.

Conclusion

Although new therapeutic approaches based on pancreatic cancer biology are in early stages of development, much progress has been made in the preclinical arena and in the development of new drugs and reagents for clinical investigation. With continued emphasis on the importance of hypothesis-driven clinical research in pancreatic cancer, it is likely that some of these strategies will become the standard management of the future.

References

1. Crist DW, Cameron JL (1994) The current status of the Whipple operation for periampullary carcinoma. Adv Surg 25:21–49
2. Kalser MH, Ellenberg SS (1985) Pancreatic cancer: adjuvant combined radiation and chemotherapy following curative resection. Arch Surg 120:899–903
3. Landis SH, Murray T, Bolden S, Bolden S, Wingo PA (1998) Cancer Statistics, 1998. CA Cancer J Clin 48:6–29
4. Moertel CG, Frytak S, Hahn RG, et al (1981) Therapy of locally unresectable pancreatic carcinoma: a randomized comparison of high-dose (6000 rads) radiation alone, moderate-dose radiation (4000 rads+5-fluorouracil), and high-dose radiation+5-fluorouracil. Cancer 48:1705–1710
5. Burris HA, Moore MJ, Andersen J, et al (1997) Improvements in survival and clinical benefit with gemcitabine as first-line therapy for patients with advanced pancreatic cancer: a randomized trial. J Clin Oncol 15:2403–2413
6. Ahlgren JD (1996) Chemotherapy for pancreatic carcinoma. Cancer 78:654–663
7. Keating JJ, Johnson PJ, Cochrane AMG, et al (1989) A prospective randomised trial of tamoxifen and cyproterone acetate in pancreatic carcinoma. Br J Cancer 60:789–792
8. Philip PA, Carmichael J, Tonkin K, Buamah PK, Britton J, Dowsett M, Harris AL (1993) Hormonal treatment of pancreatic carcinoma: a phase II study of LHRH agonist goserelin plus hydrocortisone. Br J Cancer 67:379–382
9. Glimelius B, Hoffman K, Sjödén PO, et al (1996) Chemotherapy improves survival and quality of life in advanced pancreatic and biliary cancer. Ann Oncol 7:593–600
10. Palmer KR, Kerr M, Knowles G, Cull A, Carter DC, Leonard CF (1994) Chemotherapy prolongs survival in inoperable pancreatic carcinoma. Br J Surg 81:882–885
11. Mallinson CN, Rake MO, Cocking JD (1980) Chemotherapy in pancreatic cancer. Br Med J 281:1589–1591
12. Frey C, Twomey P, Keehn R, Elliott D, Higgins G (1981) Randomized study of 5-FU and CCNU in pancreatic cancer. Cancer 47:27–31
13. Almoguerra C, Shibata D, Forrester K, Martin J, Arnheim N, Perucho M (1988) Most human carcinomas of the exocrine pancreas contain mutant c-K-ras genes. Cell 53:549–554
14. Hruban RH, van Mansfeld ADM, Offerhaus GJA, et al (1989) K-ras oncogene activation in adenocarcinomas of the human pancreas: a study of 82 carcinomas using a combination of mutant-enriched polymerase chain reaction analysis and allele-specific oligonucleotide hybridization. Am J Pathol 143:545–554
15. Ito T, Kawata S, Tamura S, et al (1996) Suppression of human pancreatic cancer growth in BALB/c nude mice by manumycin, a farnesyl protein transferase inhibitor. Jpn J Can Res 87:113–116
16. Gibbs JB, Kohl NE, Koblan KS, et al (1996) Farnesyl transferase inhibitors and anti-Ras therapy. Breast Cancer Res Treat 38:75–83
17. Hohl RJ, Lewis K (1995) Differential effects of monoterpenes and lovastatin on RAS processing. J Biol Chem 270:17508–17512
18. Stark MJ, Burke YD, McKinzie JH, et al (1995) Chemotherapy of pancreatic cancer with monoterpene perillyl alcohol. Cancer Lett 96:15–21
19. Ripple G, Gould M, Arzoomanian R, et al (1998) Phase I trial of perillyl alcohol administered four times a day. ASCO Proc 17:231a, Abstr 885

20. Liotta LA, Tryggvason K, Garbisa S, et al (1980) Metastatic potential correlates with enzymatic degradation of basement membrane collagen. Nature 284:67–68
21. Liotta LA, Stetler-Stevenson WG (1991) Tumor invasion and metastasis: an imbalance of positive and negative regulation. Cancer Res 51:5054–5059
22. Bramhall S (1997) The matrix metalloproteinases and their inhibitors in pancreatic cancer. Int J Pancreatol 21:1–12
24. Shichinohe T, Senmaru N, Furuuchi K, et al (1996) Suppression of pancreatic cancer by the dominant negative ras mutant, N116Y. J Surg Res 66:125–130
25. Moelling K, Strack B, Radziwill G (1996) Signal transduction as target of gene therapy. Rec Res Cancer Res 142:63–71
26. Clayman GL, el Naggar AK, Roth JA, et al (1995) In vivo molecular therapy with p53 adenovirus for microscopic residual head and neck squamous carcinoma. Cancer Res 55:1–6
27. Bischoff JR, Kirn DH, Williams A (1996) An adenovirus mutant that replicates selectively in p53-deficient human tumor cells. Science 274:373–376
28. Mulvihill SJ, Warren RS, Fell S, et al (1998) A phase I trial of intratumoral injection with an E1B-attenuated adenovirus, ONYX-015, into unresectable carcinomas of the exocrine pancreas. ASCO Proc 17:211a, Abstr 815
29. Joshi US, Dergham ST, Chen YQ, et al (1998) Inhibition of pancreatic tumor cell growth in culture by p21WAF1 recombinant adenovirus. Pancreas 16:107–113
30. Barton CM, Lemoine NR (1995) Antisense oligonucleotides directed against p53 have antiproliferative effects unrelated to effects on p53 expression. Br J Cancer 71:429–437
31. Aoki K, Yoshida T, Matsumoto N, et al (1997) Gene therapy for peritoneal dissemination of pancreatic cancer by liposome-mediated transfer of herpes simplex virus thymidine kinase gene. Hum Gene Ther 8:1105–1113
32. Ohashi M, Kanai F, Tanaka T, et al (1998) In vivo adenovirus-mediated prodrug gene therapy for carcinoembryonic antigen-producing pancreatic cancer. Jpn J Cancer Res 89:457–462
33. Evoy D, Hirschowitz EA, Naama HA, et al (1997) In vivo adenoviral-mediated gene transfer in the treatment of pancreatic cancer. J Surg Res 69:226–231
34. Green NK, Youngs DJ, Neoptolemos JP, et al (1997) Sensitization of colorectal and pancreatic cancer cell lines to the prodrug 5-(aziridin-1-yl)-2,4-dinitrobenzamide (CB1954) by retroviral transduction and expression of the E. coli nitroreductase gene. Cancer Gene Ther 4:229–238
35. Thor A, Ohuchi N, Szpak CA, Johnson WW, Schlom J (1986) The distribution of oncofetal antigen TAG-72 defined by monoclonal antibody B72.3. Cancer Res 46:3118–3124
36. Buchsbaum DJ, Lawrence TS, Roberson PL, et al (1993) Comparison of ^{131}I- and ^{90}Y-labeled monoclonal antibody 17-1A for treatment of human colon cancer xenografts. Int J Radiat Oncol Biol Phys 25:629–638
37. Juweid M, Sharkey RM, Swayne LC, Griffith GL, Dunn R, Goldenberg DM (1998) Pharmacokinetics, dosimetry and toxicity of rhenium-188-labeled anti-carcinoembryonic antigen monoclonal antibody, MN-14, in gastrointestinal cancer. J Nucl Med 39:34–42
38. Welt S, Scott AM, Divgi CR, et al (1996) Phase I/II study of iodine 125-labeled monoclonal antibody A33 in patients with advanced colon cancer. J Clin Oncol 14:1787–1797
39. Alisauskus R, Wong GY, Gold DV (1995) Initial studies of monoclonal antibody PAM4 targeting to xenografted orthotopic pancreatic cancer. Cancer Res 55:5743–5748
40. Molinolo A, Simpsom JF, Thor A, Schlom J (1990) Enhanced tumor binding using immunohistochemical analyses by second generation anti-tumor-associated glycoprotein 72 monoclonal antibodies versus monoclonal antibody B72.3 in human tissue. Cancer Res 50:1291–1298
41. Tempero MA, Leichner P, Dalrymple G, et al (1997) High dose therapy with ^{131}I labeled monoclonal antibody CC49: a phase I trial. J Clin Oncol 15:1518–1528
42. Leichner PK, Akabani G, Colcher D, et al (1997) Patient-specific dosimetry of indium-111/yttrium-90-labeled monoclonal antibody CC49. J Nucl Med 38:512–516
43. Kashmiri SVS, Shu L, Padlan EA, et al (1995) Generation, characterization, and in vivo studies of humanized anticarcinoma antibody CC49. Hybridoma 14:461–473
44. Beresford GW, Pavlinkova G, Booth BJM, Batra SK, Colcher D (1998) Binding characteristics and tumor targeting of a covalently linked divalent CC49 single-chain antibody
45. Okazaki S, Tempero MA, Colcher D (1998) Combination radioimmunotherapy and chemotherapy using ^{131}I-B72.3 and gemcitabine. AACR Proc 39:310, Abstr 2119

46. Marani G, Molea N, Bacciardi D, et al (1995) Initial tumor targeting, biodistribution, and pharmacokinetic evaluation of the monoclonal antibody PAM4 in patients with pancreatic cancer. Cancer Res 55:5911–5915
47. Kotera Y, Fontenot JD, Pecher G, Metzgar RS, Finn OJ (1994) Humoral immunity against a tandem repeat epitope of human mucin MUC-1 in sera from breast, pancreatic, and colon cancer patients. Cancer Res 54:2856–2860
48. Karanikas V, Hwang LA, Pearson J, et al (1997) Antibody and T-cell responses of patients with adenocarcinoma immunized with mannan-MUC2 fusion protein. J Clin Invest 100:2783–2792
49. Gjertsen MJ, Bakka A, Breivik J, et al (1996) Ex vivo ras peptide vaccination in patients with advanced pancreatic cancer: results of a phase I/II study. Int J Cancer 65:450–453
50. Reddish MA, MacLean GD, Poppema S, Berg A, Longnecker BM (1996) Pre-immunotherapy serum CA27.29 (MUC-1) mucin level and CD69+ lymphocytes correlate with effects of Theratope sialyl-Tn-KLH cancer vaccine in active specific immunotherapy. Cancer Immunol Immunother 42:303–309
51. Clary BM, Coveney EC, Philip R, et al (1997) Inhibition of established pancreatic cancers following specific active immunotherapy with interleukin-2 gene-transduced tumor cells. Cancer Gene Ther 4:97–104
52. Jaffee EM, Pardoll DM (1997) Considerations for the clinical development of cytokine gene-transducted tumor cell vaccines. Methods 12:143–153

Pancreatic Cancer: Preclinical Development of an Experimental Treatment Strategy Using Retinoids and Interferon-alpha

ST. ROSEWICZ

Pancreatic Cancer: The Therapeutic Dilemma

Human adenocarcinoma of the pancreas is currently the fifth most common cause of cancer death in Western countries [1]. At the time of diagnosis more than 80% of the patients have advanced regional disease or distant metastases [2]. Therefore, curative resection cannot be considered for a vast majority of pancreatic cancer patients. Despite multiple clinical trials using a large panel of chemotherapeutic regimens, the prognosis of advanced pancreatic cancer has not significantly improved over the past 30 years. The median survival varies between 4 and 6 months and the 5-year survival is less than 2% (reviewed in [3, 4]). A recent survey of 27 randomized trials for advanced pancreatic cancer revealed median survivals of 1.3–11 months for patients receiving active treatment, with a median overall survival between 150 and 160 days under therapy [5]. The authors of this study concluded that there is currently no standard treatment available for advanced pancreatic cancer with the objective of prolonging disease-free survival or overall survival. Given that considerable toxicities were associated with the majority of the evaluated chemotherapeutic regimens, it appears questionable whether the relatively small gains in survival justify the side effects, hospitalization, and the potential reduction in quality of life. Furthermore, it seems unlikely that conventional chemotherapy will significantly improve the current therapeutic dilemma.

Based on these observations, the development of new drugs for palliative treatment of pancreatic cancer, in our opinion, should meet the following criteria: (a) new mechanism of action; (b) preclinical evidence of antitumor activity; (c) low toxicity profile; (d) administration of the drug on an outpatient basis to minimize hospitalization associated with treatment-related procedures.

Given that conventional chemotherapy is relatively ineffective in the treatment of advanced pancreatic cancer, new therapeutic strategies focusing on inhibition of tumor cell proliferation paralleled by induction of tumor cell

This work was supported by the Deutsche Krebshilfe and the Maria-Sonnenfeld-Gedächtnisstiftung.

differentiation offer a promising therapeutic approach. In this context numerous in vitro and in vivo studies in a variety of malignancies and experimental tumor models have shown that natural and synthetic derivatives of vitamin A, biochemically summarized as retinoids, are capable of inhibiting tumor cell proliferation and inducing cellular differentiation. In subsequent clinical trials, retinoids have been demonstrated to be an effective treatment modality for quite diverse malignancies such as cervical cancer, squamous cell carcinoma of the skin, and promyelocytic leukemia (for review see [6]).

The goal of our studies was therefore to develop an experimental treatment strategy with retinoids and interferon-alpha (IFN-α) for advanced human pancreatic carcinoma.

Preclinical Studies

Retinoids Regulate Growth and Differentiation

Our initial studies were performed using an in vitro system of a broad panel of human pancreatic carcinoma cell lines of ductal phenotype [7]. Using this in vitro system as well as xenotransplanted tumors derived from these cell lines, we found that retinoid treatment results in a time- and dose-dependent growth inhibition in vitro and in vivo of ductal but not acinar pancreatic tumor cells. Retinoid treatment induces a more differentiated phenotype in ductal tumor cells, as evidenced by morphological criteria and increased expression of carbonic anhydrase II [7, 8]. These findings were later independently confirmed by other groups in a variety of pancreatic carcinoma cell lines [9, 10]. The antiproliferative effects of retinoic acid can be augmented by IFN-α in some epithelial cell lines, as well as in the clinical treatment of squamous cell cancer of the skin and cervix (for review see [11, 12]) and in renal cell carcinoma. With respect to pancreatic carcinoma [13], we have been able to demonstrate antiproliferative effects of IFN-α in a subset of pancreatic carcinoma cell lines and synergistic antiproliferative effects of RA with IFN-α in vitro (Rosewicz et al., unpublished data).

Retinoids Inhibit Metastatic Potential

The fate of pancreatic cancer patients is critically determined by local tumor growth and infiltration as well as by the presence of distant metastases. These processes are determined at least partly by a complex interplay of tumor cells with extracellular matrix components of the basement membrane. For infiltrative growth, tumor cells have to penetrate the basement membrane of the organ; in the process of metastasis, tumor cells traverse the vascular basement membrane on their way from the circulation to the target organ. Adhesion to basement membrane components therefore represents the initial step in the cascade of infiltrative growth and metastasis. Accordingly, the ability to metastasize has been correlated with the extent of tumor cell adhesion to basement membrane components. The major constituents of basement membranes are type IV collagen, heparan-sulfate proteoglycan, nidogen/entactin, and laminin. Laminin has been of particular interest, because it has been shown to modulate tumor cell adhesion, growth, and differentiation; furthermore, the ability of tumor cells to interact with laminin has been shown to correlate with their tumorigenicity and their metastatic potential. Because the interaction of tumor cells with laminin and other basement membrane components plays a critical role in the control of local growth and metastasis of pancreatic carcinoma, we analyzed the effects of retinoids on pancreatic carcinoma cell adhesion to basement membrane components, with a particular focus on tumor cell adhesion to laminin [14]. Treatment with retinoids results in a time- and dose-dependent inhibition of DAN-G cell adhesion to fibronection and laminin, but not to collagens I, IV, and VI. The adhesion of DAN-G cells to laminin was completely blocked by anti-α_6 and anti-β_1 antibodies, but not by the synthetic peptide YIGSR. Flow-cytometric analysis of DAN-G cells revealed no quantitative difference of α_6 integrin expression in retinoid-treated and untreated DAN-G cells. Furthermore, radioimmunoprecipitation showed no difference in the appearance of $\alpha_6\beta_1$ integrin expression after retinoid incubation. Retinoids therefore decrease pancreatic carcinoma cell adhesion to laminin via specific alteration of the $\alpha_6\beta_1$-integrin receptor function and thereby open interesting perspectives for the modulation of infiltrative growth and metastasis in pancreatic cancer [14].

Retinoids: Mechanism of Action

Over the past few years, much has been learned about the molecular mechanisms by which retinoids can exert such pleiotropic effects as inhibition of proliferation and induction of tumor cell differentiation. Retinoids exert these intriguing effects through interaction with specific nuclear receptors. Based on molecular cloning studies so far, two families of nuclear retinoid receptors have been described, each consisting of three receptor subtypes α, β, and γ: the retinoic acid receptors (RAR) which bind the naturally occurring retinoid all-*trans* retinoic acid (ATRA) with high affinity [15, 16], and the retinoid X receptors (RXR), whose naturally occurring, biologically active ligand is 9-*cis* retinoic acid, a geometric isomer of ATRA [17]. The ligand-binding domains between these two retinoid receptor families share only 29% sequence homology [18]. In addition, each RAR/RXR gene generates multiple isoforms by either differential use of internal promotors or alternative splicing of exons [19]. Both receptor families act as ligand-dependent transcription factors, controlling gene transcription initiated from promotors of retinoid regulated genes by interacting with *cis*-acting DNA elements, the so-called RAREs (retinoic acid responsive elements) (reviewed in [19, 20]). This multiplicity of receptors and gene pathways explains the diverse effects of retinoids on a wide range of cellular processes.

Retinoid Receptor Subtype-specific Biological Functions

Tissue-specific restricted expression of RAR/RXR subtypes and isoforms during embryogenesis and in the adult organism suggests that each RAR and RXR subtype has a unique biological function [21]. Furthermore, disruption of the intracellular retinoid pathway via interference with specific RAR subtypes can result in carcinogenesis [22–24]. Based on this, and on our observation that retinoids exert antiproliferative effects and induce differentiation in human pancreatic carcinoma cells, we hypothesized that a deregulation of RAR subtype expression might be involved in the propagation of the malignant phenotype of human pancreatic cancer. In a subsequent in situ hybridization study we therefore analyzed RAR subtype expression in the human pancreatic carcinoma tissue of 24 patients [25]: while there was no difference between normal and malignant tissue in the expression of RARα and -γ, we observed that approximately one third of all pancreatic tumors completely lost the expression of RARβ when compared with their nontransformed counterparts. Furthermore, the remaining tumors expressed significantly fewer RARβ mRNA transcripts than did adjacent normal pancreatic ductal cells. Moreover, we observed a tight correlation between the loss of RARβ expression and the degree of cellular dedifferentiation [25]. These data suggested that loss or decreased expression of RARβ either could be an innocent epiphenomenon associated with malignant transformation or might indeed play a central role in the propagation of the malignant phenotype in human pancreatic adenocarcinoma. To dissect this problem we chose a reverse approach by overexpressing RARβ in the human pancreatic tumor cell line DAN-G. Overexpression of RARβ in DAN-G cells by stable transfection inhibits cellular proliferation in vitro and in vivo [26]. Furthermore, RARβ overexpression results in induction of cellular differentiation in xenografted tumors as evidenced by increased tumor cell expression of duct cell differentiation markers CEA, CA19-9, and cytokeratin 7 [26]. These data suggest that expression of RARβ plays a key role in the maintenance of a malignant phenotype in human pancreatic adenocarcinoma and might therefore represent a novel target for experimental strategies in the treatment of pancreatic cancer patients.

When we examined the expression pattern of retinoid receptor subtypes in a broad panel of pancreatic carcinoma cell lines by reverse-transcriptase polymerase chain reaction (RT-PCR), the most surprising observation was the expression of RARγ in all retinoid-sensitive pancreatic ductal tumor cell lines [7], because this receptor isoform has not been observed in any other gastrointestinal tissue; RARγ expression was thought to be restricted to keratinocytes of the skin, the classical highly sensitive target tissue of retinoid action. In contrast, RARγ was not detected by Northern blotting or the sensitive RT-PCR technique in the retinoid-resistant pancreatic amphicrine cell line AR42J [27]. This intriguing observation suggests that RARγ might play a key role in retinoid action on human pancreatic ductal tumor cells. This hypothesis is further supported by experiments using targeted gene disruption of both RARγ alleles; these genetically engineered RARγ-deficient cells lose their responsiveness to retinoids and fail to exhibit a differentiated phenotype upon retinoid treatment [28]. In addition, null mutant mice for RARγ, created by homologous recombination, exhibited marked growth deficiency and early death, suggesting a crucial role for RARγ in the regulation of growth and differentiation in vivo [29]. Experimental proof for the hypothesis that RARγ confers retinoid sensitivity of human pancreatic ductal carcinoma cells and that the lack of RARγ expression is furthermore responsible for retinoid resistance of pancreatic acinar tumor cells requires the stable transfection of RARγ into AR42J cells or targeted RARγ gene disruption of ductal tumor cells; preliminary experiments using ballistomagnetic gene transfer revealed that RARγ expression indeed confers retinoid sensitivity to AR42J cells (Rosewicz et al., manuscript in preparation).

Interaction of Retinoids with Protein Kinase C (PKC)

In addition to nuclear receptors, recent experimental evidence suggests that retinoids can interfere at the intersection of other intracellular signaling systems essential for the regulation of cellular growth, a phenomenon which has been commonly described as "cross-talking". One such example of cross-talking which has recently been discovered is the interference of retinoids with protein kinase C (PKC). PKC is a phospholipid-dependent serine/threonine kinase implicated in essential cellular processes such as regulation of gene expression, cellular proliferation, and differentiation (for review see [30–32]). PKC constitutes the naturally occurring receptor for the mitogenic phorbol esters, which act as tumor promotors. The naturally occurring activators of PKC in vivo are diacylglycerol and arachidonic acid, which are generated as second messengers upon cellular binding of many mitogenic stimuli, such as hormones, growth factors, and other extracellular ligands [33]. Based on biochemical purification and molecular cloning studies, PKC represents a multigene family which can be divided into two subgroups, depending on whether the enzymes require calcium for activation (PKC-α, -βI, -βII, and -γ) or not (PKC-δ, ε, ζ, η, and L). These PKC isoforms differ in their cofactor requirement, substrate specificity, subcellular distribution, and tissue-restricted expression, suggesting that each isoform might serve a distinct biological function.

We have established an in vitro system in which retinoic acid exerts opposite effects on anchorage-independent growth in two cell lines derived from an identical histological origin, a human pancreatic adenocarcinoma [34]. This system can therefore serve as a valuable model to explore the interplay of various PKC isoenzymes in the differential growth regulation by retinoic acid. RA treatment results in dose-dependent stimulation of anchorage-independent growth in AsPc1 cells and growth inhibition in Capan 2 cells. Both cell lines express an identical pattern of nuclear RARs and RXRs, as determined by reverse-transcriptase PCR. Western blotting using monospecific antibodies revealed that both cell lines express PKC isoenzymes *α* and *ζ*, while *β*, *γ*, *δ*, and *ε* were not detected. Incubation with RA in the growth-stimulated AsPc1 cell line resulted in induction of PKC *α* expression, whereas

PKC α expression was decreased by RA in the growth-inhibited Capan 2 cell line. In contrast, PKC ζ expression was not affected by RA in either cell line. Incubation of AsPc1 cells with the phorbolester TPA resulted in a time- and dose-dependent selective down-regulation of PKC α but not ζ. The dose-dependent decrease of intracellular PKC α concentration correlated well with the anchorage-independent growth rate of AsPc1 cells. Furthermore, selective down-regulation of PKC α blocks subsequent growth stimulation by RA in AsPc1 cells. When PKC α concentration was decreased by stably transfecting AsPc1 cells with a PKC α cDNA antisense construct, RA-stimulated growth was also partially blocked. These data therefore suggest that differential regulation of PKC α expression plays a central role in determining the bidirectional effects of retinoids on growth in pancreatic carcinoma cells [34].

Clinical Studies

Based on the results of our preclinical experiments, we conducted a phase-II trial of 13-*cis* retinoic acid and IFN-α in patients with advanced pancreatic carcinoma [35]. The purpose of this trial was to examine feasibility and tolerability of a combination therapy of 13-*cis* RA and IFN-α in patients with advanced, unresectable pancreatic carcinoma. Twenty-two patients (median age 62 years) with histologically confirmed, unresectable pancreatic adenocarcinoma of UICC stage III (5/22) or IV (17/22) were included. Patients received 1 mg/kg body wt. 13-*cis* RA p.o. and 6 million IU IFN-α s.c. daily. Restaging by ultrasound, CT scan, and chest X-ray was performed every 2 months. No complete and one partial remission (PR: 4.5%) were observed; 14 patients (63.6%) demonstrated stable disease with a median duration of 5.0 months (range 2.3–17.7+). Toxicity was mainly IFN-α related and predominantly hematologic (no grade 4, 13.6% grade 3). Nonhematological toxicity did not exceed grade 2 (skin, oral mucosa) and was related mainly to 13-*cis* RA. Median survival of stage III cancer patients was 8.7 months (range 6.8–23.9+), that of stage IV patients 7.4 months (range 0.9–19.9+), resulting in a median overall survival of 7.7 months (range 0.9–23.9+). These data indicated that combination therapy with 13-*cis* RA and IFN-α is feasible and well tolerated in patients with advanced pancreatic carcinoma. In view of the median survival rates observed in this study, this combination should be further investigated in phase-III trials.

Future Directions

Based on our preclinical studies regarding retinoid receptor subtype-specific biological functions, it may be possible to further optimize the clinical treatment protocol. By screening pancreatic cancer biopsies for RARγ expression by in situ hybridization and RT-PCR we might be able to select a "retinoid-sensitive" subgroup of pancreatic cancer patients before initiating therapy.

With the current development of synthetic retinoid receptor subtype-specific agonists, we might be able to amplify the desired therapeutic effects such as growth inhibition and induction of differentiation (mediated by the RARβ) and to minimize undesired side effects potentially mediated by other receptor subtypes. In addition, we are currently in the process of identifying retinoid-regulated genes responsible for the growth-inhibitory effects observed in pancreatic carcinoma. These molecules might serve as novel therapeutic targets for antiproliferative treatment of pancreatic cancer.

References

1. Silverberg E, Boring CC, Squires TS (1990) Cancer statistics, 1990. CA Cancer J Clin 40:9–26
2. Bakkevold KE, Arnesjo B, Kambestag B (1992) Carcinoma of the pancreas and papilla of Vater: presenting symptoms, signs, and diagnosis related to stage and tumor site. A prospective multicentre trial in 472 patients. Scand J Gastroenterol 27:317–325
3. Arbuck SG (1990) Chemotherapy for pancreatic cancer. Baillieres Clin Gastroenterol 4:953–964
4. Rosewicz S, Wiedenmann B (1997) Pancreatic carcinoma. Lancet 349:485–489
5 Lionetto R, Pugliese V, Bruzzi P, Rosso R (1995) No standard treatment is available for advanced pancreatic cancer. Eur J Cancer 31A:882–887
6. Bollag W, Holdener EE (1992) Retinoids in cancer prevention and therapy. Ann Oncol 3:512–526
7. Rosewicz S, Stier U, Brembeck F, Kaiser A, Papadimitriou CA, Berdel WE, Wiedenmann B, Riecken EO (1995) Retinoids: effects on growth, differentiation and nuclear receptor expression in human pancreatic carcinoma cell lines. Gastroenterology 109:1646–1660
8. Rosewicz S, Riecken EO, Stier U (1995) Transcriptional regulation of carbonic anhydrase II by retinoic acid in the human pancreatic tumor cell line DANG. FEBS Lett 368:45–48
9. Egawa N, Maillet B, vanDamme B, DeGreve J, Klöppel G (1996) Differentiation of pancreatic carcinoma induced by retinoic acid or sodium butyrate: a morphological and molecular analysis of four cell lines. Virchows Arch 429:59–68
10. Bold RJ, Ishizuka J, Townsend CM, Thompson JC (1996) All-trans retinoic acid inhibits growth of human pancreatic cancer cell lines. Pancreas 12:189–195
11. Moore DM, Kalvakolanu DV, Lippman SM, Kavanagh JJ, Hong WK, Borden EC, et al (1994) Retinoic acid and interferon in human cancer: mechanistic and clinical studies. Semin Hematol 31[Suppl 5]:31–37
12. Eiscnhauer EA, Lippman SM, Kavanagh JJ, Parades-Espinoza M, Arnold A, Hong WK, et al (1994) Combination 13-cis-retinoic acid and interferon alpha-2a in the therapy of solid tumors. Leukemia 8:1622–1625
13. Rosewicz S, Weder M, Kaiser A, Riecken EO (1996) Antiproliferative effects of interferon alpha on human pancreatic carcinoma cell lines are associated with differential regulation of protein kinase C isoenzymes. GUT 39:255–261
14. Rosewicz S, Wollbergs K, v Lampe B, Matthes H, Kaiser A, Riecken EO (1997) Retinoids inhibit adhesion to laminin in human pancreatic carcinoma cells via the $\alpha_6\beta_1$-integrin receptor. Gastroenterology 112:532–542
15. Petkovich M, Brand NJ, Krust A, Chambon P (1987) A human retinoic acid receptor which belongs to the family of nuclear receptors. Nature 330:444–450
16. Zelent A, Krust A, Petkovich M, Kastner P, Chambon P (1989) Cloning of murine and retinoic acid receptors and a novel receptor predominantly expressed in the skin. Nature 339:714–717
17. Heyman RA, Mangelsdorf, DJ, Dyck JA, Stein RB, Eichele G, Evans RM, Thaller C (1992) 9-cis retinoic acid is a high affinity ligand for the retinoid X receptor. Cell 68:397–406
18. Leid M, Kastner P, Chambon P (1992) Multiplicity generates diversity in the retinoic acid pathway. Trends Biol Sci 17:427–433

19. Giguere V (1994) Retinoic acid receptors and cellular retinoid binding proteins: complex interplay in retinoid signaling. Endocrin Rev 15:61–79
20. Hashimoto Y (1991) Retinobenzoic acids and nuclear retinoic acid receptors. Cell Struct Funct 16:113–123
21. Dolle P, Ruberte E, Leroy P, Morriss-Kay G, Chambon P (1990) Retinoic acid receptors and cellular retinoid binding proteins. A systematic study of their differential pattern of transcription during mouse organogenesis. Development 110:1133–1151
22. Houle B, Rochette-Egly C, Bradley WEC (1993) Tumor-suppressive effect of the retinoic acid receptor β in human epidermoid lung cancer cells. Proc Natl Acad Sci USA 90:985–989
23. de The H, Chomienne C, Lanotte M, Degos L, Dejean A (1990) The t(17:15) translocation of acute promyelocytic leukemia fuses the retinoic acid receptor α gene to a novel transcribed locus. Nature 347:558–561
24. Gebert JF, Moghal N, Frangioni JV, Sugarbaker DJ, Neel BG (1991) High frequency of retinoic acid b receptor abnormalities in human lung cancer. Oncogene 6:1859–1868
25. Xu XC, Stier U, Rosewicz S, El-Naggar AK, Lotan R (1996) Differential suppression of nuclear retinoic acid receptor beta in pancreatic carcinomas. Int J Oncol 8:445–451
26. Kaiser A, Herbst H, Fisher G, Koenigsmann M, Berdel WE, Riecken EO, Rosewicz S (1997) Retinoic acid receptor β regulates growth and differentiation in human pancreatic carcinoma cells. Gastroenterology 113:920–929
27. Rosewicz S, Vogt D, Harth N, Grund C, Franke WW, Ruppert S, Schweitzer S, Riecken EO, Wiedenmann B (1992) An amphicrine pancreatic cell line: AR42J cells combine exocrine and neuroendocrine properties. Eur J Cell Biol 59:80–91
28. Boylan JF, Lohnes D, Taneja R, Chambon P, Gudas LJ (1993) Loss of retinoic acid receptor γ function by gene disruption results in aberrant Hoxa-1 expression and differentiation upon retinoic acid treatment. Proc Natl Acad Sci U S A 90:9601–9605
29. Lohnes D, Kastner P, Dierich A, Mark M, LeMeur M, Chambon P (1993) Function of retinoic acid receptor γ in the mouse. Cell 73:643–658
30. Kikkawa U, Kishimoto A, Nishizuka Y (1989) The protein kinase C family: heterogeneity and its implications. Annu Rev Biochem 58:31–44
31. Basu A (1993) The potential of protein kinase C as a target for anticancer treatment. Pharmacol Ther 5:257–280
32. Hug H, Sarre TF (1993) Protein kinase C isoenzymes: divergence in signal transduction? J Biochem 291:329–343
33. Nishizuka Y (1992) Intracellular signaling by hydrolysis of phospholipids and activation of protein kinase C. Science 258:607–613
34. Rosewicz S, Brembeck F, Kaiser A, v Marschall Z, Riecken EO (1996) Differential growth regulation by all-trans retinoic acid is determined by protein kinase C in human pancreatic carcinoma cells. Endocrinology 137:3340–3347
35. Brembeck FH, Schoppmeyer K, Leupold U, Gornistu C, Keim V, Mössner J, Riecken EO, Rosewicz S (1998) A phase II pilot trial of 13-cis retinoic acid and interferon-α in patients with advanced pancreatic carcinoma. Cancer 83:2317–2323

CHAPTER 23

Aspects of Radical Surgery for Exocrine Cancer of the Pancreatic Head

Åke Andrén-Sandberg, Dag Hoem, and Hjörtur Gislason

Introduction

Although almost exactly a century has elapsed since Alessandro Codivilla performed the first pancreaticoduodenectomy in Bologna in 1898 [1], and it has been only 16 years less since Walter Kausch succeeded with a partial pancreaticoduodenectomy in Germany 1912 [2], this remains a most complex operation that carries a substantial operative risk and limited long-term success. In 1942, A. O. Whipple stated that "Many more cases with 5-year survival will be required before valid claims can be made for the operation (i.e., pancreaticoduodenectomy) as done at present. But, it must be remembered that those patients untreated have an average risk of 6 months' survival from onset of symptoms until death... The considerable risk of 30%–35% is justified if they can be made comfortable for even a year or two" [3].

Perioperative mortality after pancreatic resections remained high up until the 1970s [4], but surgical resection of pancreatic cancer continued to be practiced, as it was the only potentially curative therapy. However, in critical reviews of the literature [5, 6], Gudjonsson has pointed out that pancreatic resections have had a minimal impact on survival rates in the total population of patients with pancreatic carcinoma. This is undoubtedly a correct statement but it is nevertheless misleading, as only the actually resected can influence the survival rates and survival times of this subset of patients. Gudjonsson – frequently cited – reports 5-year survivals of 0%–55% in his collection of 340 papers dealing with survival rates and containing apparently adequate confirmation of the diagnosis of exocrine pancreatic cancer. He reports on survivors who have been resected, but he points out the probability that some patients are rereported up to six times by authors from different countries in different articles. He claims that survivors who were not resected are frequently overlooked, which further implies that the actuarial statistics used may exaggerate the results. After correction for repetitions, approximately 300 survivors were found, 10% of whom had not undergone resection, among the estimated 80 000 patients reported. In his summaries the overall survival rate is therefore less than 0.4%; he gives the best overall survival rate in surgical studies reported in detail as only 3.6% and in a nonsurgical study as 1.7%. He therefore claims that the average excess cost for each resection is at least US$ 150000, which gives a cumulative cost per "successful" resection of approximately US$ 4.5 million.

Even though the Gudjonsson figures may be challenged both from a statistical and from an academic point of view, and while they might reflect a time period with difficulties that have now been overcome, they should make also the most optimistic surgeons humble enough to address the questions regarding resection for pancreatic cancer in a most critical way.

Current Strategy for Radical Surgery

The evaluation of a patient with pancreatic carcinoma aims first to establish the diagnosis and then to assess the stage of disease and the fitness of the patient with regard to the possibility of resection. The patient should be sufficiently fit not only to survive a major operation and to participate in the first postoperative period, but also to survive possible complications. The combination of these demands makes only 15%–20% of pancreatic cancers in western Europe and the USA resectable at the time of diagnosis [7–10], and even resection of overgrowth on the portal vein does not change that in more than a very few cases.

Most clinicians will no longer perform pre- or perioperative core biopsy or cytology (fine needle aspiration biopsy, FNAC) while resection for potential cure remains a possibility. The reasons for this are two. First, even though the specificity is almost 100%, the sensitivity is about 80% [11]. This implies that one of five patients with a resectable cancer will be missed, and most probably the smallest cancers with the best prognosis have the greatest risk of being overlooked. Second, even if it is "only" chronic pancreatitis, a resective procedure is a good choice for the patient if the complication rate can be kept at a minimum, which makes pancreaticoduodenectomy today also indicated for selected benign and inflammatory pancreatic diseases [12].

The standard pancreaticoduodenectomy (Whipple resection) has for many years continued to be the most widely performed operation for pancreatic cancer around the world. When resections are performed today, operative mortality should be less than 2% and there should be a tolerable, even though not insignificant, long-term morbidity [13–19]. Unfortunately, the overall 5-year survival is only approximately 10%, at least in unselected, larger groups [13–19]. The Japanese results are often considerably better [14, 20–31], but there are indications that Japanese surgeons are more reluctant to publish less good results, which leads to a positive selection bias.

It is obvious that surgeons must continue to modify the surgical procedures in efforts to further reduce the mortality and morbidity and to cure more patients. One of the more important modifications in recent years has been the pylorus-preserving pancreaticoduodenectomy (PPPD) [32]. The choice between a "standard Whipple" and a PPPD cannot, however, be made today on the basis of medical evidence alone. Preservation of the antrum and pylorus was proposed to avoid the postgastrectomy symptoms such as dumping, diarrhea, distention, and dyspepsia associated with the standard

Whipple procedure without increasing the risk of marginal ulceration [32–34]. The reintroduction of the pylorus-preserving procedure embodied an appealing concept, also because processing and absorption of food appears to be more physiologic than if an antiulcer antrectromy – or vagotomy – has to be added to the pancreaticoduodenectomy. Omitting these parts of pancreaticoduodenectomy may also decrease the risk of postoperative diarrhea compounding the problems of possible pancreatic insufficiency [35]. In an early series of eight patients with PPPD the mean time required to resume a full and independent oral diet was more than 6 days longer than in a group of eight patients who had a standard Whipple operation with vagotomy [35]. From an early collected review [36] of 252 PPPDs the disquieting incidence of 30% for early delayed postoperative gastric emptying was reported. In yet another group of 15 patients delayed gastric emptying was seen in 61% after PPPD compared with 41% of 52 patients who underwent a standard Whipple operation [37]. Due to this and other reports, the incidence of early delayed gastric emptying was initially thought to be increased after pylorus-preserving resections [35]. Nowadays this statement is questioned, and at most centers the incidence of delayed gastric emptying as well as of other complications is recognized to be about equal after standard and after pylorus-preserving pancreaticoduodenectomies [16, 17, 38–42].

For a time, some surgeons advocated total pancreatectomy [43, 44], but it is currently agreed that the long-term survival rate was not improved after this more extensive resection. Moreover, the perioperative morbidity was probably higher, and it produced a "brittle" diabetes mellitus that is often difficult to manage. Total pancreatectomy is nowadays not an option for "ordinary" cancer of the head of the pancreas [18]. However, under special circumstances there may also be a place for this procedure. Analysis of 458 patients who had undergone the Whipple procedure in Mannheim between 1972 and 1994 revealed that 16 patients with malignant tumors (seven of them pancreatic) subsequently required completion pancreatectomy due to complications or a delayed report of cancer at the margin of the pancreatic transection (n=1). Completed pancreatectomy was often difficult and there was considerable postoperative morbidity (41%) and mortality (24%). Patients who survived lived a mean of nearly 4 years (median 2.6 years), and tumor recurrence led to death in ten of 13 patients. Three patients remained alive and free of recurrence more than 8 years after resection [45].

On the other hand, even though it is not a part of the standard procedure, portal vein involvement should no longer be considered an indication that patients have unresectable disease [14, 25, 46, 47]. Patients with isolated portal vein resection had perioperative mortality and overall median survival similar to that of a group with no vascular involvement who underwent standard pancreatic resection [15].

Improving Results by Extended Resections?

The prognostic determinants for pancreatic cancer surgery are the tumor's tendency to extension and metastasis, i.e., the high incidence of local invasion, lymphatic metastasis, transperitoneal and hematogenous spread. In 1978, Cubilla et al. [48] published a classic study of lymph node involvement by pancreatic cancer. They showed that specimens from more extensive pancreatic resections contained more than twice as many lymph nodes as those from standard pancreaticoduodenectomies (70 versus 33). Moreover, 33% of patients had metastases present in nodes not usually removed in the standard operation. Nagai et al. [21] examined eight autopsy specimens from patients with pancreatic cancer. They found that half of the patients had metastatic tumors in the lymph nodes located between the superior and the mesenteric arteries. This tissue is not routinely included in the field of dissection in the standard pancreaticoduodenectomy. Examination of pancreaticoduodenectomy specimens by others has revealed an incidence of retroperitoneal invasion in 89% of patients and involvement of the extrapancreatic neural plexuses in 62% [23, 49]. This occurred even with small tumors. These findings, and the fact that approximately 75% of patients who die from pancreatic cancer are found to have a local recurrence in the pancreatic bed [10, 22, 50], stimulated a trial of a more radical operative approach. The first attempt to improve the poor prognosis of pancreatic carcinoma was therefore logically to perform more aggressive procedures such as primary total pancreatectomy [51, 52]. However, total pancreatectomy has failed to yield a better survival rate than pancreaticoduodenectomy in patients with pancreatic cancer [18, 43, 44, 53].

In an attempt to improve survival in patients with pancreatic carcinoma, Fortner introduced an approach termed "regional pancreatectomy" [52, 54], in which, in addition to the standard Whipple operation, he removed adjacent soft tissue, lymphatics, and a segment of the superior mesenteric-portal vein and superior mesenteric artery. Although operative mortality was only slighter higher (8%), morbidity was increased and 5-year survival rates were not improved. Indeed, an evaluation by the National Cancer Institute of 20 patients treated with regional pancreatectomy found a higher operative morbidity (55%) and mortality (20%), with no improvement in survival over historical controls treated with standard pancreaticoduodenectomy [55]. Thus, the first attempts made it obvious that regional pancreatectomy failed to improve the long-term survival rate and carried a high operative mortality [55, 56]. Recently, however, Fortner et al. [57] have reported a 5% operative mortality (4% for subtotal regional pancreatectomy) and 33% 5-year survival after regional pancreatectomy for pancreatic lesions smaller than 2.5 cm. In the early 1980s, Japanese surgeons adopted the extended pancreaticoduodenectomy, which owes its popularity to the fact that the poor prognosis of pancreatic cancer after resection is related to local recurrence and distant metastases [20, 58, 59].

Later, Japanese surgeons proposed a technique referred to as "extended pancreaticoduodenectomy", which combined pancreaticoduodenectomy with extended lymphadenectomy and clearance of the neural plexuses and connective tissue of the celiac trunk, superior mesenteric axis, aorta, and inferior vena cava from the diaphragm to the inferior mesenteric artery, based on a detailed clinicopathologic study of the manner in which pancreatic cancer spreads [60, 61].

The extended pancreaticoduodenectomy technique starts with isolation of the portal vein, the proper hepatic artery, the superior mesenteric artery and vein, and the splenic vein, and the dorsal pancreatic artery is ligated and divided. The inferior mesenteric vein is identified and isolated to the left of the superior mesenteric artery. The resection line is 2–3 cm to the left of the origin of the splenic artery, but if cancer is seen in frozen section, more pancreatic tissue is removed. Following pancreatic transection, the lymph nodes and nerve plexuses located around the celiac artery and over the root of the superior mesenteric artery are dissected sharply by exposing the arterial wall from the patient's left side to the anterior surface. The portal vein, superior mesenteric vein, and splenic vein are occluded with vascular clamps and divided. Following resection of veins of the portal system, the pancreatic plexus is displayed as a cord-like structure running between the pancreas and the superior mesenteric artery. Once the inferior pancreaticoduodenal artery is ligated and sectioned at its origin, en bloc resection of the tumor in the pancreatic head is performed, with portal vein, retroperitoneal connective tissue, extra pancreatic nerve plexuses, and lymph nodes attached. Reconstruction of the portal vein is performed by end-to-end anastomosis with 5/0 nonresorbable suture. If needed, additional dissection of extrapancreatic nerve plexuses, celiac ganglia, and para-aortic lymph nodes is performed. Finally, the splenic vein is anastomosed end-to-side to the superior mesenteric vein. The additional dissection, including the vascular reconstructions, adds no more than 1 h to the operation. Reconstruction of the gastrointestinal tract is similar to that in the standard Whipple resection. In the experience of Hanyu et al. [24], the morbidity and mortality of extended resection (20% and 4%, respectively) were similar to those of the standard operation (morbidity 22%, mortality 12%), using their own historical controls. The most common postoperative complications of the extended operation were pancreatic fistula (7%) and intra-abdominal bleeding and abscess (2%), also not different than after the standard Whipple resection.

The European, mostly German, experience with extended pancreaticoduodenectomy has revealed some interesting differences. Large series of standard pancreaticoduodenectomies have been performed with low operative mortalities [13]. Trede and Schwall [13] reported on 76 patients undergoing extended pancreaticoduodenectomy with no deaths and a low morbidity of 18%. In the 44 patients undergoing curative resections, 5-year survival was 25%, with an actuarial survival in 76 patients of 36%. Another group recently analyzed 101 patients with pancreatic cancer [62], 86 of whom were treated with extended pancreaticoduodenectomy and 15 with the standard Whipple procedure. Their data suggest that after an R0 resection (histologically free margins), even in those patients with locally advanced disease but with nodal involvement, the extended resection confers a survival benefit (35% versus 0% 5-year survival in stage I and II disease; extended versus standard pancreaticoduodenectomy. If lymph nodes were involved, the radical resection did not offer any survival benefit. Unfortunately, the status of lymph nodes is usually not known until after resection, so this may not help the surgeon to decide whether an extended resection should be performed.

The influence of the extent of the nodal and soft-tissue resection was studied retrospectively by Ishikawa et al. [61]. A total of 53 patients undergoing resection between 1971 and 1983 were evaluated. Thirty-two patients underwent standard pancreaticoduodenectomy, 21 underwent the extended operation. The 3-year cumulative survival for the two groups was 13% and 38%, respectively. For patients with positive nodes, there were no 3-year survivors in the first group, but four (27%) node-positive patients in the second group survived. These data suggested that the more extensive resection improved survival in patients subsequently shown to have involved nodes. Similar results from other Japanese surgeons have appeared in the literature [33, 35–40]. Tashiro et al. [46] reported on 14 patients with pancreatic cancer who underwent the extended pancreaticoduodencetomy and received 30 Gy of intraoperative radiation. The 5-year survival was 33%. Ozaki [22] reported on 16 patients, four of whom had cancers of the body and tail of the gland. Survival at 1 year was 88%, at 3 years 53%. Manabe et al. [25] performed 42 standard Whipple operations with a 10% operative mortality and no 3-year survivors. Thirty-two patients underwent extended pancreaticoduodenectomy with a 6% operative mortality and a 5-year survival of 34%. Nagakawa et al. [26] recently reviewed their experience with 134 pancreatic cancer patients treated since 1973. Sixty-one patients underwent the extended pancreaticoduodenectomy, a 46% resectability rate. Forty-nine of these patients had an R0 resection, with an operative mortality of 14% at 60 days. In the subgroup of 13 patients without lymph node metastases, the 5-year survival was 66%. Lymph nodes adjacent to the pancreas were involved in 21 patients, of whom only two (9%) survived for 5 years. Other pathologic factors were analyzed to determine their prognostic significance. The 5-year survival for patients with small cancers (less than 2 cm in diameter) was 67%, compared with 37% in the 14 patients with tumors between 4 and 6 cm in diameter. The presence of invasion of the retroperitoneal tissue was also important; its absence conferred a 73% chance of surviving 5 years. When the tissue was involved, the 5-year survival was 14%. There are also reports of more extensive retropancreatic vessel resections with good outcome [63] as well as on combinations with advanced cytotoxic drugs [64].

Both extended and standard pancreatic resection appeared to increase the postoperative survival period without impairment of the physical performance status, even in patients with advanced cancer [29]. It is clear that the extended operation can be performed safely, with little additional morbidity, and with an operative mortality similar to that of standard resection. With this more aggressive approach, resectability rates of 50% or more are common, which is higher than with the standard operation (15%–20%). However, there is currently little published evidence for the fact that extended pancreatic resections (including segments of the portal venous system and wide lymphatic and soft-tissue dissections) prolong survival in most patients with pancreatic cancer, compared with the standard Whipple operation. The apparent differences in survival between the extended and standard operation in a few reports may result from the different pathologic staging systems used at different centers; i.e., the patients being compared may not have the same stage of disease. Moreover, all the available data are retrospective, using historical controls, and none of the studies has randomized patients between the standard and the extended operations. Further randomized studies are eagerly awaited.

Improving Surgical Results by Centralizing Surgery?

Surgical resections for pancreatic cancer can be accomplished today with very low mortality – at most one or two percent – although the majority of patients are still diagnosed at an incurable stage of the disease. Concerns about the morbidity and mortality of surgery for pancreatic cancer have been quieted by results from specialized centers showing low mortality. Prior to 1980, the in-hospital mortality for this procedure exceeded 20% [65, 66]. Since then it has decreased substantially, with specialized centers reporting rates of 0 to a few percent [16, 17, 19, 67].

Regionalization includes formulation of treatment protocols and critical pathways for the procedure, as well as standardization of diagnostic work-ups, technical operative details, and the management of the postoperative course. It must also include a continuing presentation of the outcome of the treatment in different media, from highly specialized scientific reports to the establishment of a home page on the Internet. If possible, there should also be reports on readmission rates, functional status, and quality of life.

In a study carried out in the state of New York [65], using data on 1972 patients who underwent pancreatic resection for malignancy between 1984 and 1991, the mortality was 16% in patients operated on by surgeons performing fewer than nine operation per year. This should be compared with a mortality of less than 5% for those performing more than 40 cases per year. In addition, mortality and hospital caseloads were negatively correlated. In a logistic regression analysis of factors contributing to mortality, individual surgeon caseload was significant but became insignificant when hospital caseload was controlled.

Cameron and co-workers [68] defined high-volume hospitals concerning pancreaticoduodenectomies as those performing 20 such procedures or more per year for at least 6 of 12 consecutive years and an average volume during the 12-year period of >12 pancreaticoduodenectomies per year. Three major studies have shown that the in-hospital mortality for the complex, high-risk pancreaticoduodenectomy is lower when performed in high-volume settings than when performed in low-volume settings [65, 69, 70], suggesting that regionalization could result in a substantial decrease in mortality, and probably morbidity, for the procedure.

In the study covering 12 years in Maryland, USA [68], it was found that the in-hospital mortality for pancreaticoduodenectomy decreased for both the high-volume and the low-volume hospitals during the study period, but the adjusted relative risk of death at the low-volume institutions more than doubled compared with the high-volume institutions during the time period. The authors estimated that the concentration of the procedure to one high-volume center accounted for nearly 61% of the observed reduction in postoperative in-hospital mortality for pancreatectomies in that state. The remaining decrease was due to the overall improvement in the mortality for pancreaticoduodenectomies during the study period.

A recent survey of experience in the West Midland region of England, relating to the experience of general surgeons in 28 district general hospitals situated within a region of 5.5 million population [71], used Cancer Registry data to identify all cases of resected and nonresected pancreatic cancer in the period 1957–1986, comprising 13,560 patients. In the recent period from 1977 to 1986 postoperative mortality was 28%; it was 45% in the earlier period. The 5-year survival also improved to 9.7% from 2.6%.

In summary, recent well-reviewed [72] data strongly suggest that regionalization, or the concentration of services at one or a few high-volume centers, could lower the in-hospital mortality for pancreatectomy.

Palliative Surgical Resection?

The question of whether extensive palliative cancer resections are worthwhile can be discussed from three viewpoints. The first is economics: Here it becomes clear that calculations of cost-effectiveness – important as they are – are meaningless for individual cases. Second, the quality of life must be considered: Of 1200 oncological procedures performed in the period 1993–1994, Trede and Schwab [73] found 138 palliative operations for extensive cancer. With an overall operative mortality of 9%, 59 of these patients were still alive after a mean follow-up period of 15 months; of the 49 who could be reached, 60% rated their quality of life as "satisfactory" or "very good". In the end, however, quality-control figures are also of little help in the individual case. Third, selected individual case histories concerning surgery for metastases make it abundantly clear that the answer to the question of palliative resection must be found anew by each individual patient and his surgeon.

Future Prospects

It is obvious that during 100 years of pancreatic cancer surgery we have learned much; however, there are many more issues still to be addressed. Today we know that a standard Whipple operation can be done with almost zero mortality and with a steadily decreasing rate of major complications. Despite this, the long-term results are still far from acceptable, with a 5-year survival of usually less than 20%.

From a surgical point of view there are two major questions to be answered. First, are extended resections better for the patients' long-term survival than the standard procedure? Today, it is clearly shown that the extended procedures can be done with a mortality equal to that of the standard procedures, and with limited complications and side effects. But we do not know if survival is prolonged more than in anecdotal cases. To answer the question we need randomized prospective studies.

Second, most exocrine pancreatic cancers are presently diagnosed at an advanced stage. Because of their failure pattern, a major need for adjuvant therapy has been clearly established. There is now considerable evidence that these cancers are sensitive to chemotherapy and radiotherapy. For the small group of pancreatic cancer patients who have resectable tumors, postoperative radiation plus 5-FU or other adjuvant treatment is reasonable [74, 75]. A major effort, however, must be made to develop new treatments for the vast majority of patients, both the resected and the nonresectable. All surgeons should be encouraged to include their patients in adjuvant protocols after pancreaticoduodenectomy, since only through tenacious and structured research can progress be made.

References

1. Codivilla A (1898) Rendiconto statistico della sezione chirurgica dell'Ospedala di Imola. (Bologna, Italy)
2. Kausch W (1912) Das Carcinoma der Papilla Duodeni und seine radikale Entfernung. Beitr Klin Chir 78:439–486
3. Cheever D (1942) Presentation of the (Bigelow) medal. N Engl J Med 226:514–515
4. Peters JH, Carey LC (1991) Historical review of pancreaticoduodenectomy. Am J Surg 161:219–225
5. Gudjonsson B (1995) Carcinoma of the pancreas: critical analysis of costs, results of resections, and the need for standardized reporting. J Am Coll Surg 181:483–503
6. Gudjonsson B (1996) Pancreatic cancer. The need for critical reassessment (editorial). J Clin Gastroenterol 23:2–6
7. Reber HA, Gloor B (1998) Radical pancreatectomy. Surg Oncol Clin N Am 7:157–163
8. Trede M (1985) The surgical treatment of pancreatic carcinoma. Surgery 97:28–35
9. Connolly MM, Dawson PJ, Michaelassi F, Moossa AR, Lowenstein F (1987) Survival in 1001 patients with carcinoma of the pancreas. Ann Surg 122:827–829
10. Andrén-Sandberg Å, Ihse I (1997) Pattern of recurrence after pancreaticoduodenectomy for exocrine pancreatic cancer: correlation with survival. In: Hanyu F, Takasaki K (eds) Pancreatoduodenectomy. Springer, Tokyo, pp 417–423
11. Carter CR, Imrie CW (1998) Is histological diagnosis essential before resection of suspected pancreatic carcinoma? In: Johnson CD, Imrie CW (eds) Pancreatic disease. Towards the year 2000, 2nd edn. Springer, London, pp 377–384
12. Barnes SA, Lillemoe KD, Kaufman HS, Sauter PK, Yeo CJ, Talamini MA, Pitt HA, Cameron JL (1996) Pancreaticoduodenectomy for benign disease. Am J Surg 171:131–135
13. Trede M, Schwall G (1988) The complications of pancreatectomy. Ann Surg 207:39–47
14. Hanyu F (1997) One thousand pancreatoduodenectomies at a single institution. In: Hanyu F, Takasaki K (eds) Pancreaticoduodenectomy. Springer, Tokyo, pp 13–21
15. Owyang C (1998) Pancreas (editorial overview). Curr Opin Gastroenterol 14:359–361
16. Cameron JL, Pitt HA, Yeo CJ, Lillemoe KD, Kaufman HS, Coleman J (1987) One hundred and forty-five consecutive pancreaticoduodenectomies without mortality. Ann Surg 217:430–438
17. Crist DW, Sitzman JV, Cameron JL (1987) Improved hospital morbidity, mortality and survival after the Whipple procedure. Ann Surg 206:358–365
18. Ihse I, Andersson H, Andrén-Sandberg Å (1996) Total pancreatectomy for cancer of the pancreas: is it appropriate? World J Surg 20:288–294
19. Friess H, Uhl W, Beger HG, Büchler MW (1994) Surgical treatment of pancreatic cancer. Dig Surg 11:378–386

20. Kayahara M, Nagakawa T, Ueno K, Otha T, Takeda T, Miyazaki I (1993) An evaluation of radical resection for pancreatic cancer based on the mode of recurrence as determined by autopsy and diagnostic imaging. Cancer 72:2118–2123
21. Nagai H, Kuroda A, Morioka Y (1986) Lymphatic and local spread of T_1 and T_2 pancreatic cancer. Ann Surg 204:65–71
22. Ozaki H (1992) Improvement of pancreatic cancer treatment. Int J Pancreatol 12:5–9
23. Kayahara M, Nagakawa T, Konishi I, et al (1991) Clinicopathological study of pancreatic carcinoma with particular reference to the invasion of the extrapancreatic neural plexus. Int J Pancreatol 10:105–111
24. Hanyu F, Suzuki, Imaizumi T (1993) Whipple operation for pancreatic carcinoma: Japanese experience. In: Beger HG, Büchler MW, Malfertheiner P (eds) Standards in pancreatic surgery. Springer, Berlin Heidelberg New York, pp 654–662
25. Manabe T, Suzuki T, Tobe T (1985) Evaluation of en bloc radical pancreatectomy for carcinoma of the head of the pancreas involving the adjacent vessels. Dig Surg 2:27–30
26. Nagakawa T, Konishi I, Ueno K, Ohta T, Akiyama T, Kayahara M, Miyazaki I (1991) Surgical treatment of pancreatic cancer. The Japanese experience. Int J Pancreatol 9:135–143
27. Satake K, Nishiwaki H, Yokomatsu H, Kawazoe Y, Kim K, Haku A, Umeyama K, Miyazaki I (1992) Surgical curability and prognosis for standard versus extended resection for T_1 carcinoma of the pancreas. Surg Gynecol Obstet 175:259–265
28. Tsuchiya R, Tsunoda T, Yamaguchi T (1990) Operation of choice for resectable carcinoma of the head of the pancreas. Int J Pancreatol 6:295–306
29. Miyata M, Nakao K, Takao T, et al (1990) An appraisal of pancreatectomy for advanced cancer of the pancreas based on survival rate and postoperative physical performance. J Surg Oncol 45:33–39
30. Tsuchiya R, Noda T, Harada N, Miyamoto T, Tomioka T, Yamamoto K, Yamaguchi T, Izawa K, Tsunoda T, Yoshino R (1986) Collective review of small carcinomas of the pancreas. Ann Surg 203:77–81
31. Nakayama T, Kinoshita H, Saitsu H, lmayama H, Okuda K, Hara M, Fukuda S, Saitoh N (1997) Surgical result of pancreatoduodenectomy for disease in pancreatic head region. In: Hanyu F, Takasaki K (eds) Pancreaticoduodenectomy. Springer, Tokyo, pp 93–106
32. Traverso LW, Longmire WP (1978) Preservation of the pylorus in pancreaticoduodenectomy. Surg Gynecol Obstet 146:959–962
33. Traverso LW, Longmire WP (1980) Preservation of the pylorus in pancreaticoduodenectomy. A follow-up evaluation. Ann Surg 192:306–310
34. Newman KD, Braasch JW, Rossi RL, Campo-Gonzales S (1983) Pyloric and gastric preservation with pancreaticoduodenectomy. Am J Surg 145:152–156
35. Warshaw AL, Torchiana DL (1985) Delayed gastric emptying after pylorus-preserving pancreaticoduodenectomy. Surg Gynecol Obstet 160:1–4
36. Itani KMF, Coleman RE, Meyers WC, Akwari OE (1986) Pylorus-preserving pancreaticoduodenectomy: a clinical and physiologic appraisal. Ann Surg 204:655–664
37. Patel AG, Toyama MT, Kusske AM, Alexander P, Ashiey SW, Reber HA (1995) Pylorus-preserving Whipple resection for pancreatic cancer. Is it any better? Arch Surg 130:838–842
38. Miedema BW, Sarr MG, van Heerden JA, Nagorney DM, McIllrath DC, Ilstrup D (1980) Complications following pancreaticoduodenectomy: current management. Arch Surg 127:945–950
39. Yeo CJ, Barry MK, Sauter PK, Sostre S, Lillemoe KD, Pitt HA, Cameron JL (1993) Erythromycin accelerates gastric emptying after pancreaticoduodenectomy. A prospective, randomized placebo-controlled trial. Ann Surg 218:229–238
40. Grace PA, Pitt HA, Longmire WP (1980) Pylorus-preserving pancreatoduodenectomy: an overview. Br J Surg 77:968–974
41. Pitt HA, Grace PA (1990) Pylorus-preserving resection of the pancreas. Baillieres Clin Gastroenterol 4:917–930
42. Grace PA, Pitt HA, Longmire WP (1986) Pancreatoduodenectomy with pylorus preservation for adenocarcinoma of the head of the pancreas. Br J Surg 73:647–650
43. Brooks JR, Brooks DC, Levin DJ (1989) Total pancreatectomy for ductal cell carcinoma of the pancreas. Ann Surg 209:405–410
44. van Heerden JA, McIllrath DC, Ilstrup DM, et al (1988) Total pancreatectomy for ductal adenocarcinoma of the pancreas: an update. World J Surg 12:658–662
45. Farley DR, Schwall G, Trede M (1996) Completion pancreatectomy for surgical complications after pancreaticoduodenectomy. Br J Surg 83:176–179

46. Tashiro S, Uchino R, Hiraoka T, Tsuji T, Kawamoto S, Saitoh N, Yamasaki K, Miyauchi Y (1991) Surgical indication and significance of portal vein resection in biliary and pancreatic cancer. Surgery 109:481–487
47. Takahashi S, Ogata Y, Tsuzuki T (1994) Combined resection of the pancreas and portal vein for pancreatic cancer. Br J Surg 81:1190–1193
48. Cubilla AL, Fortner J, Fitzgerald PJ (1978) Lymph node involvement in carcinoma of the pancreas area. Cancer 41:880–887
49. Nagakawa T, Kayahara M, Ohta T, et al (1991) Patterns of neural and plexus invasion of human pancreatic cancer and experimental cancer. Int J Pancreatol 10:112–119
50. Griffin JF, Smaley SR, Jewell W, et al (1990) Patterns of failure after curative resection of pancreatic carcinoma. Cancer 66:56–61
51. Brooks JR, Culebras JM (1976) Cancer of the papilla: palliative operation, Whipple procedure or total pancreatectomy? Am J Surg 131:516–520
52. Moossa AR, Scott MM, Lavelle-Jones M (1984) The place of total and extended total pancreatectomy in pancreatic cancer. World J Surg 8:895–899
53. Sarr MG, Behrns KE, van Heereden JA (1993) Total pancreatectomy. An objective analysis of its use in pancreatic cancer. Hepatogastroenterology 40:418–421
54. Fortner JG (1973) Regional resection of cancer of the pancreas: a new surgical approach. Surgery 73:307–320
55. Sindelar WF (1989) Clinical experience with regional pancreatectomy for adenocarcinoma of the pancreas. Arch Surg 124:127–132
56. Fortner JG (1984) Regional pancreatectomy for cancer of the pancreas, ampulla, and other related sites. Ann Surg 199:418–425
57. Fortner JG, Klimstra DS, Senie RT, MacLean BJ (1996) Tumor size is the primary prognosticator for pancreatic cancer after regional pancreatectomy. Ann Surg 223:147–153
58. Tepper T, Nardi G, Suit H (1976) Carcinoma of the pancreas: review of MGM experience from 1963 to 1973. Analysis of surgical failure and implications for radiation therapy. Cancer 37:1519–1524
59. Westerdahl J, Andrén-Sandberg Å, Ihse I (1993) Recurrence of exocrine pancreatic cancer – local or hepatic? Hepatogastroenterology 40:384–387
60. Nagakawa T, Kurachi M, Konishi K, Miyazaki I (1982) Translateral retroperitoneal approach in radical surgery for pancreatic cancer. Jpn J Surg 12:229–233
61. Ishikawa O, Ohigashi H, Sasaki Y, Kabuto T, Fukoda I, Furukawa H, Imaoka S, Iwanaga T (1988) Practical usefulness of lymphatic and connective tissue clearance for carcinoma of the pancreatic head. Ann Surg 208:215–220
62. Gall FP, Zirngibl H (1993) Cancer of the pancreas – extended lymph node dessection. In: Beger HG, Büchler MW, Malfertheiner P (eds) Standards in pancreatic surgery. Springer, Berlin Heidelberg New York, pp 654–662
63. Manabe T, Baba N, Setoyama H, et al (1991) Venous bypass grafting for celiac occlusion in radical pancreaticoduodenectomy. Pancreas 6:368–371
64. Ishikawa O, Ohigashi H, Sasaki Y, Furukawa H, Kabuto T, Kameyama M, Nakamori S, Hiratsuka M, Imaoka S (1994) Liver perfusion chemotherapy of both the hepatic artery and portal vein to prevent hepatic metastasis after extended pancreatectomy for adenocarcinoma of the pancreas. Am J Surg 168:361–364
65. Lieberman MD, Kilburn H, Lindsey M, Brennan MF (1995) Relation of preoperative deaths to hospital volume among patients undergoing pancreatic resection for malignancy. Ann Surg 222:638–645
66. Andrén-Sandberg Å, Ihse I (1983) Factors influencing survival after total pancreatectomy in patients with pancreatic cancer. Ann Surg 198:605–610
67. Al-Sharaf K, Ihse I, Dawiskiba S, Andrén-Sandberg Å (1997) Characteristics of the gland remnant predict complications after subtotal pancreatectomy. Dig Surg 14:101–106
68. Gordon TA, Bowman HM, Tielsch JM, Bass EB, Burleyson GP, Cameron JL (1998) Statewide regionalization of pancreaticoduodenectomy and its effect on in-hospital mortality. Ann Surg 228:71–78
69. Gordon TA, Burleyson GP, Tielsch JM, Cameron JL (1995) The effects of regionalization on cost and outcome for one general high-risk procedure. Ann Surg 221:43–49
70. Glasgow RE, Mulvhill SJ (1996) Relation of hospital volume to outcome in patients undergoing Whipple resections for adenocarcinoma in Northern California hospitals in 1993. Presented at the Thirtieth Annual Meeting of Pancreas Club Inc, San Fransisco, Calif., May 19

71. Bramhall SR, Allum WH, Jones AG, Allwood A, Cummins C, Neoptolemos JPN (1995) Treatment and survival in 13,560 patients with pancreatic cancer, and incidence of the disease, in the West Midlands: an epidemiological study. Br J Surg 82:111–115
72. Finch MD, Neoptolemos JP (1998) Pancreatic resection for pancreatic cancer: outcome in specialist units. In: Johnson CD, Imrie CW (eds) Pancreatic disease. Towards the year 2000, 2nd edn. Springer, London, pp 385–396
73. Trede M, Schwab M (1996) Extensive palliative carcinoma operation – is it really worthwhile? What are the aims? Langenbecks Arch Chir Suppl Kongressbd 113:89–90
74. Andrén-Sandberg Å, Bäckman PL, Andersson R (1997) Results of adjuvant therapy in resected pancreatic cancer. Int J Pancreatol 21:31–38
75. Yeo CJ, Abrams RA, Grochow LB, Sohn TA, Ord SE, Hruban RH, Zahurak ML, Dooley WC, Coleman J, Sauther PK, et al (1997) Pancreaticoduodenectomy for pancreatic adenocarcinoma: postoperative adjuvant chemoradiation improves survival. A prospective, single-institution experience. Ann Surg 225:621–633

Part V
Epidemiology

CHAPTER 24

Lessons Learned about Pancreatitis and Pancreatic Cancer from Epidemiological Studies

A. B. Lowenfels, P. Maisonneuve, and P. G. Lankisch

Introduction

Acute pancreatitis, chronic pancreatitis, and pancreatic cancer are the three acquired pancreatic disorders most commonly encountered by physicians and surgeons. In addition, about 90% of persons with cystic fibrosis, an autosomal regressive disorder, suffer from severe pancreatic insufficiency. The etiology of these diseases is becoming clearer, and we are beginning to understand the interrelationships between all of these serious disorders. In this chapter we will review current thinking about benign and malignant exocrine pancreatic disease, discuss risk factors, and consider what is known about the natural history of these diseases.

The Epidemiological Method

Clinicians are skilled at diagnosing and treating individual patients with pancreatic disorders. The experience of a busy clinician treating a few hundred patients with benign or malignant pancreatic disease during a professional lifetime has provided valuable clues about the etiology of pancreatic disease.

Additional insight into pancreatic disease can be obtained from an epidemiological approach. Epidemiology was originally defined as the study of outbreaks of disease; a current broader definition focuses on causation and control of benign and malignant disease in populations. The epidemiological approach requires three separate types of information: (a) a listing and description of cases, i.e., a "numerator"; (b) information about the population at risk for the disease, i.e., a "denominator;" and (c) the length of time during which the observations were made – often a year.

Supported by grants from the C.D. Smithers Foundation, Mill Neck, NY.

The main difference between the clinical approach and the epidemiological approach is that the epidemiologist requires information about the background population, the denominator, whereas the clinician does not. Without this information it is not possible to calculate disease rates. Without rates, it is impossible to calculate changes in the frequency of disease, sex distribution, or risk factors for development of disease.

Cancer registry data, available now for many countries, provide accurate epidemiological information about pancreatic cancer [28]. For benign pancreatic disease there are few reliable sources of epidemiological data, and the limited amount of information is usually regional rather than national. Furthermore, there is disagreement about the diagnostic criteria for benign pancreatic disease, making it difficult to compare different reports. Despite these limitations, epidemiological studies have provided valuable information about pancreatic disease which has helped physicians and their patients.

Acute Pancreatitis

Although the list of diseases capable of causing acute pancreatitis is extensive, we know that the between two thirds and three quarters of all cases are caused by either biliary tract disease or alcoholism. About 10% of cases are related to definitive but rare causes, and for about 20% of cases, despite a careful search, the cause remains obscure.

Acute Biliary Pancreatitis

The simplest explanation for biliary pancreatitis is that it is related to obstruction of the pancreatic ductal system from stones which become lodged in the sphincter of Oddi. This explanation is controversial, because impacted stones are found in only a minority of cases of biliary pancreatitis. We do know that the epidemiology of biliary pancreatitis resembles that of gallstones. Both diseases are more common in women than in men, and the frequency of both diseases increases with age. Small gallstones are more likely than large gallstones to cause biliary pancreatitis [11, 17].

Compared with the frequency of acute cholecystitis, gallstone-related pancreatitis is rare. The relative frequency of the two diseases has not been accurately documented, but it is unlikely that gallstone pancreatitis accounts for more than 5% of the total burden of benign complications of gallstones. Because of the popularity of laparoscopic cholecystectomy, cholecystectomy rates are increasing. As a result, we can anticipate a gratifying reduction in the frequency of gallstone pancreatitis.

Acute Alcoholic Pancreatitis

In men, the most common cause of acute pancreatitis is alcohol. Despite an enormous amount of animal and human research, the mechanism of alcohol-induced pancreatic injury is still not clear. We know that a single bout of heavy drinking does not induce acute pancreatitis, implying that the pathogenesis must be related to cumulative damage induced by multiple, frequent exposure to large amounts of alcohol. To develop acute pancreatitis, a person must consume large quantities of alcohol – four or more drinks per day over a period of several years. Despite the strong association between alcohol consumption and glandular damage, it is still unclear whether the major site of damage is ductal, acinar, or vascular. For patients who continue to drink, longitudinal studies [1, 2] suggest that, over time, acute alcoholic pancreatitis gradually progresses to chronic pancreatitis.

Chronic Pancreatitis

Prolonged, heavy drinking is the leading cause of chronic pancreatitis. The mean age at onset of chronic pancreatitis is about 45 years, or nearly 20–25 years after the age when drinking usually begins.

The incidence of this disease has been estimated in only a few regions. During the 1970s, the overall frequency of all types of chronic pancreatitis in Copenhagen was estimated to be 7–10/100 000 per year, similar to a recent estimate of about 7/100 000 per year in Lüneburg, Germany [10, 20]. As with alcoholic cirrhosis, it appears that only a small fraction of alcoholics ever develop this particular complication, implying that, in addition to alcohol, there are other causative or protective factors involved in the pathogenesis of chronic pancreatitis.

Hospital discharge data for the United States (Table 1) provide useful epidemiological information about the relative frequency of benign pancreatic disease. Acute pancreatitis is more common than chronic pancreatitis. Women are more prone to acute pancreatitis, whereas men are more likely to develop chronic pancreatitis. Acute pancreatitis is seen with nearly equal frequency in young, middle-aged, and older individuals; chronic pancreatitis is infrequent in older individuals.

Table 1. Number of hospital discharges (in thousands) for acute and chronic pancreatitis in the United States, 1993[a]

Type of pancreatitis	Total cases (*n*)	Sex (*n*)		Age-group (years)		
		Male	Female	15–44	45–64	≥65
Acute	215	110	105	72	72	70
Chronic	87	48	35	31	29	11

[a] Data from Vital and Health Statistics. Series 13, publication date 1995. Detailed diagnoses and procedures, National Hospital Discharge Survey, 1993.

Other Risk Factors Leading to Chronic Pancreatitis

Are there suspected risk factors other than alcohol that might cause chronic pancreatitis? Smoking has been implicated in several studies as a probable risk factor for chronic pancreatitis [22, 31, 32]. Most heavy drinkers are heavy smokers, so it is difficult to determine the independent impact of smoking. If smoking is related to chronic pancreatitis, it might help to explain the increased risk of pancreatitis in African-Americans compared with whites. African-Americans have recently been determined to be less able to detoxify highly reactive substances in tobacco smoke [30]. Accumulation of active products from tobacco within the pancreas plus exposure to alcohol could lead to pancreatitis.

Cohn and co-workers have investigated a small group of patients with idiopathic chronic pancreatitis [9]. There was a highly significantly increased number of patients carrying one or more copies of genes usually associated with cystic fibrosis. These patients had no recognizable pulmonary symptoms – the most common manifestation of cystic fibrosis. If confirmed, this suggests either that cystic fibrosis carriers are at increased risk for idiopathic pancreatitis, or that some idiopathic chronic pancreatitis patients (perhaps a third) have a previously unrecognized mild form of cystic fibrosis.

Pancreatic Cancer

Although a relatively rare tumor, pancreatic cancer is one of our most lethal forms of cancer – usually listed among the top five causes of death from cancer. In the United States and in most European countries, the cumulative lifetime risk of pancreatic cancer is about 1%. As with nearly all forms of cancer, the risk rises exponentially with age: nearly three quarters of all patients are 65 years or older at the time of diagnosis.

Time Trends

Only in the past few decades have we been able to diagnose pancreatic cancer with a high degree of accuracy. It is possible, therefore, that some of the recent increases in the frequency of pancreatic cancer are due simply to improved diagnosis. However, since pancreatic cancer is related to smoking, most of the observed increase is probably related to the smoking epidemic. For the United States, time trends are intriguing: male rates appear to be decreasing, while female rates are either steady or slightly increasing (Fig. 1). These trends are consistent with changes in male and female smoking patterns.

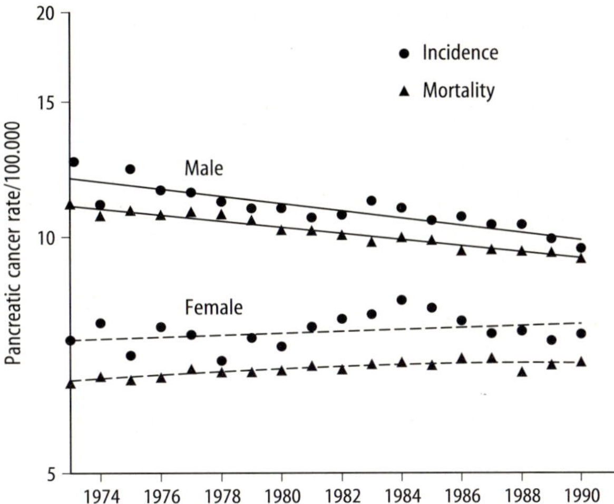

Fig. 1. Sex-specific incidence and mortality of pancreatic cancer in the United States during the period 1974–1990. (Data from Seer Cancer Statistics Review, 1973–1994. U.S. Department of Health and Human Services, Bethesda, Maryland. NIH Publication No. 97–2789)

Smoking and Pancreatic Cancer

Experimental and epidemiological data conclusively support a strong relationship between smoking and pancreatic cancer [4, 5, 13, 15, 18, 19, 34]. Perhaps the strongest evidence for this relationship comes from the remarkable cohort study of British physicians, which has been conducted for approximately 50 years [12]. This study was originally designed to study the relationship between smoking and lung cancer, but it also contains mortality data for pancreatic cancer. The main findings with respect to smoking and pancreatic cancer include: (a) There is a clear dose response, the risk of pancreatic cancer increasing with the cumulative increase in smoking exposure. (b) Heavy smokers have about a threefold risk of pancreatic cancer compared with nonsmokers.

Diet and Pancreatic Cancer

Numerous epidemiological studies have examined the relationship between diet and cancer. The results support a link between diet and pancreatic cancer, but individual studies do not always agree on which particular dietary item increases or decreases the risk of cancer [3, 6, 13–16, 21, 27, 33].

Much of the confusion is understandable, because most studies designed to investigate the diet–cancer hypothesis rely on accurate dietary recall by patients with cancer and control subjects without cancer. Another problem is that cancer develops only after a long latent period, so that current dietary intake may not reflect consumption patterns one or two decades prior to the appearance of cancer. For pancreatic cancer there is another problem: because the tumor is so aggressive, the patient may have died before dietary information can be obtained. If so, then the only source of dietary information would be from a family member. Despite these limitations, several dietary items are suspected to be risk factors for pancreatic tumors. These include: high fat and high carbohydrate diets and diets that are deficient in fruits, fiber, and vegetables. The list of suspected items is similar to findings for other cancers.

Race and the Risk of Pancreatic Cancer

Race is a strong predictor of pancreatic cancer. In the United States, the risk of developing pancreatic cancer is about 50% higher for blacks than for whites. This finding is similar to other smoking related tumors, including those of the lung, larynx, and esophagus. Excessive smoking in blacks compared with whites does not seem to be the entire explanation. There are racial and ethnic differences in serum cotinine levels after cigarette smoking, perhaps because of differential pharmacokinetics. Racial differences in the ability to detoxify tobacco-related carcinogens would help to explain the excess risk of pancreatic cancer in blacks [7].

Relationship Between Acute and Chronic Pancreatitis and Pancreatic Cancer

What is the relationship between pancreatitis and pancreatic cancer? Acute pancreatitis is not thought to cause pancreatic cancer, but chronic pancreatitis causes progressive pathologic changes within the pancreas. Several studies suggest that any form of longstanding chronic pancreatitis increases the risk of pancreatic cancer.

In a multicenter cohort study of 1552 patients with well-documented chronic pancreatitis followed for a minimum of 2 years, 29 pancreatic cancers were observed. The expected number was only 1.8, yielding a risk ratio of 16.5 ($p=0.001$) [23]. The elevated risk was not confined to any single risk group, but was observed in all centers, in both men and women, and in both alcoholic and nonalcoholic pancreatitis. A more recent cohort study of chronic pancreatitis patients from a single French hospital revealed the same high risk of pancreatic cancer [25]. The findings in case-control studies and record linkage studies have generally been similar, but somewhat weaker, perhaps because of less strict inclusion criteria.

Hereditary pancreatitis is rare, accounting for approximately 1% of all cases of chronic pancreatitis. It now appears that patients with hereditary pancreatitis have an exceptionally high risk of developing pancreatic cancer – about 50 times greater than background rates [24]. The cumulative risk to age 70 has been estimated to be at least 30%. The high risk of pancreatic cancer may be explained by the early age of onset of pancreatitis.

Tropical pancreatitis is another rare form of chronic pancreatitis, characterized by pancreatic insufficiency, diabetes, and calcification. Only a few patients have a family history of pancreatitis, suggesting that the disease is not inherited. This disease also has been associated with an elevated risk of pancreatic cancer [8].

The available evidence implies that chronic pancreatitis is a risk factor for pancreatic cancer. This is not entirely surprising, because in other digestive organs such as the esophagus, the stomach, and the colon, benign disease often precedes malignant disease. The mechanism may be related to increased cell turnover [29]. Despite this probable link, chronic pancreatitis explains no more than about 2 or 3% of all pancreatic cancer cases.

Cystic Fibrosis and Pancreatic Disease

Cystic fibrosis (CF) is the most common autosomal recessive genetic disorder of white populations. In the United States there are approximately 20 000–30 000 living persons with CF, with about an equal number in Europe. Only about 10% of CF patients are pancreatic sufficient and do not require enzyme replacement. These patients usually have one of the milder genetic mutations, and they sometimes develop attacks of acute pancreatitis.

Approximately 90% of CF patients have pancreatic insufficiency, requiring pancreatic enzyme replacement therapy. Pancreatic insufficiency develops early in life and, although severe, is not associated with attacks of pain, so characteristic of other forms of chronic pancreatitis. Much of the damage to the pancreas occurs in utero.

The risk of all types of digestive tract cancer, including pancreatic cancer, is elevated in patients with CF [26]. Again, the excess risk is probably related to the widespread pathologic changes found throughout the digestive tract in CF. The relationship between acute pancreatitis, chronic pancreatitis, and pancreatic cancer can be conceptualized as shown in Fig. 2.

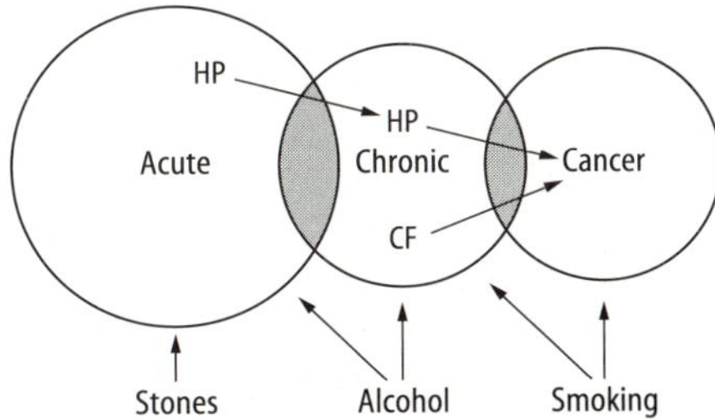

Fig. 2. Relationship between acute pancreatitis, chronic pancreatitis, and pancreatic cancer. Size of *circles* approximates the relative frequency of these three diseases. *Shaded portions* represent estimated overlap between acute and chronic pancreatitis, and between chronic pancreatitis and pancreatic cancer. Hereditary pancreatitis (*HP*) shows progression of disease from acute to chronic phase, and then in some patients, to pancreatic cancer. Cystic fibrosis (*CF*) usually begins as chronic pancreatitis with pancreatic insufficiency. A few patients eventually develop pancreatic cancer. *Arrows* illustrate the suspected connections between the main risk factors and pancreatic disease

Epidemiology of Pancreatic Disease: Unsolved Problems

The previous sections emphasize what we know about disorders of the pancreas. Despite significant progress during the latter part of this century, there are still many vexing epidemiological problems that remain unsolved, limiting our ability to treat patients with pancreatic disease. Some current questions related to *benign pancreatic disease* are:

- Why does heavy drinking cause some persons to develop pancreatitis? Are there additional risk factors, such as smoking, that increase the risk?
- Why do some heavy drinkers develop pancreatitis, while others develop liver cirrhosis? Only a few patients develop both diseases. Is this just chance, or are there specific environmental or genetic factors that determine which organ will be damaged?
- What is the natural history of alcoholic pancreatitis? Does chronic alcoholic pancreatitis develop in patients who have sustained prior attacks of acute pancreatitis? If so, what factors predict progression of acute to chronic pancreatitis? How much overlap is there between acute and chronic alcoholic pancreatitis?
- What is the role of the sphincter of Oddi in the causation of pancreatic disease?
- How frequent are benign pancreatic disorders among the general population?
- What causes idiopathic pancreatitis? What is the relationship between idiopathic pancreatitis and cystic fibrosis?

Some unanswered questions relating to *pancreatic cancer* are:

- Why is pancreatic cancer so aggressive?
- What are the intermediate steps between a normal pancreatic cell and pancreatic malignancy?
- Can we predict which patients with pancreatitis are at risk for pancreatic cancer?
- What screening procedures are suitable for detection of early, potentially curable pancreatic cancers in high-risk populations?

Summary

During the past 50 years, the epidemiology of pancreatic disease has become much more clearly defined. Gallstones or alcohol cause most attacks of acute and chronic pancreatic cancer. Because of the widespread acceptance of laparoscopic cholecystectomy, more patients with cholelithiasis are now being operated on, implying that the frequency of acute pancreatitis should decrease, particularly among women. In some countries, such as the United States, alcohol consumption has decreased, which, after a lag period of one or two decades, could lead to a modest reduction in chronic pancreatitis.

Two risk factors for pancreatic cancer – smoking and diet – have been identified, affording an opportunity for control of this aggressive malignancy.

However, we still lack an effective screening program to detect potentially curable cancers in high-risk populations.

References

1. Ammann RW, Abovbiantz A, Largiader F, Schueler G (1984) Course and outcome of chronic pancreatitis. Longitudinal study of a mixed medical-surgical series of 245 patients. Gastroenterology 86:820–828
2. Ammann RW, Heitz PU, Kloppel G (1996) Course of alcoholic chronic pancreatitis: a prospective clinicomorphological long-term study Gastroenterology 111:224–231
3. Baghurst PA, McMichael AJ, Slavotinek AH, Baghurst KI, Boyle P, Walker AM (1991) A case-control study of diet and cancer of the pancreas. Am J Epidemiol 134:167–179
4. Boyle P, Hsieh CC, Maisonneuve P, La Vecchia C, Macfarlane GJ, Walker AM, et al (1989) Epidemiology of pancreas cancer (1988). Int J Pancreatol 5:327–346
5. Bueno de Mesquita HB, Maisonneuve P, Moerman CJ, Runia S, Boyle P (1991) Lifetime history of smoking and exocrine carcinoma of the pancreas: a population-based case-control study in The Netherlands. Int J Cancer 49:816–822
6. Bueno de Mesquita HB, Maisonneuve P, Runia S, Moerman CJ (1991) Intake of foods and nutrients and cancer of the exocrine pancreas: a population-based case-control study in The Netherlands. Int J Cancer 48:540–549
7. Caraballo RS, Giovino GA, Pechacek TF, et al (1998) Racial and ethnic differences in serum cotinine levels of cigarette smokers. Third national health and nutrition examination survey, 1988–1991. JAMA 280:135–139
8. Chari ST, Mohan V, Pitchumoni CS, Viswanathan M, Madanagopalan N, Lowenfels AB (1994) Risk of pancreatic carcinoma in tropical calcifying pancreatitis: an epidemiologic study. Pancreas 9:62–66
9. Cohn JA, Friedman KJ, Silverman LM, et al (1998) Abnormalities of the CFTR gene predispose to idiopathic chronic pancreatitis. Gastroenterology 114:449 Abstr
10. Copenhagen Pancreatitis Study Group (1981) Copenhagen Pancreatitis Study. An interim report from a prospective epidemiological multicentre study. Scand J Gastroenterol 16:305–312
11. Diehl AK, Holleman DRJ, Chapman JB, Schwesinger WH, Kurtin WE (1997) Gallstone size and risk of pancreatitis. Arch Intern Med 157:1674–1678
12. Doll R, Peto R, Wheatley K, Gray R, Sutherland I (1994) Mortality in relation to smoking: 40 years' observations on male British doctors. Br Med J 309:901–911
13. Falk RT, Pickle LW, Fontham ET, Correa P, Fraumeni JFJ (1988) Life-style risk factors for pancreatic cancer in Louisiana: a case-control study. Am J Epidemiol 128:324–336
14. Ghadirian P, Simard A, Baillargeon J, Maisonneuve P, Boyle P (1991) Nutritional factors and pancreatic cancer in the francophone community in Montreal, Canada. Int J Cancer 47:1–6
15. Ghadirian P, Simard A, Baillargeon J (1993) A population-based case-control study of cancer of the bile ducts and gallbladder in Quebec, Canada. Rev Epidemiol Sante Publ 41:107–112
16. Gold EB, Gordis L, Diener MD, et al (1985) Diet and other risk factors for cancer of the pancreas. Cancer 55:460–467
17. Houssin D, Castaing D, Lemoine J, Bismuth H (1983) Microlithiasis of the gallbladder. Surg Gynecol Obstet 157:20–24
18. Howe GR, Jain M, Burch JD, Miller AB (1991) Cigarette smoking and cancer of the pancreas: evidence from a population-based case-control study in Toronto, Canada. Int J Cancer 47:323–328
19. Kalapothaki V, Tzonou A, Hsieh CC, Toupadaki N, Karakatsani A, Trichopoulos D (1993) Tobacco, ethanol, coffee, pancreatitis, diabetes mellitus, and cholelithiasis as risk factors for pancreatic carcinoma. Cancer Causes Control 4:375–382
20. Lankisch PG, Assmus D, Pflichthofer D, Maisonneuve P, Lowenfels AB (1998) The burden of pancreatic disease in a well-defined population. Gastroenterology 114:A24 Abstr
21. La Vecchia C, Negri E, D'Avanzo B, Ferraroni M, Gramenzi A, Savoldelli R, et al (1990) Medical history, diet and pancreatic cancer. Oncology 47:463–466
22. Lowenfels AB, Zwemer FL, Jhangiani S, Pitchumoni CS (1987) Pancreatitis in a native American Indian population. Pancreas 2:694–697

23. Lowenfels AB, Maisonneuve P, Cavallini G, Ammann RW, Lankisch PG, Andersen JR, et al (1993) Pancreatitis and the risk of pancreatic cancer. International Pancreatitis Study Group. N Engl J Med 328:1433–1437
24. Lowenfels AB, Maisonneuve P, DiMagno EP, Elitsur Y, Gates LKJ, Perrault J, et al (1997) Hereditary pancreatitis and the risk of pancreatic cancer. International Hereditary Pancreatitis Study Group. J Natl Cancer Inst 89:442–446
25. Madeira I, Pessione F, Malka D, Hammel P, Ruszniewski P, Bernades P (1998) The risk of pancreatic adenocarcinoma in patients with chronic pancreatitis: myth or reality? Gastroenterology 114:A481 Abstr
26. Neglia JP, FitzSimmons SC, Maisonneuve P, Schoni MH, Schoni-Affolter F, Corey M, et al (1995) The risk of cancer among patients with cystic fibrosis. N Engl J Med 332
27. Negri E, La Vecchia C, Franceschi S, D'Avanzo B, Parazzini F (1991) Vegetable and fruit consumption and cancer risk. Int J Cancer 48:350–354
28. Parkin DM, Muir C, Whelan SL, et al (1992) Cancer incidence in five continents. IARC Scientific Publications No. 120. IARC Sci Publ 1–1033
29. Preston-Martin S, Pike MC, Ross RK, Jones PA, Henderson BE (1990) Increased cell division as a cause of human cancer. Cancer Res 50:7415–7421
30. Richie JP, Carmella SG, Muscat JE, Scott DG, Akerkar SA, Hecht SS (1997) Differences in the urinary metabolites of the tobacco-specific lung carcinogen 4-(methynitrosamino)-1-(3-pyridyl)-1-butanone in black and white smokers. Cancer Epidemiol Biomarkers Prev 6:783–790
31. Talamini G, Bassi C, Falconi M, Frulloni L, Di Francesco V, Vaona B et al. (1996) Cigarette smoking: an independent risk factor in alcoholic pancreatitis. Pancreas 12:131–137
32. Yen S, Hsieh C, MacMahon B (1982) Consumption of alcohol and tobacco and other risk factors for pancreatitis. Am J Epidemiol 116:407–414
33. Zatonski W, Przewozniak K, Howe GR, Maisonneuve P, Walker AM, Boyle P (1991) Nutritional factors and pancreatic cancer: a case-control study from south-west Poland. Int J Cancer 48:390–394
34. Zatonski WA, Boyle P, Przewozniak K, Maisonneuve P, Drosik K, Walker AM (1993) Cigarette smoking, alcohol, tea and coffee consumption and pancreas cancer risk: a case-control study from Opole, Poland. Int J Cancer 53:601–607

Subject Index

A
AAC (asparagine) 4
abscess, pancreatic 78
acceleration 117
acidic fibroblast growth factor (aFGF) 210
acid-resistant microsphere preparations of porcine pancreatin 182
acinar cell, pancreatic
- in acute pancreatitis 14–23
- - autodigestion 14, 68
- - calcium release 14, 19–22
- - cellular injury 36
- - dehydration 14
- - rehydration 19
- - secretory blockade 14
- - trypsinogen activation 14–18, 22
- - vacuolization 18
- in chronic pancreatitis 116
acinus 102
acute pancreatitis (AP) 14–89, 133, 160, 254
- acinar cell (*see there*) 14–23
- alcoholic (*see there*) 37, 255
- *algorithm* in AP 50
- cell injury 1–13
- epidemiology 254
- extracellular matrix 133
- severe 78
adenocarcinoma 222
adenovirus
- AdCMV.lip (adenovirus vector-mediated transfer of human pancreatic complimentary DNA) 128
- AAV (adenovirus-associated virus) 174
- vectors 174
African-Americans 256
alcoholism 15, 37, 66, 93–95, 142, 255
- chronic pancreatitis, alcohol-induced 93–95, 112, 142
- epidemiology 255
- etiology 112
- risk factor alcohol 94
alleles, complex alleles 171
amitriptyline 143
amphiregulin 208
amylase 103, 113, 122, 128
- salivary 114
- secretion 22
analgesia, interpleural 143
anatomical variations 93
animal models 16, 26
antagonists
- H2-antagonists 18
- IL-8 31
- PAF antagonists 29
antibiotics 44–47, 71, 87
- prophylactic 44–47, 71, 87
- treatment 71
antibodies
- neutralizing antibody 136
- to TNFα 32
anticytokines 27, 29
- strategies 29
antifibrotic agents / treatment 135–139
- gene therapy 136
- TGFβ as a therapeutic target 136
antiinflammatory drugs 143
α_1-antitrypsin deficiency 96
AP (*see* acute pancreatitis) 14–89, 133, 160, 254
APACHE II (acute physiology and chronic health evaluation II) 56–59, 83
apolipoprotein C-II 10
apoptosis 21, 22, 215
aprotinin 69
arginine (CGC) 4
asparagine (AAC) 4
ATC (isoleucine) 4
Atlanta criteria 55
ATP conduction 170
ATP-binding cassette (ABC) transporters 169
ATRA (retinoid all-trans retinoic acid) 232
atropine 18, 69
autodigestion 6, 14, 68
- pancreatic acinar cell 14
autoimmune pancreatitis / autoimmunological reaction 96
autophagic phenomena 18
autophagocytosis 18

B
bacterial (*see also* infection)
- frequency 44

- infected pancreatic necrosis, bacterial spectrum of 81
- lipase 127
- translocation (*see also* infection) 39–54
Balthazar score 57
beatcellulin 208
bicarbonate 102, 113, 114
- concentration 102
- output 113, 114
bile/biliary
- acid 113, 114, 118
- - inhibition of 118
- - precipitation of 114
- biliary pancreatitis
- - epidemiology 254
- - treatment 72–74
- common bile duct stricture/stenosis 151, 156
- focal biliary cirrhosis 180
- salts 127
- secretion 114
blood flow, pancreatic 142
BMI (body mass index) 56–59
bombesin 105
brush border
- oligosaccharidase 114
- peptidase 114
Burkholderia plantasii 127

C
C22–C157 disulfide 9
CAC (histidine) 4
calcifications 156
calcitonin 18, 69
calcium (Ca^{2+}) 7, 8
- chelators, pancreatic acinar cell 14, 22
- hypercalcemia 10, 19
- increases 21
- intracellular 19, 20
- oscillations 21
- release, pancreatic acinar cell 14, 19–22
- and trypsinogen 8
camostate 15
cancer, pancreatic (*see also* tumor) 155, 203–249
- acute and chronic pancreatic cancer, relationship 258
- biological approaches to therapy 222–229
- chemotherapy 222, 230, 246
- diet and pancreatic cancer 257, 258
- epidemiology 253, 256
- extracellular matrix components 231
- gene therapy 223–225
- growth factors 205–212
- malignant phenotype 233
- median survival 235
- palliative resection 245
- race and the risk of pancreatic cancer 258
- regionalization 244
- retinoids regulate growth and differentiation (*see there*) 231, 232–234
- RT-PCR (reverse-transcriptase polymerase chain reaction) 233
- smoking and pancreatic cancer 257
- stable transfection 233
- survival, five-year 243
- transcription factors 212–221
- tumor cell proliferation 230
carbohydrate 115
carbonic anhydrase 231
carcinoma, pancreatic (*see also* tumor) 96
- adenocarcinoma 222
- carcinoma cell lines 231
cathepsin B 6, 7, 18
causes of AP 66
CBAVD (congenital bilateral absence of the vas deferens) 168
CCK (cholecystokinin) 18, 20, 22, 104, 106, 116
- CCK hyperstimulation 7
- CCK-releasing peptide/-factor (CCK-RF) 104, 106
CCR1, β chemokine receptor 28
celiac plexus block 143
cell(s)
- acinar cells
- - in acute pancreatitis (*see there*) 14–23
- - in chronic pancreatitis 116
- apoptosis 21, 22, 215
- calcium, intracellular 19, 20
- cellulary injury, mechanisms 36, 37
- damage 22
- death 20, 21
- dehydration 22
- inflammatory cells 95, 155
- mechanisms of cell injury 1–13
- necrosis (*see there*) 21, 22
- proliferation 134
- PSC (pancreatic stellate cells) 133, 135
- shrinkage 14, 22
cephalic phases, pancreatic secretion 107
cephalosporines 71
c-erbB-2, c-erbB-3 and c-erbB-4 207
cerulein 20, 22
CF (cystic fibrosis) 94, 95, 165–202
- assessment of pancreatic function 181
- enzyme treatment, side-effects 183
- epidemiology 253, 256, 259
- fat balance study 182
- genetic and molecular pathology 167–179
- genotype-phenotype correlations 181
- large bowel manifestations 184
- liver disease 186
- nutritional management 181
- somatic gene therapy 189
- transmembrane conductance regulator gene (*see* CFTR) 95, 167–171, 193–195
- treatment of gastrointestinal manifestations in 180–192
- ultrasonographic studies 185
- ursodeoxycholic acid (UDCA), cystic fibrosis 181, 186
c-fos 213, 214

CFTR (cystic fibrosis transmembrane conductance regulator) gene 95, 167–171, 193–195
- functions 169
- genotypes 196, 198
- genotype-phenotype correlation 194
- molecular pathology 171
- mutations 195–197
- phenotypes 198
- post-translational maturation and trafficking 168
- preclinical evaluation of CFTR gene transfer 174
- promotor 168
CGC (arginine) 4
chemokines
- β chemokine receptor CCR1 28
- in the gland 25–27
- rats 26
chemotherapy 222, 230, 246
chinolons 71
cholangiopancreatography, endoscopic retrograde (ERCP) 6, 15, 16, 72–74, 156
cholecystectomy 55
cholecystokinin (*see* CCK) 7, 18, 20, 22, 104, 106, 116
cholestasis 156
cholinergic enteropancreatic reflex 108
chromosome
- artificial chromosomes 174
- chromosome 7q35 region 9
chronic pancreatitis (CP) 91–164
- acinar cell 116
- alcohol-induced CP 93–95, 112, 142, 255
- clinical outcome in relation to etiology of CP 97
- complications 146–154
- epidemiology 255
- exocrine pancreatic insufficiency, treatment of 121–131
- extracellular matrix 133
- frequency 155
- ICP (idiopathic chronic pancreatitis) 193–201
- obstructive CP 93, 96, 97
- pathogenesis 93
- stages of 115
- surgical treatment of 155–164
chyme
- intestinal transite of chyme and its regulatory role 112–120
- postprandial 113, 114
chymotrypsin 15, 114
chymotrypsinogen 4
cirrhosis
- focal biliary 180
- multilobular 180
c-jun 213, 214
classification of AP 78
c-met 206
c-myc 213, 214
colipase 103
collagen
- synthesis 132, 135–137
- type IV collagen 232
colocalization 18
colonic
- flora 115
- wall thickness 185
colonopathy, fibrosing 180, 183, 184
common bile duct (*see* bile)
comostate 69
complications 67
- of chronic pancreatitis 146–154
- local 155
contamination (*see also* infection) 39–54
- SDD (selective bowel decontamination) 47, 48
contrast-enhanced CT scanning 56
CP (*see* chronic pancreatitis) 91–164
C-reactive protein 27, 56
crinophagy 18
cryptic splice site mutation 171
CT (computer tomography) 56, 71
- contrast-enhanced CT scanning 56
- fine-needle aspiration (FNA), CT-guided 71
- interventional drainage, CT-guided 158
CTGF (connective tissue growth factor) 134
cysts
- cystic fibrosis (*see* CF) 94, 95, 165–202
- enlarging pseudocysts, pain 141
cytokines 25–33, 36
- anticytokines 27, 29
- and chemokines in the gland 25–28
- consequences for diagnosis and treatment 29–33
- as effectors of systemic inflammation 27–29
- research 33

D
débridement 84, 85
- conventional 84
- surgical 85
dehydration 22
- pancreatic acinar cell 14, 19
denaturation 114
diabetes mellitus
- insulin-dependent 156
- pancreatic 110
diagnose on AP 66
- cytokines, consequences for diagnosis and treatment 29–33
- FNA (*see* fine-needle aspiration) 71, 82, 239
diclofenac 143
diets
- exocrine pancreatic insufficiency 125
- pancreatic cancer 257, 258
digestive
- enzymes 15
- secretory and motor responses 115
- trypsin 5
DNA fragmentation 21

documentation, standardized protocol 147
Doppler ultrasonography studies 186
doxepin 143
drainage
- CT-guided interventional drainage 158
- endoscopic 146
- of pancreatic pseudocysts 158
- *Puestow* drainage 157
- transpapillary 146
drug treatment
- antiinflammatory drugs 143
- exocrine pancreatic insufficiency 123
ductal hypertension 93
duodenal stenosis 156
duodenoileal transit 113
duodenum
- pancreatic head resection, duodenum-preserving 159
- survives 113

E
ECM 132, 134
EGF (epidermal growth factor) 97, 206, 207
- HB-EGF 208
- human EGF receptor (EGFR) type 2, type 3 and type 4 (HER-2, HER-3 and HER-4) 207
elastase, pancreatic 14, 15, 182
electrolyte secretion 95
endogenous stimulation 115
endoprosthesis, plastic 151
endoscopic
- cystogastrostomy 150
- drainage 146
- interventional therapy 146
- sphincterectomy 55
- treatment of pain 146–154
- ultrasonography 143, 149
endothelial cells 25
endotoxin 61, 62
enteral nutrition (*see also* nutrition)
- infective prevention 48
- staging and nasoenteral feeding 55–65
enterokinase 103
enzyme/enzymatic activities 112, 113
- compensating enzyme systems 113
- cystic fibrosis, side-effects of enzyme treatment 183
- digestive enzymes 15
- enteric-coated mini-dose-unit preparations 123
- fate of pancreatic enzymes during small intestinal transit 112
- futures studies 126, 127
- proteolytic enzymes 103, 128
- replacement therapy 112
- supplementation 115, 118
- - symptom-relieving effects 118
- treatment of exocrine pancreatic insufficiency 123–126
- trypsin-like enzymes 9

epidemiology 251–262
- acute pancreatitis 254, 255
- cystic fibrosis 253
- gallstones/gallstone pancreatitis 254
- pancreatic cancer 253
epidermal growth factor (EGF) 97, 206, 207
- receptor (EGFR) 207
epithelial cells 25
ERC/EPT 72
ERCP (endoscopic retrograde cholangiopancreatography) 6, 15, 16, 72–74, 156
ERM-binding phosphoprotein EBP50 169
ERP, post-ERP pancreatitis 27
estrogens 20
ethanol 20
etiology of chronic pancreatitis 97
eudragit 184
exogenous stimulation 116
exocrine
- pancreatic insufficiency 121–131, 173
- - cystic fibrosis 181
- - pathophysiology 122
- - treatment 121, 123
- secretion 19, 103, 104, 116
exocytosis 21
extracellular matrix 97, 132

F
fasting state 115
fat 95
- cystic fibrosis, fat balance study 182
- necrosis 1
fatty
- degeneration 93
- free fatty acids 15
feeding (*see* nutrition) 48, 55–65, 71
fibroblast 25, 97, 134
- activation/fibroblasts 97
- growth factor (*see* FGFs) 97, 134, 206, 210, 211
- - acidic (aFGF) 210
- - basic (bFGF) 135, 210
- - receptors (FGFRs) 206, 210
fibronectin 132
fibrosis
- antifibrotic agents/treatment (*see there*) 135–139
- collagen synthesis and deposition 136
- colonopathy, fibrosing 180, 183, 184
- cystic fibrosis (*see* CF) 94, 95, 165–202
- mechanisms of 132–135
- TGFβ in development of pancreatic fibrosis 134
fine-needle aspiration (FNA) 71, 82, 239
- CT-guided 71
- ultrasound-guided 82
fluorouracil 69, 222
food intake, oral 19
free
- fatty acids 15
- radicals 20, 94
fresh-frozen plasma 69

G
gabexate 15, 69
galanin 105
gallstones 15, 55, 66, 72
- epidemiology, gallstones / gallstone pancreatitis 254
gastric
- acid secretion 116
- emptying 116, 124, 240
- - delayed emptying 240
- outlet syndrome 157
- phases, pancreatic secretion 106
gastrin 105
gastrointestinal
- functions 115
- - upper gastrointestinal regulation 115
- secretion and motility 116
- transit 117
gene therapy 128, 129, 136, 174
- gene agents 136
- exocrine pancreatic insufficiency 128, 129
- perspectives 174
genetic
- factors / risk factors 1–13, 94
- heterogeneity 171
genotype-phenotype associations 172, 194
- CFTR 194
Gibson-Cooke pilocarpine iontophoresis sweat test 173
Glasgow prognostic score 57
glucagon 18, 69, 106
- GLP-1 (glucagon-like pepide-1) receptors 116
- intestinal glucagon 106
glutathione 170
Golgi apparatus 6, 18
grading (*see also* scores) 56–60
- early accurate 56
growth factors 97, 132–134, 205–221
- pancreatic cancer 205–221
- protein 43 expression, growth-associated 142
guanylin 169

H
H2-receptor antagonists 18, 69
HB-EGF 208
hemodilution 70
- isovolemic 70
hemofiltration 70
HGF (hepatocyte growth factor) 206, 212
histidine (CAC) 4
HOE-077 137
homocystinuria 10
hormones / hormonal mechanisms 116
- distal intestinal hormones 116
- pain hormones 160
hypercalcemia 10, 19
hyperlipemia 9, 10, 15, 20
hyperparathyroidism 10, 19
hypertension, ductal 93

I
idiopathic cases 66, 97
- early-onset idiopathic 97
- ICP (idiopathic chronic pancreatitis) 193–201
- - diagnostic implications 199
- - pathogenesis 198
- late-onset idiopathic 97
IGFs (insulin-like growth factors) 206, 211, 212
- IGF-I and IGF-II 211
- IGF-IR and IGF-IIR 211, 212
ileal lipid perfusion 115
ileum 113
ileus 19
imipenem 44, 71
IMMC (interdigestive migrating motor complexes) 107
immunological mechanisms 24–35
- autoimmunological reaction 96
- chemokines (*see there*) 25–28
- cytokines (*see there*) 25–27
- mediators in inflammation 24, 25, 36
immunoreactivities 113
in situ hybridization 233
infection / infectious diseases (*see also* bacterial translocation) 39–54, 79–82
- bacteria (*see also there*) 43, 44, 81
- clinical significance 42, 43, 80
- incidence 80
- infection rate 43
- necrosis (*see there*) 21, 22, 49–51, 66, 79–84
- pathogenesis 40
- possible pathways 39–42
- prevention (*see there*) 44–48
- sepsis, abdominal / pancreatic 32, 85
- surgical methods, infectious diseases 49, 79–84
- systemic complications 79
- treatment 48, 49
inflammation
- mediators in 24, 25, 36
- septic inflammatory response syndrome 24
- systemic inflammatory response syndrome 37, 55, 62
inflammatory cells / -mass 95, 155
inhibition of secretion 113
inhibitory mechanisms 116
insecticides, organophosphorous 20
insulin-dependent diabetes mellitus 156
insulin-like growth factors (*see* IGFs) 206, 211, 212
integrin 232
intensive care / ICU 56, 67, 82, 86
interferones (IFNs) 136, 231
- IFNα 231
interleukin (IL)
- IL-1 24, 25
- - IL-1-receptor antagonist 27
- IL-6 25

- IL-8 25
- - antagonist 31
- IL-10 28, 36
intestinal
- distal intestinal
- - hormones 116
- - obstruction 180
- ICM (intestinal current measurements) 173
- phases, pancreatic secretion 106
- small intestinal transit 117
- transit of chyme and its regulatory role 112–120
ischemia, pancreatic 142
isoleucine (ATC) 4
isosorbite mononitrate 142

J
jejunum 113
- feeding, jejunal 71
- nasojejunal feeding 63

K
Kalfarentzos study 63
ketoprofen 143
knockout 28
K-ras 213, 214

L
laminin 232
lavage
- *Lesser* sac, closed lavage and necrosectomy 85, 86
- peritoneal 49, 70
- - continuous local 49
leakage of lipase-rich fluid 1
lecithin 16
- lysolecithin 16, 17
lentivirus 174
Lesser sac, closed lavage and necrosectomy 85, 86
leukocyte scintigraphy 25
lexipafant 61, 70
life expectancy 155
lipases 9, 10, 15–17, 103, 112, 122, 127, 128
- apolipoprotein C-II 10
- bacterial lipase 127
- colipase 103
- hyperlipemia 9, 10, 15, 20
- impairment of pancreatic lipase synthesis and secretion 113
- inactivation of 113, 127
- leakage of lipase-rich fluid 1
- lipoprotein lipase 9, 10
- phospholipase A_2 14–17, 69
lipid
- digestion 113
- ileal lipid
- - concentrations 115
- - perfusion 115
lipoproteins 20
- lipoprotein lipase 9, 10
liposomes 174
lithiasis 94
lithostathines 94
lithotripsy 149, 156
- electrohydraulic and laser 149
liver disease, cystic fibrosis 186
long-term follow-up 155
lymph node dissection 242
lymphocytes 25
lysolecithin 16, 17
lysosomes 6

M
macrophages, monocytes / macrophages 25
malabsorption 110, 112–114
- nutrients, malabsorbed 114
- overt malabsorption 115
- pathophysiologic regulatory role of malabsorbed nutrients in pancreatic insufficiency 116, 117
- physiologic 115
- regulatory role of physiologically malabsorbed nutrients 116
maldigestion 117, 121
malignant phenotype 233
malnutrition (tropical chronic pancreatitis) 95
matrix metalloproeteases (MMPs) 133, 134
mechanoreceptors 108
medical and endoscopic treatment 66–77
- antibiotics 71
- assessment of severity 66, 68
- biliary pancreatitis, treatment of 72–74
- clinical studies 70
- conservative treatment 68–70
- management of pain 72
- nutritional support 71
menadione 22
meperidine 143
mesotrypsinogen 5
metastases 231
metronidazole 71
microcirculation 37
missense mutations 171
MMPs (matrix metalloproteases) 133, 134
MODS (multiorgan dysfunction syndrome) 60
molecular
- conjugates 174
- defect 4
- mechanism, early 1
monitoring, therapy 182
monocytes / macrophages 25
motility 19, 116
- gastrointestinal 116
motor function, abnormal 117
MRCP 156

N
N21I mutation, cationic trypsinogen 8
nadione 21
nafamostate 15
nasal potential difference (NPD) 173

nasoenteral feeding 55–65
nasogastric
- feeding 63
- tube 18
nasojejunal feeding 63
nasopancreatic probe 150
natrium, NHERF (Na^+/H^+ exchanger regulator factor) 169
NDFs 207
necrosis / necrotizing pancreatitis 1, 21, 22, 49–51, 66, 79–86, 93, 94
- chronic pancreatitis 93
- continuous local lavage 49
- fat necrosis 1
- infected necrosis (*see also* infection) 79–82
- surgical management (*see there*) 49, 82–86
- TNF (tumor necrosis factor) 26, 28, 32, 36
nerve
- damage to pancreatic nerves 141, 142
- intra- and interlobular nerve bundles 142
- splanchnic nerve denervation 143
neural mechanisms 116
neuritis, pancreatitis-associated 160
neurolytic treatments for pain 143
neurotensin 105
neurotransmitters 142
neutralizing antibody 136
NF-K*β* 26
NHERF (Na^+/H^+ exchanger regulator factor) 169
nicotine, risk factor 94
nonparallel secretion 104
nonsense mutations 171
NPD (nasal potential difference) 173
nuclear receptors 232
nutrient 113–116
- fate of nutrients during small intestinal transit 115
- hydrolysis 113
- malabsorbed nutrients 114
- pathophysiologic regulatory role of malabsorbed nutrients in pancreatic insufficiency 116, 117
- regulatory role of nutrients
- - in distal small intestine 115
- - of physiologically malabsorbed nutrients 116
nutrition
- cystic fibrosis, nutritional management 181
- enteral (*see there*) 48, 55–65
- hypercaloric 182
- jejunal feeding 71
- nasogastric feeding 63
- nasojejunal feeding 63
- parenteral 62, 71
- risk factor 94, 95
- therapeutic nutritional support 71

O
obesity 57
obstruction / obstructive
- chronic pancreatitis 93, 96, 97, 146
- distal intestinal obstruction 180
obturation of duct lumen 148
octreotide 69, 143
open and semiopen packing 85
oral food intake 19
organophosphorous insecticides 20
oxygen / oxidative
- damage 22
- free radicals, oxygen-derived 94
- reactive oxygen species 22
- stress 22

P
p53 213, 215
p55 and p75 soluble receptors 28
PAF (platelet-activating factor) 29, 36, 70
- antagonists 29
pain 72, 109, 140–145, 156
- abdominal 72, 156
- celiac plexus block 143
- chronic pancreatic pain 109
- endoscopic treatment of pain 146–154
- hormones 160
- management of 72, 140–145
- neurolytic treatments 143
- pancreatic extracts 143
- pancreaticogastrostomy for pain 143
- pseudocysts, enlarging 141
- TENS (transcutaneous electric nerve stimulation), pain treatment 143
palliative resection 245
pancreas divisum 96
pancreatectomy 240, 241
- extenede 241
- total 240
pancreatic
- abscess 78
- acinar cell (*see there*) 14–23
- carcinoma (*see also* tumors) 96
- diabetes 110
- duct
- - prosthesis 146
- - sphincterectomy 146, 152
- - stones 148, 149
- - stricture 146–148
- elastase, pancreatic 14, 15, 182
- exocrine secretion 19, 102–111, 116
- ischemia 142
- nerves, damage to 141, 142
- polypeptide 18, 106
- PSTI (pancreatic secretory trypsin inhibitor) 6, 9
pancreaticoduodenectomy
- pylorus-preserving (PPPD) 162, 239
- *Whipple* resection 239
pancreaticogastrostomy for pain 143
pancreaticojejunostomy, lateral 157
pancreatitis
- acute (*see there*) 14–89, 133, 160, 254

- autoimmune pancreatitis 96
- biliary pancreatitis (*see there*) 72–74, 254
- characterization 132
- chronic (*see there*) 19, 91–164, 255
- classification 78
- cystic fibrosis (*see there*) 165–202
- diffuse 161
- hereditary 4–10, 17, 258
- ICP (idiopathic chronic pancreatitis) 193–201
- necrosis/necrotizing pancreatitis 1, 21, 22, 49–51, 66, 79–86, 93, 94
- neuritis, pancreatitis-associated 160
- obstructive 146
- post-ERP pancreatitis 27
- segmental 161
- tropical pancreatitis 95, 259

parasympathetics 105
parenchymal pH 142
parenteral nutrition 62, 71
pathology of AP (*overview*) 60
PDGF (platelet-derived growth factor) 97, 206
- receptor (PDGFR) 206

pentazocine 143
peptide YY (PYY) 106, 116
peritoneal lavage 49, 70
peroxynitrite 21, 22
pH
- intraduodenal 114, 126
- intragastric 127
- parenchymal 142

phagocytosis, autophagocytosis 18
phase-II trial, retinoids in pancreatic cancer 235
phospholipase A_2 inhibitors 14–17, 69
phosphoprotein EBP50, ERM-binding 169
phytopharmacon silymarin 136
pilocarpine iontophoresis sweat test, *Gibson-Cooke* 173
PKC (protein kinase C), interaction with retinoids 234
plasma
- exchange 70
- fresh-frozen 69

plasminogen activator 97
platelet-activating factor (*see* PAF) 29, 36, 70
platelet-derived growth factor (PDGF) 97, 206
plexus block, celiac 143
polymerase chain reaction (PCR), reverse-transcriptase (RT-PCR) 233
porcine pancreatin, acid-resistant microsphere preparations of 182
portal
- compression of the portal vein 156
- hypertension 156, 180

post-ERP pancreatitis 27
postprandial chyme 113, 114
PPPD (pylorus-preserving pancreaticoduodenectomy) 162, 239
precipitation 113
predictive value 29
pressure, pain occation 140
- intraductal pressure 109, 140
- interstitial pressure 140

prevalence 102
preventive strategies 1
- infectious prevention 44–48
- - antibiotics, prophylactic intravenous 44–47
- - enteral nutrition 48
- - selective bowel decontamination (SDD) 47, 48

procollagen type III peptide 133
prognosis 57, 68
- Glasgow prognostic score 57

proline hydroxylation 137
prophylactic antibiotics 44–47, 71, 87
proteases 14, 22, 113
protein 14, 95
- growth-associated protein 43 expression 142
- PKC (protein kinase C) 234
- secretion 14

proteoglycans 132
proteolytic
- degradation 114
- destruction 113
- enzymes 103, 128
- intragastric proteolytic activity 114
- potential 22

protocol, standardized 147
pseudocysts of pancreas 141, 143, 149, 157, 158
- drainage 158
- enlarging pseudocysts, cause of pain 141

pseudohypoaldosteronism 171
pseudomonas glumae 127
PSTI (pancreatic secretory trypsin inhibitor) 6, 9
pylorus-preserving
- partial pancreaticoduodenectomy 162
- *Whipple* 162

R

R117H mutation, cationic trypsinogen 4–9
race and the risk of pancreatic cancer 258
radical surgery for exocrine cancer of the pancreatic head 238–249
Ranson score 60
RAR (retinoic acid receptors) 232
RAREs (retinoic acid responsive elements) 232
rat chemokines 26
recurrence 159
rehydration, pancreatic acinar cell 19
retinoids, pancreatic cancer 231–234
- ATRA (retinoid all-trans retinoic acid) 232
- inhibiting metastatic potential 231
- interaction with protein kinase C (PKC) 234

- mechanism of action 232
- phase-II trial 235
- RAR (retinoic acid receptors) 232
- RAREs (retinoic acid responsive elements) 232
- receptor subtype-specific biological function 233
- regulating growth and differentiation 231
- RXR (retinoid X receptors) 232
- surgical treatment (*see there*) 239, 240

ribonuclease 103
rodent models 7
RT-PCR (reverse-transcriptase polymerase chain reaction) 233
RXR (retinoid X receptors) 232

S

salivary amylase 114
scintigraphy, leukocyte 25
scoring 56–60, 83
- APACHE II (acute physiology and chronic health evaluation II) 56–59, 83
- *Balthazar* score 57
- BMI (body mass index) 56–59
- early accurate grading 56
- Glasgow prognostic score 57
- *Ranson* score 60

scorpions 20
SDD (selective bowel decontamination) 47, 48
secretin 104
secretory
- blockade, pancreatic acinar cell 14, 22
- digestive 115
- granules 18, 103
- PSTI (pancreatic secretory trypsin inhibitor) 6, 9
- vacuoles 18

sepsis, abdominal/pancreatic 32, 85
- septic inflammatory response syndrome 24

severity 66, 68
shrinkage 14, 22
silymarin, phytopharmacon 136
small intestinal transit 117
smoking and pancreatic cancer 257
soluble receptors 28
- P55 28
- P75 28

somatic gene therapy, cystic fibrosis 189
somatostatin 18, 69, 106
sphere size 124
sphincterectomy 55, 73, 146, 152
- endoscopic 55
- pancreatic duct sphincterectomy 146

splanchnic nerve denervation 143
stable disease 235
- transfection 233

staging and nasoenteral feeding 55–65
starch 115
steatorrhea 110, 112–114, 121, 127
- development of 112–114

steatosis 180
stellate cells, pancreatic (PSC) 133, 135
stenosis/stricture
- common bile duct 151, 156
- duodenal 156
- pancreatic main duct 156

stents, plastic and metal stents 148
- self-expanding 151

surgical treatment 49, 55, 73, 78–89
- cholecystectomy 55
- chronic pancreatitis 155–164
- closed labage of the *Lesser* sac (closed management) 85, 86
- débridement (*see there*) 84, 85
- endoscopic
- – cystoduodenostomy 150
- – cystogastrostomy 150
- future trends 87
- indications 79, 156
- infection relevance 49, 79–84
- intensive care/ICU, postoperative 56, 67, 82, 86
- lymph node dissection 242
- necrosectomy 49, 85, 86
- necrosis, sterile, surgical management 82–86
- open and semiopen management 85
- pancreatectomy (*see there*) 240, 241
- pancreatic
- – head resection, duodenum-preserving 159
- – left resection 161
- pancreaticoduodenectomy (*see there*) 162, 239, 240
- pancreaticogastrostomy for pain 143
- pancreaticojejunostomy, lateral 157
- pylorus-preserving *Whipple* 162
- radical surgery for exocrine cancer of the pancreatic head 238–249
- sphincterectomy 55, 73, 146, 152
- stent, plastic and metal stents 148
- techniques of surgical treatment 83–86
- timing of operative intervention in necrotizing pancreatitis 83

sympathetic innervation 105
symptom-relieving effects of pancreatic enzyme supplementation 118
syntaxin 1A 170
systemic inflammatory response syndrome 37, 55, 62

T

TAP (trypsinogen activation peptide) 6, 17, 18
TENS (transcutaneous electric nerve stimulation), pain treatment 143
TGF (transforming growth factor)
- TGFα 135, 207
- TGFβ (transforming growth factor β) 97, 132–134, 206, 209
- – acute and chronic pancreatitis 133, 134
- – antifibrotic treatment 136

– – development of pancreatic fibrosis 134
– TGFβ_1 135, 209
– TGFβ_1 209
therapy
– *algorithm* of decisionmaking and therapeutic strategies 73
– antibiotics 71
– antifibrotic agents/treatment 135–139
– biliary pancreatitis 72–74
– cancer therapy, biological approaches 222–229
– chemotherapy 222, 230, 246
– chronic pancreatitis, therapeutic concepts 118
– conservative treatment 68–70
– cytokines, consequences for diagnosis and treatment 29–33
– enzyme replacement therapy 112
– exocrine pancreatic insufficiency, treatment of 121–131
– gene therapy 223–225
– infection 48, 49
– medical and endoscopic treatment 66–77
– monitoring 182
– nutritional support 71
– pain
– – endoscopic treatment 146–154
– – neurolytic treatments 140–145
– problem-oriented treatment 68
– surgical treatment (*see there*) 49, 55, 73, 78–89
thiazides 20
thyroid, hyperparathyroidism 10, 19
time trends 256
TIMP2 133
TMB-8 20
TNF (tumor necrosis factor) 26, 28
– TNFα 26, 32, 36
– – antibodies to 32
transcription factors, pancreatic cancer 205–221
transfection, stable 233
transforming growth factor β (*see* TGFβ) 97, 132–134
trauma 93
treatment (*see* therapy)
triglycerides 113, 126
– long-chain (LCTs) 126
– medium-chain (MCTs) 126
trioleoin 16
tropical chronic pancreatitis (malnutrition) 95, 259
trypsin 5, 6, 14, 15, 22, 36, 113, 122
– autodigestion 6
– autolysis 5
– chymotrypsin 15, 114
– in digestion 5
– enzymes, trypsin-like 9
– inhibitors 14–16
– – PSTI (pancreatic secretory trypsin inhibitor) 6, 9
– premature trypsin activation 6
– radical-induced activation 21
trypsinogen
– activation 5, 14–18, 22, 36, 96
– – animal models 6
– – pancreatic acinar cell 14–18, 22, 36
– – TAP (trypsinogen activation peptide) 6, 17, 18
– anionic 5–9
– α_1-antitrypsin deficiency 96
– calcium and trypsinogen 8
– cationic 4–9, 96
– – N21I mutation 8
– – R117H mutation 4–9
– gene 17
– mesotrypsinogen 5
tumor
– cancer, pancreatic (*see there*) 155, 203–249
– carcinoma, pancreatic (*see there*) 96, 222, 231
– chemotherapy 222, 230, 246
– growth factors and transcription factors 205–221
– metastases 231
– tumor cell proliferation 230
– tumor invasion 93
– tumor necrosis factor (*see* TNF) 26, 28, 32, 36

U
ultrasound examination 55, 82
– cystic fibrosis, several ultrasonographic studies 185
– Doppler ultrasonography studies 186
– endoscopic ultrasonography 143, 149
– fine-needle aspiration 82
urokinase activator 97
ursodeoxycholic acid (UDCA), cystic fibrosis 181, 186

V
vaccine 226
vagovagal pathway 105
vasoconstriction 105
VIP fibers 105
viscosity 95
vitamins 126

W
wall thickening, submucosal 180, 184, 185
weight
– increase 159
– loss 109, 158
Whipple, A.O. 238
– pancreaticoduodenectomy (*Whipple* resection) 239, 240
– pylorus-preserving *Whipple* (PPPD) 162, 239

X
xanthine oxidase (XOD) 20, 22
XOD (xanthine oxidase) 20, 22

Z
zymogen granules 6, 7, 18, 22

Printing and Binding: Druckhaus Beltz, Hemsbach